KEY FACTS
in
PATHOLOGY

KEY FACTS
in
PATHOLOGY

Para Chandrasoma, M.D., M.R.C.P.(U.K.)

Assistant Professor
Department of Pathology
University of Southern California
 School of Medicine
Director of Surgical Pathology
Los Angeles County–University of
 Southern California Medical Center
Los Angeles, California

Clive R. Taylor, M.D., D. Phil., M.R.C. Path.

Professor and Chairman
Department of Pathology
University of Southern California
School of Medicine
Director of Laboratories and Pathology
Los Angeles County–University of
 Southern California Medical Center
Los Angeles, California

Churchill Livingstone
New York, Edinburgh, London, Melbourne   1986

Library of Congress Cataloging-in-Publication Data

Chandrasoma, Para.
  Key facts in pathology.

  Includes index.
  1. Pathology—Outlines, syllabi, etc. I. Taylor,
C.R. (Clive Roy) [DNLM: 1. Pathology—outlines.
QZ 18 C456k]
RB32.C48   1986   616.07   86-12891
ISBN 0-443-08270-7

Distributed in the United Kingdom by Churchill Livingstone, Robert Stevenson
House, 1–3 Baxter's Place, Leith Walk, Edinburgh EH1 3AF, and by associated
companies, branches, and representatives throughout the world.

Accurate indications, adverse reactions, and dosage schedules for drugs are
provided in this book, but it is possible that they may change. The reader is
urged to review the package information data of the manufacturers of the
medications mentioned.

Acquisitions Editor: *Gene C. Kearn*
Copy Editor: *Ann Ruzycka*
Production Designer: *Charlie Lebeda*
Production Supervisor: *Jocelyn Eckstein*

Printed in the United States of America

First published in 1986

PREFACE

Most medical school curricula in the United States teach pathology in the second year, after the students have had anatomy and physiology and before they start ward (clinical) medicine. The usual course lasts one year. During this time period, the student is required to assimilate a massive volume of information. The recommended reading in pathology is overwhelming; the basic texts suggested at the University of Southern California exceed 1,500 full pages (over one million words). These textbooks cover pathology in such depth that they also serve as textbooks for pathology residents preparing for their specialty board examinations.

Presented with a 4-lb textbook and an additional load of hand-out material, we see many students lapse into a state of "data-shock." Faced with too many facts, students struggle with the minutiae without concentrating on fundamentals. We believe that it is impossible to teach a second-year medical student to become a pathologist in one year. Any course that attempts to train the student to make pathologic diagnoses based on gross and microscopic examination of tissues is doomed to failure.

It is our belief that pathology at the second-year level should provide the basic information that is necessary for the student to understand how the healthy individual with "normal" anatomy and physiology changes into the sick patient in the hospital. It is such minimum basic information that we intend to supply in this book. We hope that delineation of absolutely vital information will help the student build up a realistic knowledge of the pathologic basis of diseases.

We would like to acknowledge Cherine Chandrasoma for help with the illustrations and Ms. Betty Redmond and Ms. Vivian Lopez for their assistance with the preparation of the manuscript.

Para Chandrasoma, M.D., M.R.C.P. (U.K.)
Clive R. Taylor, M.D., D. Phil., M.R.C. Path.

CONTENTS

Part I

General Pathology

The Inflammatory Response

ACUTE INFLAMMATION

I. Definition
   A. The immediate response of a tissue to injury
   B. Types of response
      1. The response of the microcirculation
      2. The cellular response
   C. Aimed at removing the agent causing injury
   D. Harmful effects of inflammation
      1. Responsible for many clinical symptoms (disease)
      2. Sometimes dangerous: inflammatory edema in a viral infection of the brain can cause death by increasing intracranial pressure

II. The microcirculatory vascular response of acute inflammation
   A. Changes in vessel caliber
      1. Initial transient vasoconstriction
      2. Followed by sustained active vasodilatation of the entire microcirculation; produces hyperemia (increased blood) (Fig. 1-1)
      3. Arteriolar dilatation: increases the hydrostatic pressure in the capillaries and venules
   B. Changes in vessel permeability
      1. Permeability of capillaries and venules increases.
      2. This is due to active contraction of actomyosin filaments in endothelial cells, causing separation of intercellular junctions (Fig. 1-2).
      3. Increased permeability permits outward passage of
         a) increased amounts of fluid.
         b) plasma proteins, including immunoglobulins and complement.
         c) fibrinogen. This is converted to fibrin by tissue thromboplastins. Fibrin appears as pink strands and clumps on microscopy (Fig. 1-3).

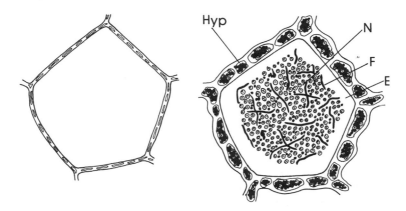

Fig. 1-1. Acute inflammation (right) compared with normal (left) lung alveolus. Hyp = hyperemia, E = fluid exudate containing neutrophils (N) and fibrin (F).

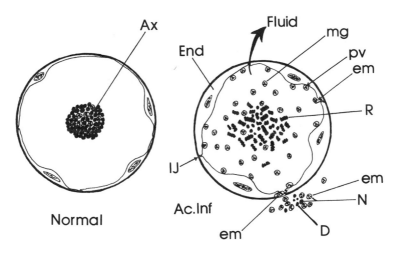

Fig. 1-2. Microcirculation in acute inflammation (Ac. Inf) compared with normal. Ax = normal axial stream of cells. Endothelial cells (End) are swollen and have widened junctions (IJ). Neutrophils (N) marginate (mg), pavement (pv) and emigrate (em). R = erythrocyte rouleaux. D = diapedesis (see III.F).

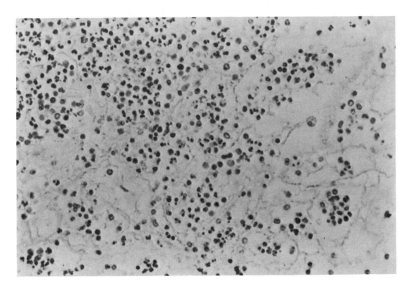

Fig. 1-3. Acute inflammatory exudate showing neutrophils, strands of fibrin and scattered macrophages.

C. Changes in blood flow rate
  1. Initially blood flow volume and rate are greatly increased due to arteriolar dilatation.
  2. As capillary permeability increases and exudation of fluid begins
    a) hemoconcentration occurs, increasing viscosity of the blood.
    b) the rate of flow in the dilated vessels decreases.
D. Changes in lymphatic flow
  1. As fluid collects in the interstitial space, lymphatic flow increases.
  2. This is beneficial in that it
    a) transfers antigens to lymph nodes, where they are exposed to large numbers of lymphocytes, promoting the immune response.
    b) exposes the injurious agent to the "filter" action of the phagocytic macrophages in the lymph nodes.
  3. Lymphatic drainage may be harmful in that it provides a

means by which the injurious agent gains access to the rest of the body.

E. Inflammatory edema
   1. Edema (swelling) is an increase in the amount of fluid in the interstitial space.
   2. Edema may result from
      a) transudation: increased filtration of fluid at a capillary of normal permeability.
      b) exudation: passage of fluid out of a capillary of increased permeability.
   3. Differences between transudates and exudates (Table 1-1)
      a) Transudates are like ultrafiltrates of plasma, lacking large molecules like proteins and cells.
      b) Exudates resemble plasma and contain large molecules.
      c) Exudates usually have inflammatory cells.
   4. Inflammatory edema, which is an exudate, is caused by
      a) increased permeability of the microcirculation.
      b) increased hydrostatic pressure in the microcirculation.
F. Five cardinal (clinical) signs of acute inflammation
   1. Redness (rubor): due to hyperemia
   2. Warmth (calor): due to hyperemia
   3. Swelling (tumor): due to fluid exudation
   4. Pain (dolor): due to increased tissue tension and stimulation of pain-sensitive nerve endings by prostaglandins and bradykinin
   5. Loss of normal function (functio laesa)
G. Mediators of the vascular response

Table 1-1. Characteristics of Transudates and Exudates

	Ultrafiltrate of Plasma	Transudate	Exudate	Plasma
Specific gravity	1.010	<1.015	>1.015	1.027
Small molecules (Na, K, Cl, glucose)	=	=	=	=
Large molecules				
Total protein	trace	<1.5 g/dl	>1.5 g/dl	7 g/dl
Fibrinogen	absent	absent	present	present
IgG, IgM, complement	absent	absent	present	present
Inflammatory cells	absent	absent	present	—

1. The active vasodilatation and increased permeability are mediated by chemical substances that are liberated in the area.
2. An identical vascular response occurs in denervated tissue, indicating that the neural contribution is minimal.
3. Chemicals that are capable of causing vasodilatation and increasing capillary permeability in acute inflammation include the following:
   a) Histamine
      (1) The first substance suggested as a chemical mediator (Lewis' H substance)
      (2) Released by mast cells
      (3) Present only in the early phase of vasodilatation
   b) Serotonin (5-hydroxy-tryptamine): released by mast cells
   c) Slow reacting substance (SRS): released from mast cells
   d) Bradykinin: formed by enzyme action on its precursor plasma protein kallikrein
   e) Prostaglandins
      (1) Formed by the action of cyclo-oxygenase on arachidonic acid
      (2) Found 6–24 hours after the onset
      (3) Most likely mediators of the sustained vasodilatation
   f) Cleavage products of complement: C3a and C5a
   g) Breakdown products of fibrin, neutrophils and lymphocytes

III. The cellular response of acute inflammation
   A. Inflammation is characterized by the movement of inflammatory cells from the blood into the area of injury.
      1. Neutrophils dominate the early phase.
      2. Macrophages and lymphocytes enter the area later.
   B. Emigration of neutrophils (Fig. 1-2)
      1. In a normal vessel, leukocytes tend to be in the central cellular stream separated from the endothelium by a zone of plasma.
      2. As the rate of flow decreases, the axial cellular stream is disrupted, bringing the leukocytes closer to the walls (margination).
      3. Leukocytes tend to adhere to the endothelium (pavementing).
      4. They then squeeze through the interendothelial junction (emigration).
      5. The role of neutrophils includes
         a) phagocytosis of infectious organisms and debris.

       b) bacterial killing.
- C. Chemotaxis

  The emigration of neutrophils is directed by chemotactic substances present in the area of inflammation:
  1. Fragments of complement: C3a and C5a
  2. Kinins
  3. Products of the fibrinolytic system
  4. Leukocyte breakdown products
- D. Emigration of monocytes
  1. Monocytes (=macrophages, histiocytes) emigrate in the later phase.
  2. The role of monocytes includes
     a) phagocytosis of injurious agents and debris.
     b) processing of antigens for lymphocytes, aiding the immune response.
- E. Emigration of lymphocytes
  1. Lymphocytes enter the area after the immune response occurs.
  2. They function to neutralize foreign antigens in the area.
- F. Diapedesis of erythrocytes: the passive escape of erythrocytes as neutrophils emigrate out of the vessel

IV. Variations of acute inflammation
- A. Acute inflammation without neutrophils
  1. Seen in infections by intracellular organisms like viruses
  2. Inflammatory cells: lymphocytes, plasma cells, macrophages
  3. Have all other features (i.e., vascular response, short duration, cardinal signs) of acute inflammation
- B. Variations based on the character of the exudate
  1. Acute inflammatory exudate composed of fluid, fibrin, and neutrophils
  2. Serous inflammation: when fluid dominates
  3. Fibrinous inflammation: when fibrin dominates
  4. Purulent inflammation: neutrophils are present in large numbers; exudate becomes thick and yellow (pus)
- C. Acute necrotizing inflammation
  1. Characterized by extensive necrosis of parenchymal cells due to the injurious agent
  2. Frequently associated with vascular disruption and hemorrhage: hemorrhagic inflammation
  3. Membranous inflammation: when involving a mucosal surface, the necrotic mucosa and inflammatory exudate remain attached as a surface membrane

D. Acute suppurative inflammation
 1. A necrotizing inflammation where tissue necrosis is caused by the enzymes of neutrophils
 2. Associated with an exaggerated neutrophil emigration
 3. Formation of a thick, yellow fluid (pus) from necrotic tissue and neutrophils
 4. Formation of abscess: suppurative areas become walled off by a reaction in the surrounding tissue

V. Systemic effects of acute inflammation
 A. Fever: due to pyrogens that enter the blood and act on the thermoregulatory center; prostaglandins are important
 B. Changes in the peripheral blood
  1. The number of neutrophils increases (neutrophil leukocytosis).
  2. Where neutrophils are not dominant, as in viral infections, their number may decrease (neutropenia) and lymphocytes increase (lymphocytosis).
  3. Changes in plasma proteins—increase in "acute phase reactants"—cause an elevation of the erythrocyte sedimentation rate.

VI. Purpose of acute inflammation
 A. Phagocytosis of the injurious agent by neutrophils and macrophages
  1. The particle is engulfed into a cytoplasmic vacuole (phagosome).
  2. Lysosomes fuse with the phagosome and their enzymes break down the contained particle.
  3. If the phagocytosed particle is a live organism, it is killed by microbicidal substances (hydrogen peroxide, superoxide) produced in the cell.
 B. Immunologic inactivation of the agent
  1. This is carried out by cytotoxic "killer" lymphocytes.
  2. Immunoglobulins (specific antibodies) attach to antigens, activate complement, and destroy the agent.
  3. Antibody and complement attachment to antigens promotes phagocytosis by macrophages (opsonization).

VII. Deficient responses
  Severe infections by microorganisms that are normally removed by acute inflammation are associated with deficiencies of the following:
 A. Neutrophil numbers (agranulocytosis)
 B. Neutrophil function (chronic granulomatous disease)
 C. Immunoglobulin (agammaglobulinemia)

D. Complement

CHRONIC INFLAMMATION

I. Definition
  A. The tissue response to an injurious agent that persists in the tissue for an extended period of time
  B. May follow acute inflammation or may occur without an acute phase
  C. No definable point in time at which an acute inflammation becomes chronic; distinction sometimes arbitrary
II. Morphologic differences between acute and chronic inflammation
  A. Chronic inflammation lacks the acute vascular response and exudation of fluid. Cardinal signs are absent.
  B. Neutrophils are usually absent. Chronic inflammatory cells are lymphocytes, plasma cells, and macrophages.
  C. In chronic inflammation there is proliferation of small blood vessels and fibroblasts.
  D. Fibrosis is a feature of chronic inflammation.
III. Types of chronic inflammation
  A. Nongranulomatous chronic inflammation: a diffuse proliferation of chronic inflammatory cells, fibroblasts, and collagen
  B. Granulomatous chronic inflammation
    1. Characterized by the formation of granulomas, aggregates of macrophages, usually surrounded by lymphocytes, plasma cells fibroblasts, and collagen
    2. Two major types of granuloma
      a) Epithelioid cell granuloma (Figs. 1-4, 1-5)
        (1) Characteristics
          i) Macrophages with abundant pink foamy cytoplasm known as epithelioid cells
          ii) Large multinucleated giant cells with 40–50 nuclei arranged around the periphery of the cell (Langhan's giant cell)
          iii) Central necrosis, which has a yellow, crumbling appearance on gross examination (caseous necrosis)
        (2) Causes
          i) Infectious agents: mycobacteria, fungi, etc.
          ii) Chemicals: beryllium
          iii) Diseases of unknown cause (sarcoidosis, Crohn's disease)

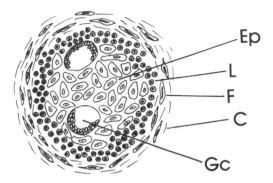

Fig. 1-4. Epithelioid cell granuloma with epithelioid cells (Ep), lympho-cytes (L), fibroblasts (F), Langhan's giant cells (Gc) and collagen (C).

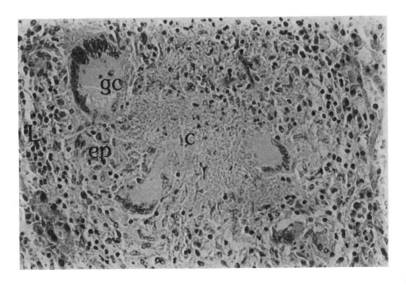

Fig. 1-5. Caseating epithelioid cell granuloma in tuberculosis. Epithelioid cells (ep), Langhan's giant cells (gc) caseation (c)

(3) Infectious granulomas are associated with caseous necrosis; noninfectious granulomas are noncaseating
b) Foreign-body granuloma (Fig. 1-6)
   (1) Differs from an epithelioid cell granuloma
      i) Giant cells are of the foreign-body type and have their numerous nuclei dispersed throughout the cell.
      ii) Foreign material (e.g., talc, sutures) can be seen.
   (2) Indicates that nondigestible foreign material has been introduced into the tissue

IV. Purpose and result of chronic inflammation
   A. Destruction of the agent by phagocytosis, aided by the cellular immune response, which arms and activates macrophages
   B. Repair of tissue necrosis by fibrosis
   C. Considerable tissue necrosis and fibrosis frequently manifests as chronic disease (e.g., pulmonary fibrosis in tuberculosis)

V. Inflammations with both acute and chronic features
   A. Chronic suppurative inflammation

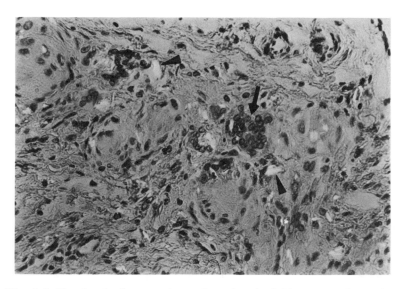

Fig. 1-6. Foreign body granuloma in a heroin "skin popper." Foreign material (talc mixed with the heroin) is refractile (arrowhead). Foreign body giant cell (arrow).

1. Suppuration may go on for long periods, eliciting chronic inflammation and fibrosis in surrounding tissue (e.g., chronic suppurative osteomyelitis).
2. If the area of suppuration is localized, a chronic abscess with a thick fibrous wall results.

B. Recurrent acute inflammation with incomplete resolution: characterized by acute and chronic inflammatory cells and fibrosis (also called "subacute" inflammation)

2

The Immune Response

INTRODUCTION

I. Activated by the entry of a substance the body recognizes as being
   A. foreign or "nonself."
   B. antigenic.
II. Highly specific for a given antigen
III. Antigens
   A. These are proteins and polysaccharides of high molecular weight.
   B. Smaller nonantigenic molecules may become antigenic when combined with larger carrier proteins. Such molecules are haptens.
   C. Antigens may be
      1. extrinsic: introduced from the outside.
      2. intrinsic: derived from altered self antigens.
IV. Recognition of antigens
   A. Macrophages phagocytose the antigen, process it, and present it to the immune cells (lymphocytes).
   B. B lymphocytes recognize some antigens directly.

CELLS OF THE IMMUNE RESPONSE

I. Lymphocytes: cells contained in lymphoid tissue, which is composed of the following:
   A. Central lymphoid tissue: thymus, bone marrow
   B. Peripheral lymphoid tissue: lymph nodes (Fig. 2-1), spleen, tonsils (Waldeyer's ring in pharynx), intestine, lung, etc.
   C. Circulating peripheral blood lymphocytes
II. Lymphocyte subpopulations
   A. All lymphocytes are derived from lymphoid stem cells in the bone marrow.
   B. Different lymphocyte subpopulations look alike.

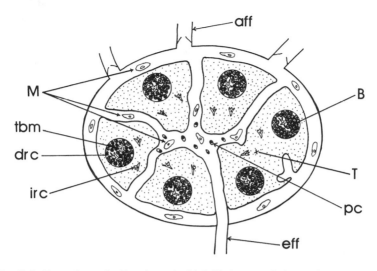

Fig. 2-1. Lymph node. B = lymphoid follicle containing B lymphocytes, dendritic reticulum cells (drc) and tingible body macrophages (tbm). T = paracortex containing T lymphocytes and interdigitating reticulum cells (irc). M = macrophages in sinuses. P = plasma cell. aff, eff = afferent and efferent lymphatics.

      C. Based on where they are primed in the fetus, lymphocytes are divided into
         1. T lymphocytes (thymus dependent).
         2. B lymphocytes (thymus independent; primed in Bursa of Fabricius in birds, fetal bone marrow in man).
  III. T lymphocytes (T cells)
      A. T lymphocytes are distributed in the T-cell domains of peripheral lymphoid tissue.
         1. Deep paracortex of lymph nodes between follicles (Fig. 2-1)
         2. 70% of lymphocytes in lymph nodes
         3. Periarterial lymphoid sheath in spleen
         4. 40% of lymphocytes in the spleen
         5. 80–90% of peripheral blood lymphocytes
      B. They continually and actively recirculate between the blood and peripheral lymphoid tissue.
      C. Following stimulation by specific antigen, T lymphocytes transform into large, actively dividing cells known as T immunoblasts (Fig. 2-2) that give rise to cytotoxic T cells.

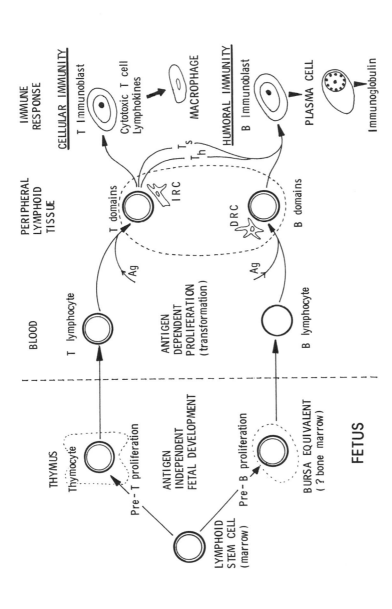

Fig. 2-2. Development and responses of immune system. Th, Ts = T helper and suppressor cells. Ag = antigen. IRC, DRC = interdigitating and dendritic reticulum cells. Postnatal lymphocyte proliferation induced by antigen constitutes the immune response.

    D. T lymphocytes are responsible for
      1. cell-mediated immunity, which is effected by
        a) cytotoxic "killer" T lymphocytes.
        b) lymphokines: a group of soluble proteins produced by activated T lymphocytes that regulate granulocyte, macrophage and lymphocyte functions.
      2. delayed hypersensitivity, the mechanism of which is unknown.
      3. regulation of B-lymphocyte activity by
        a) T helper cells (Th), which assist in B-lymphocyte activation, transformation, and immunoglobulin production.
        b) suppressor T cells (Ts), which inhibit B-cell activation and regulate immunoglobulin synthesis.
    E. Identification of T lymphocytes and T subpopulations
      1. E-Rosettes: T lymphocytes have surface receptors that bind sheep erythrocytes in the form of a rosette around the cell.
      2. Identification of T-lymphocyte antigens is by specific monoclonal antibodies developed against different subpopulations of T lymphocytes. T helper cells mark with OKT4, Leu3; T suppressor cells with OKT8, Leu2; Pre-T thymocytes with OKT6.
IV. B lymphocytes (B cells)
    A. B lymphocytes are distributed in B-cell domains of peripheral lymphoid tissue.
      1. Lymphoid follicles and medullary sinuses in lymph nodes (Fig. 2-1)
      2. 30% of lymph node lymphocytes
      3. Follicular centers in the malpighian corpuscles of spleen
      4. 40% of splenic lymphocytes
      5. 10–20% of peripheral blood lymphocytes
    B. When B cells are stimulated by antigen, they transform into B immunoblasts that give rise to plasma cells (Fig. 2-2).
    C. Plasma cells synthesize immunoglobulins and are responsible for humoral immunity.
    D. B lymphocytes are identified by
      1. presence of surface immunoglobulin.
      2. recognition of B-cell antigens, including BA-1 (early B cells) and B-1 (most mature B cells), by monoclonal antibodies.
 V. Null cells
    A. Null cells are lymphocytes that do not form E-rosettes and have no surface immunoglobulin.
    B. 5–10% of peripheral blood lymphocytes are null cells.
    C. Some null cells are cytotoxic ("natural killer cells").

    D. Some are involved in cellular destruction of antibody-coated antigens (antibody-dependent cellular cytotoxicity: ADCC).

VI. Macrophages (monocytes, histiocytes)
    A. Derived from monocyte precursors in bone marrow
    B. Location of macrophages
       1. Lymph nodes (Fig. 2-1)
         a) Subcapsular and medullary sinuses: phagocytic cells
         b) Dendritic reticulum cells in follicles: process antigen for B cells
         c) Interdigitating reticulum cells in deep paracortical zone: process antigen for T lymphocytes
       2. Spleen: lining the sinusoids in the red pulp
       3. Liver (Kupffer cells)
       4. Peripheral blood: monocytes
       5. Interstitial tissue all over the body: histiocytes
    C. Macrophage functions
       1. Nonspecific phagocytosis of particulate matter
       2. Processing of antigens
       3. Immune phagocytosis of antigens coated with immunoglobulin and complement
       4. Destruction of antigen, aided by T-cell lymphokines
    D. Identification of macrophages
       1. The presence of muramidase, lysozyme, and chymotrypsin
       2. Specific antigens demonstrated by monoclonal antibodies

IMMUNOGLOBULINS (ANTIBODIES)

I. Synthesis
    A. Synthesis is by plasma cells, which develop from transformed B lymphocytes.
    B. One clone of plasma cells synthesizes only one type of antibody with reactivity against one antigen (monoclonal).
II. Structure of immunoglobulins (Fig. 2-3)
    A. The immunoglobulin molecule is composed of two heavy chains and two light chains. Heavy chains define class (IgG, IgM, IgA, IgD, IgE). Light chains define type (kappa or lambda).
    B. Each chain has a constant and a variable region.
    C. Amino acid sequence variations in hypervariable regions of light and heavy chain determine antibody specificity.
    D. The variable end of the molecule is the antigen combining site. Each molecule has two such sites.
    E. The constant region has receptors for complement.

     F. IgM and IgA are polymeric with molecules joined by a J chain.

III. Classes of immunoglobulins

    A. IgG (gamma heavy chain; 4 sub-classes)

       1. The major circulating immunoglobulin

       2. Fixes complement

       3. Crosses the placenta in pregnancy

    B. IgM (mu heavy chain; pentameric)

       1. High-molecular-weight macroglobulin

       2. First immunoglobulin produced in a primary immune response

       3. Highly effective in fixing complement

       4. Does not cross the placenta

    C. IgA (alpha heavy chain; dimeric)

       1. Present in high concentration in gastrointestinal and respiratory secretions

       2. Minute amounts in serum

    D. IgD and IgE (delta and epsilon heavy chains)

       1. Minute amounts in serum

IV. Effects of antigen and antibody interaction

    A. Agglutination and precipitation of antigen

    B. Neutralization of toxins

    C. Opsonization with immune adherence and phagocytosis

    D. Complement activation (Fig. 2-4)

       1. Complement: nine plasma proteins making up about 10% of serum proteins

       2. Classical pathway of activation

         a) Initiated by binding of IgG or IgM to antigen

         b) Complement components are activated sequentially: C1 C4 C2 C3 C5 C6 C7 C8 C9 (note: only C4 is out of sequence).

         c) Activation sequence occurs on the surface of antigen. Some fragments of complement—C3a, C5a—are released.

       3. Alternate pathway of activation

         a) C3 activation does not require antigen–antibody interaction or early complement (C1 4 2) factors.

         b) C3 is activated directly by bacterial endotoxins, complex carbohydrates, and aggregated IgG complexes.

         c) C3 activation requires properdin (a serum globulin), two serum factors B and D and magnesium ions.

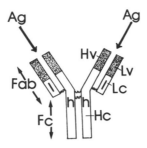

Fig. 2-3. Immunoglobulin molecule with two light (1) and two heavy (h) chains. Each chain has a constant (Hc, Lc) and variable (Hv, Lv) part. Papain digestion splits the molecule into two Fab and one Fc fragment. Ag = site of antigen binding.

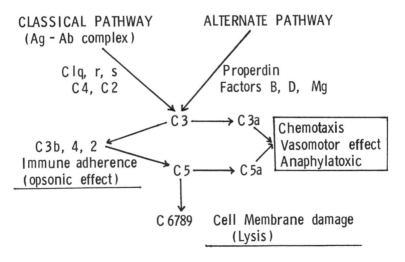

Fig. 2-4. Activation of complement. Ag-Ab = antigen-antibody complex. Mg-magnesium ions.

    d) Activation sequence after C3 is as in the classical pathway.
4. Effects of complement activation
    a) Cell membranes are lysed by C9 activation.
    b) C3b on surface of antigen is recognized by macrophages, leading to immune phagocytosis (opsonic effect).
    c) C3a and C5a produce vasodilatation, increased capillary permeability, and neutrophil chemotaxis (acute inflammation).

IMMUNE DEFICIENCY DISEASES

I. Congenital (primary) immunodeficiency
    A. Severe combined immunodeficiency (Swiss type)

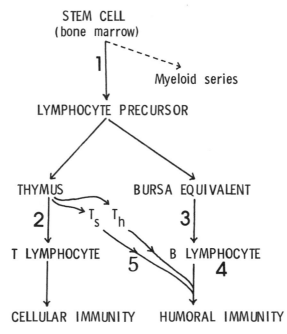

Fig. 2-5. Development of immune system. Numbers refer to points at which immune deficiency defects occur (see text).

1. The most severe form, usually fatal in infancy due to a variety of infections
2. Failure of both T and B lymphocytes (Position 1 in Fig. 2-5)
3. Lymphocytes absent in peripheral blood and lymphoid tissue
4. Immunoglobulins absent in serum
B. Thymic hypoplasia (DiGeorge's syndrome)
    1. Failure of thymic development (Position 2 in Fig. 2-5)
    2. Not inherited; may be associated with maldevelopment of other third and fourth pharyngeal arch structures (aorta, parathyroids)
    3. Failure of T lymphocytes
    4. Lack of cell-mediated immunity leading to viral, fungal, and mycobacterial infections
    5. Very low peripheral blood lymphocyte count
    6. Depletion of T-cell domains in lymph nodes and spleen
    7. Normal B-cell function and serum immunoglobulins
C. Congenital agammaglobulinemia (Bruton's syndrome)
    1. X-linked recessive inheritance; male infants affected
    2. Failure of B lymphocytes (Position 3 in Fig. 2-5)
    3. B cells absent in blood; total blood lymphocyte count normal because T cells are normal
    4. B-cell domains in lymph nodes and spleen depleted
    5. Serum immunoglobulins absent; humoral immunity absent
    6. Occurrence of recurrent pyogenic infections after passive maternal antibodies disappear (6–9 months)
D. Isolated IgA deficiency
    1. Common; occurs in 1 in 1000 individuals
    2. Failure of terminal differentiation of B cells (Position 4 in Fig. 2-5)
    3. Mostly asymptomatic; respiratory and intestinal infections occur
E. Complement deficiency (very rare)
    1. Early factor (C1 C4 C2 and C5) deficiency associated with systemic lupus erythematosus
    2. C3 deficiency resulting in recurrent pyogenic infections
    3. Late factor (C6 C7 C8) deficiency predisposing to Neisseria infections
II. Acquired (secondary) immunodeficiency
    A. Conditions associated with immune deficiency
        1. Malnutrition (kwashiorkor)
        2. Infections: viral (measles), lepromatous leprosy
        3. Chronic renal failure

    4. Malignant neoplasms
      a) B-cell lymphoma: depressed humoral immunity
      b) Hodgkin's disease: depressed cellular immunity
      c) Thymoma (hypogammaglobulinemia)
    5. Diabetes mellitus
    6. Use of immunosuppressive drugs in treating cancer, auto-immune disease, transplant rejection, and hypersensitivity diseases
    7. Idiopathic: cause unknown, often with increased suppressor cells (position 5 in Fig 2-5)
  B. Acquired immune deficiency syndrome (AIDS)
    1. First seen in 1979; has increased in epidemic fashion
    2. Has an almost 100% mortality within 3 years
    3. Occurrence
      a) Male homosexuals and bisexuals
      b) Haitian males
      c) Female sexual contacts of male bisexuals
      d) Patients receiving infected blood products
        (1) Hemophiliacs who are dependent on factor VIII preparations
        (2) Patients, mainly children, receiving blood transfusions
    4. Rarely seen in individuals other than the above
    5. Characteristics
      a) Oportunistic infections
        (1) *Pneumocystis carinii* pneumonia
        (2) Atypical mycobacterial infection: lung, intestine, and lymph nodes
        (3) Toxoplasmosis: brain
        (4) Fungal infections, particularly Candida and Cryptococcus
        (5) Herpesvirus and Cytomegalovirus infection
        (6) Cryptosporidiosis and *Isospora belli*: intestine
      b) Kaposi's sarcoma, a malignant vascular neoplasm of skin, intestine, and lymph nodes
      c) Malignant lymphoma, mainly B-immunoblastic sarcoma; primary lymphoma of the central nervous system common
      d) Squamous carcinoma of the mouth and anal canal
    6. Exact immunodeficiency not known
      a) Decreased T helper: T suppressor ratio (Position 5 in Fig. 2-5) in most patients

b) Abnormal lymphoid hyperplasia commonly present in lymph nodes (persistent generalized lymphadenopathy)
7. Probable cause: infection of lymphocytes by the human T-lymphocyte virus (HTLV: a retrovirus), which is transmitted by sexual contact and transfusion of blood products

IMMUNOLOGIC HYPERSENSITIVITY

Immunologic hypersensitivity is an immune reaction that results in injury to the host.
  I. Type I immediate hypersensitivity (Fig. 2-6)
    A. The antigen (=allergen) reacts with specific IgE immunoglobulin ("reagins") on the surface of mast cells.
    B. This leads to degranulation of mast cells with release of histamine and other vasoactive substances.

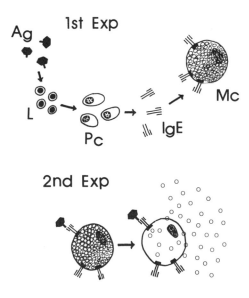

Fig. 2-6. Type I hypersensitivity. IgE is attached to surface of mast cells (Mc). Ag = allergen. L = B lymphocyte transforming into a plasma cell (Pc). First exposure (1st Exp) produces sensitization: 2nd Exp gives allergic reaction.

C. Localized type I hypersensitivity (atopy)
1. is very common, and has a familial tendency.
2. causes allergic acute dermatitis (eczema) and urticaria when involving the skin.
3. causes allergic rhinitis (hay fever) when involving the nasal mucosa .
4. causes bronchial muscle spasm (bronchial asthma) due to histamine when involving the lung .
D. Systemic type I hypersensitivity (anaphylaxis)
1. Usually a reaction to intravenously introduced allergen
2. Caused by penicillin, foreign sera and blood, and bee stings; a very small dose can cause anaphylaxis
3. Histamine release into the circulation causes
   a) generalized vasodilatation and peripheral circulatory failure (anaphylactic shock). It can cause death within minutes.
   b) increased capillary permeability, resulting in generalized edema (angioneurotic edema).
II. Type II hypersensitivity (cytotoxic) (Fig. 2-7)
A. The antigen is on the surface of a host cell.
B. The antigen may be
1. intrinsic: autoimmune disease.
2. extrinsic: commonly a drug (hapten) binding to a cell.

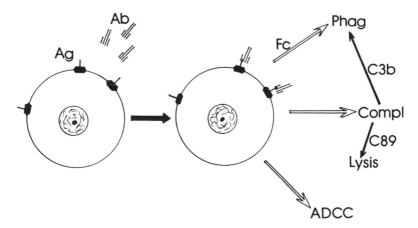

Fig. 2-7. Type II hypersensitivity. Ag = antigen on surface of cell. Antibody binding leads to immune phagocytosis (Phag), complement activation (Compl) or antibody-dependent cellular cytotoxicity (ADCC).

C. Circulating specific antibody combines with the antigen, causing
   1. immune adherence to macrophages, leading to phagocytosis.
   2. complement activation with cell lysis.
   3. antibody-dependent cellular cytotoxicity (ADCC). The antibody-coated cell is destroyed by cytotoxic null lymphocytes.
D. Type II hypersensitivity causes disease by action against
   1. erythrocyte antigens (hemolytic anemias).
      a) Transfusion incompatibility reactions
      b) Rh and ABO hemolytic disease of the newborn
      c) Drug-induced and autoimmune hemolytic anemia
   2. neutrophil antigens.
      a) Neonatal leukopenia
      b) Transfusions reactions due to leukocyte HLA antigens
   3. platelet antigens: idiopathic thrombocytopenic purpura, drug-induced, neonatal and post-transfusion thrombocytopenias.
   4. basement membrane antigens: Goodpasture's syndrome, where there is injury to glomerular and alveolar basement membrane.

III. Type III hypersensitivity (immune complex) (Fig. 2-8)
   A. Deposition of antigen–antibody complexes in tissues leads to local complement activation and injury.

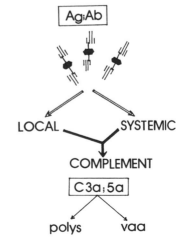

Fig. 2-8. Type III hypersensitivity. Immune complexes (Ag;Ab) activate complement, causing neutrophil chemotaxis (polys) and release of vasoactive amines (vaa).

B. Two distinct types of immune complex injury are recognized:
   1. Arthus reaction type: local
      a) Immune complexes form at the site of entry of the antigen.
      b) Precipitating antibody is present in high titer in serum.
      c) It causes disease in
         (1) lung: inhaled antigen (hypersensitivity pneumonitis).
         (2) skin: injected antigen, e.g., rabies vaccine.
   2. Serum sickness type: systemic
      a) Circulating immune compelxes are deposited in small vessels, causing complement-mediated inflammation (vasculitis).
      b) It may involve many organs (serum sickness, systemic lupus erythematosus), or single tissues (glomerulonephritis, arthritis)
      c) It may be caused by
         (1) extrinsic antigens: foreign serum, infectious agents (post-streptococcal glomerulonephritis).
         (2) intrinsic antigens: e.g., DNA is systemic lupus erythematosus.
C. Diagnosis of immune complex disease is by
   1. visualization of immune complexes by electron microscopy.
   2. demonstration of immunoglobulin and complement in the complexes by immunologic techniques.
   3. detection of immune complexes in the blood.
IV. Type IV hypersensitivity (delayed hypersensitivity) (Fig. 2-9)
   A. Type IV hypersensitivity is mediated by T lymphocytes.
   B. It causes necrosis of the cells bearing the antigen in
      1. autoimmune diseases: Hashimoto's thyroiditis, atrophic gastritis (pernicious anemia).
      2. infections causing granulomas: caseation necrosis.
      3. transplant rejection.
      4. immune reaction against neoplasms.
V. Type V hypersensitivity (stimulatory and inhibitory)
   A. Type V hypersensitivity is mediated by antibodies that react with antigens and influence the functioning of those antigens.
   B. Stimulatory antibody (Fig. 2-10): In Grave's disease (primary hyperthyroidism) binding of autoantibody to thyroid follicular cells stimulates increased hormone secretion.
   C. Inhibitory antibodies cause
      1. myasthenia gravis: antibody against acetylcholine receptors.
      2. pernicious anemia: antibodies binding with intrinsic factor interfere with vitamin B_{12} absorption.

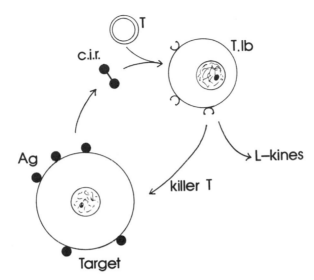

Fig. 2-9. Type IV hypersensitivity. T = T lymphocyte transforms into a T immunoblast in the cell-mediate immune response (c.i.r.). T cells may be cytotoxic (killer T) or produce lymphokines.

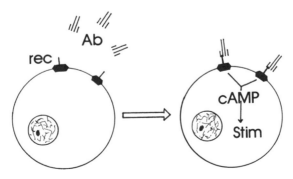

Fig. 2-10. Type V hypersensitivity. Combination of antibody (Ab) with cell receptor (rec) stimulates it via cyclic AMP (cAMP).

D. Many authorities classify this as a subset of Type II hypersensitivity.

TISSUE TRANSPLANTATION

I. Introduction
   A. The only limitation to transplantation is rejection.
   B. Rejection does not occur with
      1. autografts: transplants of the recipient's own tissue from one part of the body to another, e.g., skin, vein, and bone grafts.
      2. isografts: transplants between genetically identical twins.
      3. avascular grafts, such as corneal grafts, where the antigens are not exposed to the immune system.
   C. Rejection reaction increases as the genetic differences between donor and recipient increase.
      1. Allografts: from genetically dissimilar members of same species
      2. Xenografts: grafts from a different species. Not used in man.
   D. Currently renal allograft transplantation is routinely done and has a high success rate. Heart, lung, liver, and bone marrow transplants are still experimental.
II. Transplantation antigens
   A. Red cell antigens must always be compatible.
   B. HLA antigen complex is found on all nucleated cells in the body.
      1. It is governed by four major (A, B, C, D) loci on chromosome 6. A fifth locus (Dr) has been proposed.
      2. An individual inherits one allele at each locus from each parent.
      3. Numerous different alleles exist (20 HLA-A, 40 HLA-B, etc.)
      4. The four loci are closely linked and inherited as a haplotype. Siblings have a 25% chance of having a complete HLA match and a 50% chance of having one identical haplotype.
      5. Transplants between siblings are more successful than random-donor transplants.
      6. HLA tissue typing tests compatibility of HLA antigens between donor and recipient. The better the match, the lesser the rejection.
      7. Renal allograft survival correlates best with Dr compatibility.

III. Transplant rejection
  A. Mechanisms
    1. Humoral: due to antibodies against transplant antigens, producing injury by types II and III hypersensitivity reactions
    2. Cellular due to sensitized cytotoxic T lymphocytes
  B. Clinical types of rejection
    1. Hyperacute rejection
      a) Severe, occurring within minutes of transplantation
      b) Due to the presence in the recipient's serum of preformed antibodies reacting against donor antigens
      c) Severe necrotizing vasculitis with ischemic damage
    2. Acute rejection
      a) Occurs within days or months after transplantation
      b) Both humoral and cellular mechanisms operate
      c) Characterized by vasculitis, parenchymal cell necrosis, and lymphocytic infiltration
    3. Chronic rejection
      a) Slowly progressive over months or years
      b) Cellular mechanisms predominate
      c) Changes include progressive loss of parenchymal cells, lymphocytic infiltration, and fibrosis
IV. Graft versus host disease
  A. This occurs when immunocompetent cells are transplanted into an immunodeficient recipient. The donor lymphocytes react against host antigens.
  B. In man, it is commonly seen in bone marrow transplantation.
  C. It is usually fatal to the recipient.

AUTOIMMUNE DISEASE

I. Self-recognition
  A. Host immune cells recognize self antigens, but do not react against them (tolerance).
  B. Tolerance is due to suppression of lymphocyte clones programmed against self antigen. Suppression occurs when antigens are presented in fetal life.
  C. T suppressor cells and blocking factors are involved.
II. Autoimmunity
  A. Autoimmunity is a breakdown of tolerance to self antigens.

B. The immune system destroys self antigens by types II, III, IV and V hypersensitivity mechanisms.

C. Breakdown of self-recognition may be caused by
   1. loss of T suppressor activity, permitting emergence of suppressed ("forbidden") clones of lymphocytes.
   2. modification of self-antigens by drugs, damage, infection.
   3. cross reactivity between foreign and self antigens.
   4. emergence of previously sequestered antigens (e.g., myelin, lens protein).

III. Classification of autoimmune disease

   A. Absolutely organ specific: antigen is specific to one organ.
      1. Hashimoto's thyroiditis, primary hyperthyroidism, Addison's disease
      2. Chronic autoimmune gastritis (causes pernicious anemia)

   B. Relatively organ specific: though antigen is not limited, disease is restricted to one organ.
      1. Chronic active hepatitis: antismooth muscle antibody
      2. Primary biliary cirrhosis: antimitochondrial antibody

   C. Non-organ specific: antigens and immune injury occur at many different sites, e.g., anti-DNA antibody in systemic lupus erythematosus.

3

Necrosis and Tissue Degenerations

NECROSIS

Definitions

I. Necrosis is cell death occurring in the tissues of a living individual (Fig. 3-1).
II. It is irreversible.
III. The cells that have died are removed by liquefaction.
   A. Autolysis: liquefaction is the result of the enzymes of the cell itself
   B. Heterolysis: due to the enzymes of neutrophils
IV. Necrotic cells release their cytoplasmic contents into the blood stream. Detection of these substances (e.g., enzymes) in the blood provides evidence of cell necrosis (Table 3-1).

Mechanisms Leading to Necrosis

I. Impairment of energy (ATP) production, resulting in defective membrane transport, swelling of cells, disorganization of organelles, and finally cell death, caused by the following:
   A. Interference with enzymes involved in oxidative phosphorylation (e.g., inactivation of cytochrome oxidase by cyanide).
   B. Uncoupling of oxidation and phosphorylation due to mitochondrial damage.
   C. Lack of oxygen (hypoxia), which may result from
      1. failure of oxygenation of blood due to
         a) lack of oxygen in the environment (e.g., drowning, smoke inhalation in fires).
         b) failure of ventilation of lungs due to respiratory muscle paralysis or to respiratory airway obstruction.
      2. failure of arterial blood to reach cells due to
         a) general circulatory failure.
         b) local arterial obstruction.

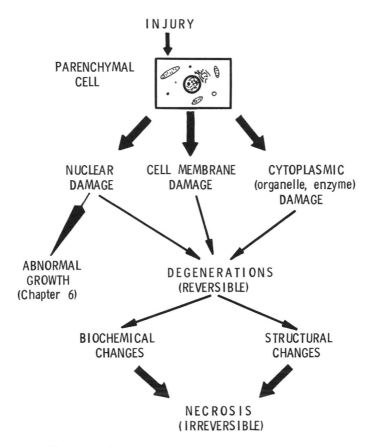

Fig. 3-1. Effect of injury on the parenchymal cell.

    3. impairment of oxygen transport in the blood due to
       a) lack of hemoglobin (anemia).
       b) presence of defective hemoglobin in the blood (e.g., carbon
          monoxide poisoning).
  D. Lack of substrate, mainly glucose (hypoglycemia).
II. Damage to the cell membrane due to the following:
  A. Free radicals
    1. High-energy particles that are extremely unstable and release
       energy by chemical reactions with nearby molecules

Table 3-1. Serum Enzyme Determinations That Indicate Cell Necrosis

Elevated levels of	=	Necrosis of
Lactate dehydrogenase		Heart, liver, muscle, erythrocytes
Creatine kinase (MB isoenzyme)		Heart
Creatine kinase (BB isoenzyme)		Brain
Creatine kinase (MM isoenzyme)		Skeletal muscle, heart
Glutamic-oxaloacetate transaminase		
(Aspartate amino-transferase)		Heart, liver, muscle
Glutamic-pyruvate transaminase		
(Alanine amino-transferase)		Liver
Amylase		Pancreas

2. Produced in the cell by
    a) external energy such as radiation
    b) abnormal electron transfer in the respiratory chain (e.g., by carbon tetrachloride)
3. Interaction between free radicals, particularly the OH$^{\bullet}$ (hydroxyl) radical and lipids in the cell membranes leading to membrane damage (lipid peroxidation)
B. Immunologic reactions leading to complement activation
    The final compounds formed in the complement cascade (C8 and C9) have phospholipase-like activity that damages cell membranes.
C. Enzymatic degradation of cell membrane
    1. By pancreatic lipase-like enzymes, which are liberated outside the pancreatic duct in acute pancreatitis
    2. Production by some microorganisms of enzymes that degrade cell membranes (e.g., *Clostridium perfringens*, which causes gas gangrene)
III. Alterations in genetic apparatus of the cell due to the following:
    A. Inherited chromosomal defects, and enzyme deficiency
    B. Viral infections, leading to introduction of the viral genome into the host cell's genetic apparatus
    C. Anticancer drugs, which interfere with DNA synthesis
    D. Radiation
IV. Miscellaneous mechanisms
    Many different toxic substances can interfere with various biochemical reactions in the cell, resulting in cell death.

Microscopic Characteristics

The following changes occur only several (6 or more) hours after irreversible cell damage has occurred. The early necrotic cell appears normal morphologically, though it is functionally dead.

I. Nuclear changes

    A. Pyknosis: clumping of the chromatin, which converts the nucleus into a small, densely basophilic structure

    B. Karyorrhexis: a later stage in which the nucleus with its clumped chromatin breaks up into several smaller particles

    C. Karyolysis: dissolution and disappearance of the nucleus from the dead cell, probably due to the action of lysosomal DNA-ases

II. Cytoplasmic changes

    A. The cytoplasm of dead cells becomes homogeneous and stains deeply pink (eosinophilic) due to loss of organelles and denaturation of the protein.

    B. Organelles are lost.

        1. Ribosomes disappear.

        2. Mitochondria swell and disappear.

        3. Glycogen granules disappear rapidly.

        4. Specific organelles, such as myofibrils in muscle cells, are lost.

        5. Vacuolation of the cytoplasm occurs due to enzymatic breakdown of organelle membranes.

    C. Lysis of the cell, with its disappearance, is the final event.

Types of Necrosis

I. Coagulative necrosis (Fig. 3-2)

    A. The necrotic cells retain their outline, appearing as ghost-like structures with no nucleus and pink homogeneous cytoplasm.

    B. It is seen typically in solid organs, such as kidney, heart, liver, and adrenals.

    C. It usually follows sudden ischemia.

II. Liquefactive (or colliquative) necrosis

    A. The lytic effect of released enzymes is the dominant change.

    B. It typically occurs in brain infarcts due to the high enzyme content of the necrotic brain cells.

    C. Suppuration is a type of liquefactive necrosis in which liquefaction is caused by enzymes released by neutrophils.

    D. Enzymes released by microorganisms may directly produce liquefactive necrosis, e.g., amebic liver "abscess."

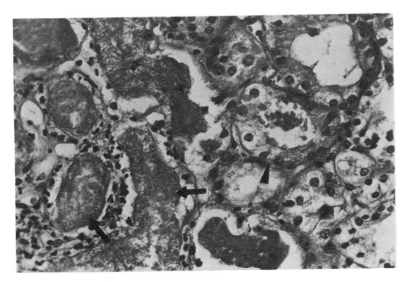

Fig. 3-2. Coagulative necrosis of renal tubular cells in a renal infarct. The dead cells (arrows) have pyknotic nuclei though the outline of the tubule is still preserved. Arrowhead shows normal renal tubule.

III. Enzymatic fat necrosis
  A. This is the classic result of action of pancreatic lipase on adipose tissue. Lipase acts on the triglycerides, forming fatty acids which complex with plasma calcium to form soaps.
  B. Grossly, fat necrosis appears as chalky white deposits.
  C. Microscopically, the deposits appear as amorphous, bluish (basophilic on account of their calcium content) masses which may retain vague outlines of necrotic fat cells.
  D. Fat necrosis may also occur in the absence of pancreatic lipase in many organs, such as breast and skin. Although there may be a history of trauma (traumatic fat necrosis), the exact pathogenesis is not certain.
IV. Caseous and gummatous necrosis
  A. Caseous necrosis (caseation) occurs in the center of epithelioid cell granulomata.
  B. Grossly, it appears as a yellowish-white, crumbling material.
  C. Microscopically, it appears as a finely granular, noncellular, pink material.

   D. Gummatous necrosis is similar and occurs in syphilis.

 V. Gangrene: tissue necrosis with secondary bacterial infection

   A. Dry gangrene

     1. Coagulative necrosis dominates over the bacterial infection.

     2. The affected tissue appears dry, shrivelled, and black.

     3. It is seen in the extremities that have undergone ischemic necrosis as a result of arterial obstruction.

   B. Wet gangrene

     1. Bacterial infection and associated acute inflammation dominate.

     2. The tissue is swollen, reddened, and odorous.

     3. It may be seen in the extremities; it is the usual form of gangrene in the intestine, appendix, gall bladder, etc.

   C. Gas gangrene

     1. This is due to clostridial infection.

     2. It is characterized by all the features of wet gangrene as well as the production of gas due to the fermentative action of the bacteria.

TISSUE DEGENERATIONS

Definition

   I. Degenerations may involve parenchymal cells or the connective tissue stroma or both.

  II. Cellular degeneration refers to a variety of *reversible* changes occurring in a cell that is damaged to a point short of necrosis.

 III. A degenerate cell remains intact, although it may function abnormally leading to disease.

 IV. Degenerations are characterized by the accumulation of abnormal substances (Table 3-2).

Classification of Degenerations by Abnormal Substance

 I. Accumulation of water

  A. Intracellular accumulation of water

    1. Occurs in any situation that impairs the energy-dependent sodium pump of the cell membrane

    2. Produces cloudy swelling and hydropic degeneration

    3. An early nonspecific cell degeneration

Table 3-2. Classification of Tissue Degenerations

Accumulated Substance	Intracellular	Connective Tissue
Water	Cloudy swelling	Edema
	Hydrophic degeneration	
Fat		
Triglyceride	Fatty change	Pathological adiposity
Cholesterol	Xanthoma	Atherosclerosis
Complex lipids	Lipid storage diseases	
Protein		Amyloidosis
Carbohydrate		
Glycogen	Glycogen storage diseases	
Mucopolysaccharide	Mucopolysaccharidosis	Myxoid degeneration
Minerals		
Calcium		Calcification
Copper	Wilson's disease	
Iron	Hemosiderosis	
	Hemochromatosis	
Pigments		
Bilirubin	Kernicterus	Jaundice
Lipofuscin/ceroid	Brown atrophy	
	Ceroid histiocytosis	
Miscellaneous		
Homogentisic acid		Ochronosis
Uric acid		Gout

B. Extracellular accumulation of water (=edema)
  1. Definition: the accumulation of water in the interstitial tissue and frequently the accumulation of fluid in body cavities
  2. Localized edema
    a) Is the occurrence of edema due to derangement of the local fluid exchange mechanism (Fig. 3-3)
    b) Occurs if there is
      (1) increased hydrostatic pressure
      (2) increased capillary permeability
      (3) obstruction to lymphatic drainage
    c) Types of localized edema

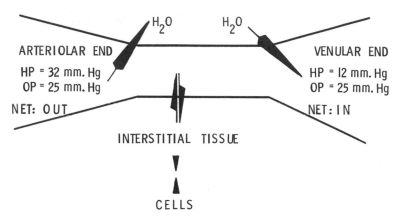

Fig. 3-3. Factors controlling fluid exchange in an idealized systemic capillary. HP = hydrostatic pressure. OP = osmotic pressure.

    (1) Inflammatory edema: due to increased hydrostatic pressure (arteriolar dilatation) and increased capillary permeability

    (2) Allergic edema: due to release of vasoactive substances (e.g., histamine) from mast cells in type I hypersensitivity that causes arteriolar dilatation and increased capillary permeability

    (3) Edema of venous obstruction: due to increase in the capillary hydrostatic pressure

    (4) Edema of lymphatic obstruction: due to the failure to remove the small amount of protein that normally escapes at the capillary

3. Generalized edema

  a) Caused by retention of sodium and water in the kidneys resulting from

    (1) decreased glomerular filtration

    (2) secondary aldosteronism due to increased renin levels which stimulate aldosterone (Fig. 3-4).

  b) Etiology of generalized edema

    (1) Cardiac edema

      i) Decreased left ventricular output causes renal vasoconstriction, renin hypersecretion and secondary aldosteronism.

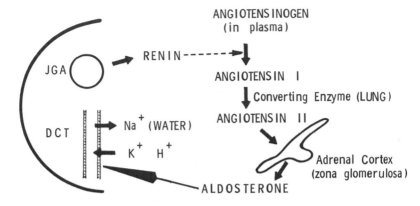

Fig. 3-4. The renin–angiotensin–aldosterone mechanism. JGA = juxtaglomerular apparatus. DCT = distal convoluted tubule.

    ii) Right ventricular failure causes increased venous and capillary hydrostatic pressure.

(2) Edema in hypoproteinemia

    i) Hypoproteinemia decreases plasma oncotic pressure, resulting in loss of fluid from capillaries, decreased effective plasma volume, secondary hyperaldosteronism, and sodium retention.

    ii) Hypoproteinemia may be caused by

        (*A*) deficient dietary intake of protein (starvation edema, kwashiorkor).

        (*B*) decreased synthesis of albumin (hepatic edema).

        (*C*) increased loss of protein in the urine (nephrotic syndrome) or from the gut (protein-losing enteropathy).

    iii) The occurrence of edema does not correlate precisely with the serum protein level.

(3) Renal edema

    i) Acute glomerulonephritis, due to sodium and water retention consequent upon diminished glomerular filtration rate

    ii) Excessive urinary protein loss with hypoproteinemia (nephrotic syndrome)

4. Clinical effects of edema
    a) Without functional significance in moderate cases
    b) Pulmonary edema
        (1) Definition: the entry of fluid into the alveolar spaces.
        (2) Causes
            i) Acute left ventricular failure, which produces a sudden increase in pulmonary venous pressure
            ii) Fluid overload
            iii) Inflammatory, toxic, and allergic diseases of the lungs, which increase permeability of alveolar capillaries
        (3) Clinical characteristics: development of acute respiratory distress and cough productive of pink frothy sputum may be rapidly fatal
    c) Cerebral edema
        (1) Definition: collection of fluid mainly in the interfibrillary extracellular space of the white matter of the brain
        (2) Complicates a large variety of brain disorders, such as traumatic lesions, infections, neoplasms, and vascular accidents.
        (3) Clinical characteristics: causes reversible neuronal dysfunction and increased brain mass with increased intracranial pressure, which threatens life
II. Accumulation of triglyceride
    A. Intracellular triglyceride accumulation (fatty change)
        1. The liver plays a central role in triglyceride metabolism (Fig. 3-5) and is the commonest site of fatty change.
        2. Fatty liver occurs in the following situations:
            a) Starvation: due to increased mobilization of peripheral adipose tissue
            b) Alcoholism: causes increased synthesis of triglyceride
            c) Presence of other toxic agents (e.g., carbon tetrachloride and phosphorus): leads to deficient production of lipid acceptor proteins
        3. Grossly, the fatty liver is enlarged, yellowish, and greasy.
        4. Microscopically, fat appears as cytoplasmic vacuoles.
        5. In acute fatty liver the fat droplets remain small (microvacuolar fatty change); this occurs in
            a) tetracycline toxicity.
            b) Reye's syndrome: a rare disease of children.
            c) acute fatty liver of pregnancy.
        6. In more chronic fatty livers, the fat globules coalesce to form

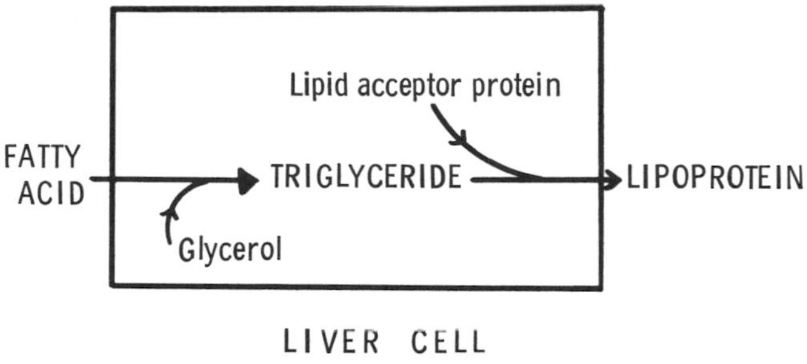

Fig. 3-5. Fat metabolism in the liver cell.

larger vacuoles. These may enlarge the liver cell and push its nucleus to one side (macrovacuolar fatty change).
7. Clinically,
    a) chronic fatty liver shows hepatomegaly and retention of normal liver function, even with extreme macrovacuolar fatty change.
    b) acute microvacuolar change is associated with acute liver failure with a high mortality.
8. Other sites of fatty change include the heart and renal tubules.
    a) In Reye's syndrome, microvacuolar fatty change in the liver is associated with fatty change in the heart and renal tubules.
    b) Fatty change of the heart occurs in severe anemia and toxic diseases. It is characterized by patchy deposition of fat in myocardial fibers.
B. Triglyceride accumulation within fat cells of interstitial tissue (pathological adiposity)
    1. This is seen in extreme obesity and is without clinical significance.
    2. Fat cells (adipocytes) accumulate in the interstitial space of many organs, such as the heart and pancreas.
III. Accumulation of other lipids
    A. Cholesterol
       1. High levels of serum cholesterol cause cholesterol deposition in the following areas:
          a) The intima of arteries (atherosclerosis)
          b) Dermal macrophages (xanthomata) and tendons (xanthoma tendinosum)

2. High serum cholesterol levels occur in the following conditions:
   a) Familial hypercholesterolemia: common
   b) Dietary hypercholesterolemia: particularly when combined with lack of exercise: common
   c) Other diseases: hypothyroidism, nephrotic syndrome, obstructive jaundice
   B. Complex lipids
   1. A large number of inborn errors of lipid metabolism have been identified (Table 3-3).
   2. Most are autosomal recessive and uncommon.
   3. Errors of lipid metabolism are associated with accumulation of a complex lipid in cells, either macrophages or parenchymal cells.
IV. Accumulation of protein
   A. Intracellular accumulation of protein: no significant diseases
   B. Extracellular accumulation of protein (amyloidosis)
   1. Definition of amyloid: by its physicochemical properties

Table 3-3. The More Common Lipid Storage Disorders

Disease	Enzyme Defect	Accumulated Material	Cells Involved
Tay-Sachs disease	Hexosaminidase A	GM2 ganglioside	CNS, retina
Metachromatic leukodystrophy	Aryl Sulfatase A	Sulfatide	CNS, kidney, gut
Krabbe's disease	Galactocerebroside Beta-galactosidase	Galactocerebroside	CNS
Fabry's disease	Alpha-galactosidase	Ceramide trihexoside	RE cells, vessels, neurons, kidneys
Gaucher's disease	Beta-glucosidase	Glucocerebroside	RE cells (liver, spleen, marrow)
Niemann–Pick disease	Sphingomyelinase	Sphingomyelin	RE cells, neurons

    a) On hematoxylin–eosin-stained sections, amyloid appears as an amorphous, pink, structureless substance.

    b) It stains red with Congo red and produces an apple-green birefringence when viewed by polarized light.

    c) It appears as nonbranching fibrils having a width of 7.5–10 nm on electron microscopy.

    d) It has a beta-pleated sheet structure on x-ray diffraction analysis.

2. Chemical composition of amyloid

    a) Amyloid of immunoglobulin origin (AIO)

      (1) AIO is seen in neoplastic proliferations of plasma cells, such as multiple myeloma, primary amyloidosis, and malignant lymphomas of B-cell origin.

      (2) Immunoglobulin fragments are produced and may be deposited in interstitial tissue as amyloid. Amyloid of immunoglobulin origin consists of either entire light chains or their amino-terminal ends.

    b) Amyloid of unknown origin (AUO)

      (1) AUO is deposited in the tissues in a large number of chronic inflammatory diseases, such as tuberculosis, lepromatous leprosy, and rheumatoid arthritis.

      (2) Many of these diseases have a prolonged increase in serum immunoglobulin levels.

      (3) AUO does not have any demonstrable immunological specificity.

3. Classification of amyloidosis

    a) Systemic amyloidosis

      (1) Primary pattern

        i) Systemic amyloidosis tends to involve heart, gastrointestinal tract, tongue, skin, and nerves.

        ii) Amyloid is of immunoglobulin origin.

        iii) It is seen in plasma cell and B-lymphocyte neoplasms, rheumatoid arthritis.

      (2) Secondary pattern

        i) Amyloidosis tends to involve kidney, liver, spleen, and adrenals.

        ii) Amyloid is of unknown origin.

        iii) It is seen in chronic inflammatory diseases.

    b) Localized amyloidosis

      (1) Localized amyloidosis forms nodular masses in organs such as the tongue, bladder, eye, lung, skin (rare).

      (2) It diffusely involves the heart: cardiac amyloidosis.

(3) It involves cerebral vessels: cerebral amyloid angiopathy.

c) Tumor amyloid

Amyloid is present in the stroma of neoplasms such as medullary carcinoma of the thyroid, islet cell tumors of the pancreas, and pheochromocytomas.

d) Heredofamilial amyloidosis

(1) Heredofamilial amyloidosis is very rare; few families are affected.

(2) Amyloid is AUO.

(3) It is classified according to sites of maximal deposition into neuropathic, nephropathic, and cardiopathic types.

4. Clinicopathologic effects of amyloidosis

a) Gross characteristics of involved organs

(1) larger (splenomegaly, hepatomegaly, enlargement of the tongue, cardiomegaly)

(2) firmer in consistency with decreased flexibility and distensibility

(3) pale gray and waxy

b) Renal amyloidosis

(1) This is the most significant clinical effect, being the common mode of death from amyloidosis.

(2) Amyloid is deposited in the glomerulus, causing increased permeability, proteinuria, and the nephrotic syndrome.

(3) With increasing deposition, the capillary lumina are obliterated, with decreased glomerular filtration rate and chronic renal failure.

c) Cardiac amyloidosis

(1) Amyloid is deposited in the subendocardial connective tissue and between the myocardial fibers.

(2) The thickened myocardium loses its distensibility, leading to impaired cardiac filling and low output failure: restrictive cardiomyopathy.

(3) With extensive amyloidosis, the conducting system may become involved, leading to heart block.

d) Hepatic amyloidosis

(1) Amyloid deposition occurs in the sinusoids.

(2) Pressure atrophy of hepatocytes occurs, but hepatic dysfunction is rare.

e) Splenic amyloidosis: occurs in two forms

(1) Localized to the splenic follicles, which become enlarged, pale gray, and waxy and stand out against the red pulp (sago spleen).

(2) Diffusely deposited in the sinusoids of the red pulp, producing a uniform waxy appearance and marked splenomegaly.

f) Gastrointestinal amyloidosis

(1) Maximal deposition is around small blood vessels in the submucosa.

(2) It is rarely associated with symptoms.

(3) It occurs both in primary and secondary distribution patterns. As such, rectal biopsy is frequently used for the diagnosis of amyloidosis.

V. Accumulation of glycogen

Glycogen accumulation occurs only intracellularly and is seen in the following conditions:

A. Hyperglycemia of uncontrolled diabetes mellitus: not associated with functional impairment

B. Glycogen storage diseases (Table 3-4)

1. These diseases are characterized by an inherited deficiency of one of the enzymes involved in glycogenolysis.

2. Symptoms depend on the type of deficiency.

a) In many of the diseases, glucose supply is impaired, leading to growth retardation.

b) Liver enzyme deficiency, if severe, leads to defective entry of glucose into the blood with hypoglycemia.

c) With muscle enzyme deficiency, muscle weakness and cramps dominate.

Table 3-4. Glycogen Storage Diseases

Type	Cells Involved	Name	Deficient Enzyme	Severity
I	Liver, kidney gut	von Gierke	Glucose-6-phosphatase	Severe
II	Systemic	Pompe	Alpha-glucosidase	Lethal
III	Systemic		Debranching enzyme	Mild
IV	Systemic		Branching enzyme	Lethal
V	Muscle	McArdle	Phosphorylase	Mild
VI	Liver		Phosphorylase	Mild

    3. Microscopically, cells with glycogen appear swollen and empty.

VI. Accumulation of mucopolysaccharide

  A. Intracellular: mucopolysaccharidoses (MPS syndromes)

    1. The mucopolysaccharidoses are a group of inherited diseases characterized by the accumulation of mucopolysaccharide in the lysosomes of affected cells.

    2. In different diseases, dermatan sulfate, heparan sulfate, keratan sulfate, and chondroitin sulfate accumulation occurs.

    3. Involvement of macrophages results in enlargement of liver and spleen and thickening of skin (gargoylism).

    4. Involvement of neurones leads to mental retardation.

    5. Peripheral blood smears show deposition of mucopolysaccharide in the cytoplasm of blood cells (Alder–Reilly bodies).

  B. Extracellular: myxoid or myxomatous degeneration

    1. Myxomatous generation is a very common degenerative change seen in many connective tissues, and is usually of little significance clinically.

    2. Myxomatous degeneration of cardiac valves, particularly the mitral valves, leads to valvular incompetence.

VII. Accumulation of calcium: calcification

  Calcification occurs extracellularly in connective tissues.

  A. Dystrophic calcification

    1. Dystrophic calcification is due to the presence in the involved tissues of abnormal material with an affinity for calcium.

    2. Calcium and phosphorus metabolism is normal and blood levels of these substances are normal.

    3. Abnormalities associated with dystrophic calcification include the following:

      a) Necrotic tissue abnormalities

        (1) Fat necrosis

        (2) Caseous necrosis in the center of granulomas

        (3) Dead parasites

      b) Abnormal blood vessels

        (1) Atheromatous plaques

        (2) Old, organized thrombi, both in arteries and veins (phleboliths)

      c) Degenerative changes of aging: associated with calcification of the media of medium-sized arteries, pineal gland, choroid plexuses, laryngeal cartilages, etc.

        d) Frequent calcification of neoplasms
          (1) Calcification may be an intrinsic feature of the neoplasm or may occur in relation to areas of necrosis.
          (2) Calcification commonly occurs in meningioma, craniopharyngioma, ovarian serous cystadenoma, papillary thyroid carcinoma, and oligodendroglioma.
        e) Tumoral calcinosis: A rare condition characterized by the presence of hard calcific masses in tissues, usually subcutaneous.

B. Metastatic calcification
   1. Metastatic calcification occurs as a result of increased blood levels of calcium and/or phosphate.
   2. It occurs in otherwise normal tissues, commonly in arterial walls, alveolar septa, and kidneys.
   3. Causes of metastatic calcification include the following:
      a) Hypercalcemia
        (1) Primary and secondary hyperparathyroidism
        (2) Metastatic malignant neoplasms in bone
        (3) Sarcoidosis, where there is increased sensitivity to the actions of vitamin D
        (4) Milk-alkali syndrome
        (5) Vitamin D intoxication
      b) Hyperphosphatemia
        (1) Hypoparathyroidism
        (2) Chronic renal failure
   4. Clinically, calcification of the renal interstitium (nephrocalcinosis) if extensive, can cause progressive chronic renal failure.
   5. Histologically, calcium deposits in tissues (both dystrophic and metastatic) appear as amorphous, granular, or crystalline masses staining deep blue (basophilic).

VIII. Accumulation of copper
  A. Wilson's disease (hepatolenticular degeneration)
   1. Inherited as an autosomal recessive
   2. characterized by decreased levels of ceruloplasmin or an abnormal ceruloplasmin in serum
   3. Decrease in total serum copper; increase in free serum copper
   4. Deposition of free copper in tissues, both intracellularly and in the interstitium
  B. Main sites affected
   1. Liver: chronic hepatitis, cirrhosis, liver failure

    2. Basal ganglia: extrapyramidal dysfunction
    3. Descemet's membrane: a green ring at the sclerocorneal junction (Kayser–Fleischer ring)

IX. Accumulation of iron

  A. Hemochromatosis (iron overload)

    1. Causes of iron overload

      a) Primary hemochromatosis: an inherited defect characterized by failure of regulation of iron absorption by the intestinal mucosal cell.

      b) Secondary hemochromatosis

        (1) Chronic hemolytic anemias like thalassemia and hereditary spherocytosis

        (2) Multiple blood transfusions

        (3) Dietary overload of iron in chronic alcoholism

        (4) Chronic liver disease due to stimulation of iron absorption

    2. Sites of iron deposition

      a) Macrophages of the reticuloendothelial system: when iron deposition is restricted to macrophages, clinical symptoms are not present. The term *systemic hemosiderosis* is sometimes used for this condition.

      b) Parencymal cells: leads to degeneration and necrosis of these cells.

        (1) Skin: increased pigmentation

        (2) Pancreas: diabetes mellitus

        (3) Liver: involvement of both hepatocytes and Kupffer cells resulting in cirrhosis and chronic liver failure

        (4) Heart: myocardial degeneration with cardiac failure

  B. Localized hemosiderosis

    1. Hemorrhage into tissue is followed by local breakdown of hemoglobin pigment, and deposition of iron in macrophages and connective tissue.

    2. It is no clinical significance.

    3. Microscopically, iron appears as granules of brown hemosiderin pigment.

X. Accumulation of bilirubin (jaundice)

  A. Metabolism of bilirubin (Fig. 3-6)

  B. Increase in serum bilirubin (jaundice or icterus)

    1. Hemolytic jaundice

      a) is caused by increased red cell breakdown.

      b) causes an increase in unconjugated serum bilirubin; it is not excreted in urine (acholuric jaundice).

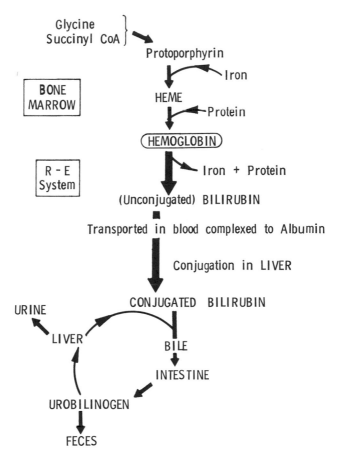

Fig. 3-6. Bilirubin synthesis and metabolism.

    c) causes an increase in excretion of bilirubin in bile, resulting in increased levels of fecal and urinary urobilinogen.

2. Hepatocellular jaundice
    a) is the failure of the hepatocyte to conjugate or excrete bilirubin.
    b) causes an increase in both conjugated and unconjugated bilirubin.

3. Obstructive jaundice
   a) is caused by obstruction of the biliary ducts.
   b) causes a reflux of conjugated bilirubin into the plasma; it is excreted in urine.
   c) causes a decrease in urinary and fecal urobilinogen since bilirubin does not enter the intestine.

C. Effects of jaundice
   1. Bilirubin deposition in the connective tissue of skin, sclera, and internal organs does not cause cellular degeneration.
   2. Kernicterus
      a) Bilirubin is deposited in the brain, mainly in the basal ganglia
      b) Unconjugated bilirubin (lipid soluble) crosses the blood-brain barrier
         (1) in neonates, particularly premature babies.
         (2) when unconjugated bilirubin levels are high, usually as a result of hemolytic jaundice.
      c) Kernicterus causes diffuse toxic injury to brain cells
      d) Infants who survive this acute episode suffer from more chronic neural dysfunction, mainly related to the extra-pyramidal system.

XI. Accumulation of hematin
   A. Hematin is a hemoglobin-derived pigment that accumulates in macrophages in malaria and massive hemolytic reactions.
   B. It is golden brown, granular, and contains iron.
   C. It has no clinical significance.

XII. Accumulation of lipofuscin
   A. Lipofuscin is a golden brown pigment commonly seen in liver cells, myocardial fibers, and neurons in elderly individuals.
   B. It is of no clinical significance.

XIII. Accumulation of urate (gout)
   A. Gout results from deposition or urate crystals in tissue, usually with elevated plasma uric acid levels (hyperuricemia).
   B. Primary gout
      1. Primary gout occurs mainly (95%) in elderly males.
      2. It has a strong familial tendency.
      3. 65% of cases have a demonstrable increase in the rate of synthesis and breakdown of purines and hence in the rate of formation of uric acid.
      4. Its basic cause is unknown.
   C. Secondary gout
      a) Hyperuricemia is the result of increased breakdown of purines associated with cell necrosis.

    b) In patients with leukemia it most frequently occurs at the start of treatment.

    c) It can be prevented by allopurinol, a xanthine oxidase inhibitor that prevents uric acid synthesis.

D. Lesch–Nyhan syndrome: A rare x-linked recessive deficiency of hypoxanthine guanine phosphoribosyltransferase (HGPRT)

E. Clinical effects of hyperuricemia

  1. Uric acid is not toxic until it is deposited in tissues as crystals of sodium urate.

  2. Acute gouty arthritis

    a) Caused by deposition of microcrystals of sodium urate in the synovial membrane of joints; the first metatarsophalangeal joints of the feet are first affected in 85% of cases.

    b) Microcrystals activate kinins and are chemotactic for neutrophils and evoke a severe acute inflammation.

    c) Recurrent attacks lead to increasing joint damage (chronic gouty arthritis).

  3. Chronic tophaceous gout

    a) Chronic tophaceous gout is characterized by deposition of sodium urate as large amorphous masses known as tophi.

    b) Tophi occur most commonly in the cartilage of the ear and around joints.

    c) Microscopically, gouty tophi appear as pale pink homogeneous masses of amorphous material surrounded by foreign body giant cells.

4

Healing of Injured Tissue

INTRODUCTION

I. The aim of the healing process is to restore injured tissue to as normal a state as possible.
II. The exact nature of the healing process depends on
   A. the type of inflammation.
   B. the amount of cell necrosis.
   C. the capacity of the parenchymal cells in the tissue for division.

METHODS OF HEALING

I. Resolution
   A. Resolution is the optimal end result of an injury that has been neutralized by an acute inflammatory response.
   B. The debris relating to the inflammatory exudate is removed by
      1. liquefaction of fibrin, dead cellular material, and inactivated injurious agent by lysosomal enzymes liberated from neutrophils.
      2. lymphatic drainage.
      3. phagocytosis by macrophages of any residual particulate matter.
   C. Removal of the exudate leaves the tissue in its normal pre-injury state.
II. Regeneration
   A. The replacement of lost parenchymal cells by similar cells by a process of cell division
   B. Restores the injured tissue to its normal pre-injured state
   C. Depends on
      1. the regenerative capacity of the cells.
      2. the presence of surviving germinative cells.
      3. the presence of a connective tissue framework.
   D. Classification of cells of the body according to their regenerative capacity
      1. Labile cells
         a) Labile cells normally divide actively throughout life to replace cells that are being continually lost, e.g.,

      (1) epithelial stem cells of the skin, gastrointestinal tract, genitourinary tract, and cells lining the ducts of glands.

      (2) blood cells: erythroblasts, myeloblasts, etc.

    b) Injury to a tissue whose parenchymal cells are labile cells results in regeneration (e.g., endometrial cells lost during menstruation or surgical curettage).

  2. Stable cells

    a) Stable cells are long-lived and have a low rate of cell turnover. They include cells of most solid glandular organs of the body such as liver, kidney, endocrine glands, pancreas, etc.

    b) Stable cells retain the capacity to divide rapidly and regenerate upon demand (e.g., the liver regenerates very rapidly after surgical or experimental removal of a lobe).

    c) The germinative cells are the differentiated parenchymal cells of the tissue at the margin of the area of cell loss.

    d) Regeneration of stable cells frequently requires that the connective tissue framework in the area of necrosis remain intact.

  3. Permanent cells

    In the adult these lack the ability to divide (e.g., neurons, muscle cells).

III. Repair by scar formation

  A. A scar is a mass of collagen that is the end result of repair.

  B. Repair by scar formation occurs

    1. when resolution does not occur in an acute inflammatory process.

    2. in chronic inflammation.

    3. when parenchymal cell necrosis cannot be replaced by regeneration; e.g.,

      a) when the cells are permanent cells.

      b) when the connective tissue framework of the area is destroyed.

      c) when all the germinative cells have been destroyed.

  C. Stages in scar formation

    1. Preparation

      a) The debris, either inflammatory exudate or necrotic tissue, is liquefied by lysosomal enzymes derived from neutrophils which migrate into the area.

      b) Liquefied debris is removed by lymphatic drainage and macrophages.

    2. Granulation

a) The capillaries at the edge of the lesion proliferate and new capillary buds grow into the involved area. Fibroblasts accompany the new capillaries. This combination of new capillaries and fibroblasts is known as granulation tissue.

b) Grossly, granulation tissue is highly vascular, soft, and fleshy.

c) Microscopically, the fibroblasts appear active with large nuclei and prominent nucleoli. Electron microscopy shows a prominent rough endoplasmic reticulum, indicating their active protein synthesis.

d) Over a period of time, the entire area of the lesion that is being repaired is replaced by granulation tissue.

3. Collagenization
   a) Collagen is the secretory protein of fibroblasts.
   b) It is fibrillar and appears pink in routine histologic sections (fibrosis; fibrous tissue).
   c) As the amount of collagen in granulation tissue increases, the tissue becomes less vascular and less cellular.
   d) A young scar contains much collagen and a modest number of vessels and fibroblasts, and because of its vascularity appears pink.
   e) A mature scar is an avascular, acellular mass of collagen.

4. Contraction
   a) Contraction is the final stage of the process.
   b) It effectively decreases the size of the scar to a fraction of the original area that was involved.
   c) It begins early in the stage of granulation and continues after the scar has matured.
   d) It is dependent on
      (1) fibroblasts, which contain myofibrils that contract.
      (2) collagen, which contracts considerably over a long period.
   e) Scar contraction is important as it permits optimal functioning of the surviving cells of the organ.

HEALING OF SKIN WOUNDS

I. Structure of skin
   A. Epidermis composed of stratified squamous epithelium (labile cells)

B. Dermis composed of collagen, blood vessels, and skin appendages such as hair follicles, sweat glands, and sebaceous glands (stable cells)

II. Injuries of skin

A. Abrasion

1. Abrasions in which there is only a removal of the superficial part of the epidermis, is the mildest skin injury.

2. Because the basal germinative cells are intact, the epithelium regenerates from below to its pre-injury state.

B. Lacerations with apposed skin edges

1. A laceration is a cutting or tearing of the skin that involves its full thickness. The optimal type of skin wound of this type is a surgical incision which has
   a) sharp edges which are closely approximated at the end of surgery with sutures or clips.
   b) no foreign material.
   c) no infection.

2. Wounds of this type heal by first intention (primary union) (Fig. 4-1).
   a) The very small gap in the epidermis and dermis is filled with blood clot.
   b) Blood clot at the surface forms a scab, which effectively seals the skin opening at an early stage.
   c) The epidermis regenerates by rapid multiplication of basal germinative cells at the edge of the wound. The regenerating epidermis grows under the scab.
   d) The dermal defect heals by granulation and formation of a thin scar.

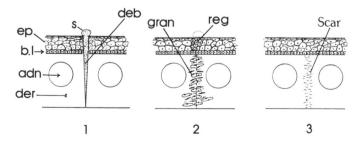

Fig. 4-1. Healing by primary intention. The epidermis (ep) regenerates (reg) from the basal layer (b.l) under the scab (s). deb = cell debris and blood clot. gran = granulation tissue. der = dermis. adn = adnexae.

3. Other kinds of lacerated wounds with lesser degrees of skin edge apposition, foreign material, necrotic tissue, or infection are associated with greater degrees of scar formation.
4. The scar is initially pink (vascular young scar), then white (mature dermal scar with thin regenerated epidermis), and finally achieves the normal skin pigmentation as the epidermis matures.

C. Lacerations with epidermal defects
1. These are severe skin injuries with denudation of large areas of epidermis and a correspondingly large amount of dermal necrosis.
2. They occur with crushing injuries and burns.
3. These wounds are allowed to remain open and heal by second intention (secondary union) (Fig. 4-2).
4. The processes involved are essentially similar, but because of the necrosis and infection, are greater in quantity and take a longer time.
5. Removal of necrotic debris occurs by enzymatic liquefaction. This process is greatly aided by surgical removal of the debris.
6. Granulation tissue grows from the healthy base, deplacing the necrotic surface upward.
7. The epidermis regenerates from the germinative epithelium at the wound edges and creeps over the granulating surface. Reepithelialization can be very slow with large defects and can be considerably aided by skin grafting.

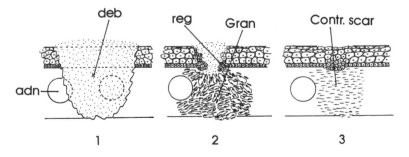

Fig. 4-2. Healing by secondary intention. Contr. scar = contracted scar. Gran = granulation tissue, reg = regeneration.

8. Surface re-epithelialization and conversion of underlying granulation tissue to a scar completes the process. Scar contraction produces a scar that is much smaller in area than the original area.

9. Skin appendages in the dermis, composed of stable cells, will regenerate unless they are completely destroyed.

III. Tensile strength of scars

   A. The initial wound is held together by the adhesive nature of blood clot and regenerating epithelium.

   B. The permanent tensile strength of wounds is provided by collagen, adequate amounts of which are present after the first week.

   C. With maturing of collagen, the tensile strength of the scar increases and reaches 75% of normal skin.

IV. Collagen

   A. Synthesis and structure

      1. Collagen is secreted by fibroblasts as tropocollagen.

      2. Tropocollagen synthesis requires
         a) hydroxylation of proline by an enzyme whose activity requires ascorbic acid (vitamin C).
         b) hydroxylation and oxidation of lysine, which permits crosslinkage between adjacent chains.

      3. In the extracellular space, these fibrillar molecules pack themselves to form collagen.

   B. Types of collagen

      1. Based on minor biochemical variations in peptide chain structure, four types of collagen (type I–type IV) are recognized.

      2. Young fibroblasts in granulation tissue initially form type III collagen.

      3. This is later replaced by type I collagen, the reason for the increased tensile strength of a mature scar.

V. Causes of impaired wound healing

   A. Vitamin C deficiency (scurvy): interferes with tropocollagen synthesis.

   B. Protein deficiency (malnutrition, hypoproteinemias)

   C. Diabetes mellitus

   D. Cushing's syndrome (hypercortisolism)

   E. Local factors

      1. Presence of foreign bodies, necrotic material, excessive amounts of blood

      2. Infection within the wound

      3. Ischemia and abnormal venous drainage

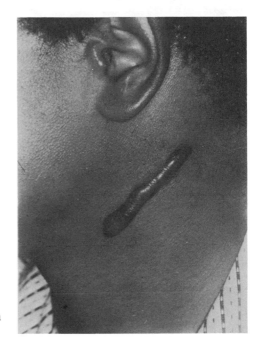

Fig. 4-3. Keloid formation in a scar.

  F. Ehlers–Danlos syndrome: an inherited disease (rare) caused by abnormal tropocollagen synthesis due to enzyme deficiencies

VI. Excessive collagen formation in scars: keloid

  A. Keloids are characterized by excessive production of collagen in relation to minor skin wounds, producing nodular masses (Fig. 4-3)

  B. The cause is unknown, they are not inherited and tend to occur in blacks.

  C. Microscopically, the collagen appears as thickened, peculiarly hyalinized bands.

HEALING OF FRACTURES

I. Types of fractures

  A. Complete vs. incomplete

    1. A complete fracture involves the full thickness of a bone.

    2. An incomplete (or *greenstick*) fracture involves only part of the thickness of the bone, and therefore there is no separation.

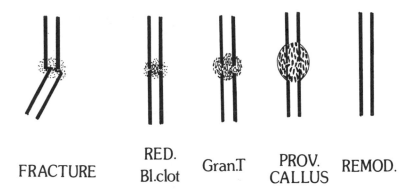

Fig. 4-4. Healing of a fracture. RED = reduced fracture. REMOD = remodelled bone, Bl. clot = Blood clot, Gran. T = granulation tissue, Prov. Callus = provisional callus.

    B. Closed (simple) vs. open (compound): Depends on whether or not the fracture site communicates with the skin surface
    C. Comminuted fracture: splintering of the bone into many fragments
    D. Depressed fracture: depressing the fractured part of a flat bone (usually skull) below the level of the rest of the bone
    E. Pathologic fracture: occurs at a site of a pre-existing disease in the bone, commonly metastatic neoplasm
  II. Healing of a simple, complete fracture (Fig. 4-4)
    A. The hematoma that forms between the fractured bone ends undergoes *organization*. The mass of granulation tissue in the fracture line is called *procallus*.
    B. After 2–3 days osteoblasts and chrondroblasts develop in the granulation tissue and begin forming bone and cartilage.
    C. By the end of 2–3 weeks the new bone and cartilage is sufficient in quantity to represent a temporary bony union of the fracture known as *provisional callus*.
    D. Over the next several weeks the bony spicules become wider and stronger and aligned along lines of muscular and weight-bearing stress in the bone (*remodeling*).
    E. The end result is a normally reconstituted bone.

5

Agents Causing Tissue Injury

FAILURE OF BLOOD SUPPLY (ISCHEMIA)

Arterial Obstruction

I. Effects of arterial obstruction
   A. When a tissue does not receive an adequate blood supply, its cells undergo necrosis (Fig. 5-1). Necrosis due to ischemia is infarction.
   B. The result of arterial obstruction on the tissue it supplies depends on the following factors.
      1. The extent of the collateral circulation. Tissues vary in this regard.
         a) Extreme 1: a free collateral circulation is available. Blood supply to such tissues is not decreased by occlusion of a single artery.
         b) Extreme 2: absence of a collateral circulation—end arteries. Occlusion of the artery will cause infarction.
         c) Between these extremes is a spectrum where some collateral circulation exists. In these cases, other factors operate.
      2. The integrity of the collateral circulation. Arterial disease, commonly atherosclerosis in the elderly, will decrease the effectiveness of the collateral supply.
      3. The rate of development of the arterial occlusion. Sudden arterial occlusion produces a more severe reduction in blood flow than gradual occlusion as there is no time to develop potential collaterals.
      4. The susceptibility of the tissue to ischemia
         a) The brain and heart are very susceptible.
         b) Skeletal muscle, bone, adipose tissue and collagen can withstand ischemia of several hours.
II. Morphologic characteristics of infarcts
   A. Types of infarcts

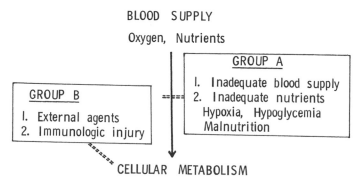

Fig. 5-1. Causes of cellular injury.

1. Pale vs red infarcts
    a) Pale infarcts occur in solid organs that do not have a free collateral circulation like heart, kidney, and spleen (Fig. 5-2).
    b) Red (or hemorrhagic) infarcts occur in organs that have
        (1) double circulations (e.g., lungs).
        (2) a collateral circulation which, though not enough to prevent infarction, permits continued flow of blood (e.g. intestine).
2. Solid vs liquefied infarcts
    a) In all tissues other than brain, infarction produces coagulative necrosis leading to a solid infarct (Fig. 5-2).
    b) In the brain, liquefactive necrosis of the cells leads to the formation of a fluid mass in the area of infarction; the end result may be a cystic cavity (Fig. 5-3).
B. Shape of infarcts
    1. Infarcts occur in the area of critical distribution of the occluded artery.
    2. Infarcts in kidney, spleen, and lung are wedge-shaped with the occluded artery situated near the apex of the wedge (Fig. 5-2).
    3. Cerebral and myocardial infarcts are irregular, following the distribution of occluded arteries (Fig. 5-3).
    4. Intestinal infarction affects loops of bowel.
C. Evolution of an infarct
    1. An infarct is an irreversible injury with necrosis of both parenchymal cells and connective tissue framework.

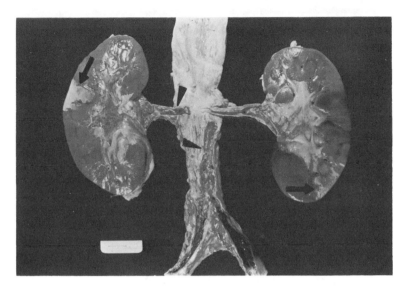

Fig. 5-2. Renal artery thrombus (arrowhead) leading to multiple pale infarcts of the kidney (arrows). Note thrombus in aorta (arrowhead) and iliac arteries.

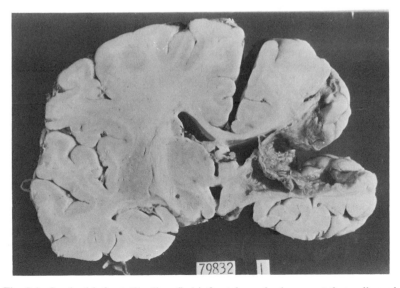

Fig. 5-3. Cerebral infarct. The liquefied infarct formed a large cyst that collapsed when the brain was cut.

2. Infiltration of neutrophils and release of lysosomal enzymes causes lysis.
3. Removal of debris is by macrophages and lymphatics.
4. Repair is carried out by granulation tissue and collagenization leading to a scar.
5. In the brain, the liquefied infarct becomes a fluid-filled cyst, walled off by gliosis (Fig. 5-3).
6. Small infarcts heal within 1-2 weeks, whereas larger infarcts take 6–8 weeks.
7. Evaluation of the gross and microscopic features of an infarct permits assessment of the time of its occurrence.

Venous Obstruction

I. Obstruction of a single vein, even when large, frequently has no effect because most areas have adequate venous collaterals.
II. When the collateral circulation is marginal, increased hydrostatic pressure in the capillaries may result in edema.
III. Congestion, an increase in the amount of blood in distended capillaries (e.g., orbital congestion in cavernous sinus thrombosis) occurs with greater obstruction.

Venous Infarction

I. Sudden and total occlusion of all venous drainage from an organ (e.g. in renal vein thrombosis, superior mesenteric vein thrombosis, superior sagittal sinus thrombosis) leads to venous infarction.
II. Venous infarcts are always red and hemorrhagic.
III. Special forms include the following:
   A. Strangulation: constriction of the neck of an abdominal hernial sac
   B. Torsion of a pedicle of an organ, commonly testis

Causes of Vascular Occlusion

I. Extramural compression: rare
II. Mural lesions
   A. Vasculitis: inflammation of the vessel
   B. Atherosclerosis
   C. Spasm of smooth muscle wall of the vessel
III. Thrombosis: common
   A. Definition: the formation of a solid mass from the constituents of the blood, within the vascular system during life
   B. Constituents of a thrombus

1. Platelets
   a) Endothelial injury causes platelet adhesion.
   b) Platelet aggregation then occurs, forming a mass that is the basis of the thrombus.
   c) Degranulation of platelets releases thromboplastic substances.
   d) Aggregated platelet masses appear microscopically as pale lines (lines of Zahn).
2. Fibrin
   a) Fibrin forms as the end result of the coagulation cascade of reactions that is activated by endothelial injury.
   b) It forms a meshwork intermingling with the amorphous platelet masses.
C. Factors in thrombus formation
   1. Endothelial damage: initiates both platelet adhesion and the coagulation cascade
   2. Decrease in the rate of blood flow: often a major factor in venous thrombosis
   3. Changes in the blood such as increased viscosity, fibrinogen, and platelet levels
D. Types of thrombi
   1. Pale thrombi
      a) Composed of platelets and fibrin with few entrapped erythrocytes
      b) Occur in vessels which have fast flowing blood (arteries)
   2. Red thrombi
      a) Composed of platelets, fibrin, and a large number of entrapped erythrocytes
      b) Occur in vessels that have a slow blood flow
E. Thrombosis in different sites
   1. Arterial thrombosis
      a) Most cases are consequent on atherosclerosis, and involve large arteries like coronary and carotid arteries.
      b) Less commonly, inflammation (arteritis) is the cause of endothelial injury.
   2. Venous thrombosis
      a) Thrombophlebitis
         (1) Thrombophlebitis is associated with inflammation of the vein.
         (2) The affected vein appears as a firm, acutely inflamed, cord-like structure.
         (3) Thrombi tend to be firmly attached to the wall and not likely to be detached as embolic fragments.

b) Phlebothrombosis
  (1) Occurs in the absence of inflammation
  (2) Occurs particularly in the deep veins of the legs, commonly in the calf (deep vein thrombosis, DVT)
  (3) Large thrombi that tend to become detached very easily, travelling in the circulation and producing pulmonary embolism
  (4) Occurrence of DVT
      i) In patients recovering from surgery and child-birth
      ii) In patients who are immobilized
      iii) In patients with cardiac failure
  (5) Factors involved in DVT
      i) Endothelial injury: a minor factor
      ii) Sluggish blood flow: important; immobilization promotes stasis in calf veins
      iii) Hypercoagulability of blood: after surgery and childbirth; oral contraceptive therapy
3. Cardiac thrombosis
  a) Inflammation of the cardiac valves (valvulitis, endo-carditis)
  b) Mural endocardial damage (as in myocardial infarction or cardiac aneurysms)
  c) Atrial chamber damage when there is stagnation of blood (e.g., in mitral valve stenosis and atrial fibrillation)
4. Disseminated intravascular coagulation (DIC)
  a) Definition: the widespread occurrence of microthrombi in the microcirculation
  b) Occurs as a complication of many diseases
  c) Causes
    (1) Diffuse endothelial injury (e.g., in gram-negative bac-teremia)
    (2) Entry of thromboplastic substances into the circulation (e.g., in amniotic fluid embolism, snake bite, and promyelocytic leukemia)
    (3) Other activation of the intrinsic pathway of coagu-lation
  d) Effects of widespread small vessel thrombosis (Fig. 5-4)
    (1) Widespread microinfarction, decreased tissue perfu-sion and "shock"
    (2) Consumption of coagulation factors (fibrinogen, factor

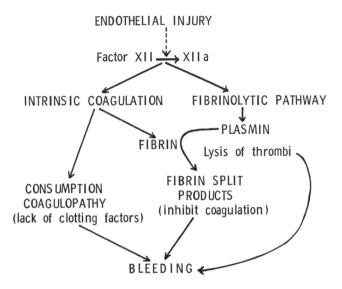

Fig. 5-4. Disseminated intravascular coagulation, leading to bleeding.

VIII, etc.) and platelets (consumption coagulopathy), causing a bleeding tendency.

(3) Activation of the fibrinolytic system, which aggravates the bleeding tendency

(4) Inhibition of coagulation by split products resulting from the action of plasmin on fibrin, which increases the bleeding tendency

F. Fate of thrombi

1. Fibrinolysis by activated plasmin

2. Organization and recanalization

a) Occurs in larger thrombi that cannot be dissolved

b) Growth of granulation tissue into the thrombus from the vessel wall leading to fibrosis

c) Frequent establishment of new channels across the thrombus by the capillaries in the granulation tissue (recanalization)

3. Thromboembolism

Fragmentation or detachment of the thrombus may cause it to travel as an embolus to a distal site.

IV. Embolism
  A. Definition
    1. Embolism is the transfer within the blood stream of a solid, liquid or gaseous mass from one site in the circulation to another.
    2. The majority of emboli are detached fragments of thrombi (thromboembolism).
  B. Thromboembolism: classified according to the site of lodgement of the thrombo-embolus
    1. Systemic embolism
      a) Occurs when the detached thrombus originates in the heart or in a large artery
      b) Of clinical consequences in the brain, heart, kidney, lower extremities, intestine, and spleen, where infarction may occur
    2. Pulmonary embolism
      a) The most common and most serious form of thrombo-embolism
      b) Over 90% of pulmonary emboli originate in phlebo-thrombosis in the deep leg veins; more rarely in pelvic veins
      c) Factors determining the effect of pulmonary embolism
        (1) Size
          i) Massive emboli obstruct the pulmonary outflow tract, causing circulatory obstruction and sudden death.
          ii) Moderate-sized emboli may lead to pulmonary infarction.
          iii) Small emboli have no immediate effect.
        (2) State of the pulmonary circulation
          i) Pulmonary infarction does not occur with moderate-sized emboli when there is a normal bronchial arterial supply.
          ii) In patients with heart failure or pulmonary vascular disease, obstruction of a medium-sized pulmonary artery leads to pulmonary infarction.
  C. Air embolism
    1. About 150 ml of air must enter the circulation to produce clinical air embolism (very rare).
    2. It occurs in the following situations:
      a) In venous injuries during neck and chest surgery or trauma

      b) During childbirth or abortion, where air may be forced into ruptured uterine venous sinuses by the contractions of the uterus

   3. Air accumulates in the right ventricle, where it effectively obstructs the circulation and causes death.

D. "Gas embolism" (decompression sickness)

   1. Gas embolism is a specific form of embolism that occurs in deep sea divers if they are decompressed too rapidly.

   2. When air is breathed under high underwater partial pressures, an increased volume of nitrogen goes into solution.

   3. Nitrogen, which is selectively soluble in fat, becomes incorporated mainly in adipose tissue and the fat of the nervous system.

   4. Rapid decompression causes the dissolved gases to come out of solution as bubbles.

   5. Involvement of muscle produces intense pain and contraction ("the bends"); bubbles in the brain and lungs may cause death.

E. Fat embolism

   1. Fat embolism is the entry of fat globules into the blood stream, which occurs in fractures of bones containing fatty marrow, like the femur.

   2. Larger globules of fat become arrested in the pulmonary capillaries, producing respiratory distress.

   3. Smaller fat globules escape the pulmonary vascular bed and pass into the systemic circulation, involving:

      a) the brain: acute neurologic dysfunction.

      b) the skin: hemorrhagic rash.

      c) the kidneys: fat globules in urine.

F. Amniotic fluid embolism

   1. Entry of amniotic fluid into ruptured uterine venous sinuses may rarely occur during childbirth.

   2. The fluid component of amniotic fluid is rich in thromboplastic substances and can cause disseminated intravascular coagulation, which may be fatal.

   3. The cellular components of amniotic fluid (fetal squames and hair) act as true emboli, lodging in the pulmonary circulation.

Shock

I. Definition

    Shock is a clinical state characterized by a generalized decrease in perfusion of tissues, due to circulatory inadequacy.

II. Causes of shock
  A. Hypovolemia: an absolute decrease in intravascular volume due to hemorrhage (external or internal) or excessive fluid loss (diarrhea, vomiting, burns, dehydration)
  B. Peripheral vasodilatation: leads to pooling of blood in the peripheral vessels (e.g., anaphylactic and gram-negative bacteremic shock)
  C. Cardiogenic shock: a reduction in cardiac output due to primary cardiac disease
III. Stages of shock
  A. Compensation
    1. The diminution of cardiac output triggers reflex increase in heart rate and peripheral resistance.
    2. Peripheral vasoconstriction is most marked in less vital tissues, such as
      a) the skin, which becomes cold and clammy.
      b) the kidneys, leading to a decreased glomerular filtration rate and oliguria (prerenal uremia).
      c) the splanchnic circulation.
    3. Maintenance of blood pressure permits adequate perfusion of vital tissues, such as brain and heart.
  B. Decompensation
    1. The compensatory vasoconstriction, when prolonged, diminishes perfusion of tissues, producing
      a) exaggeration of anaerobic glycolysis, leading to lactic acidosis.
      b) cellular damage in
        (1) the kidneys: tubular necrosis.
        (2) the liver: predominantly centrizonal necrosis.
        (3) the intestine: ischemic mucosal necrosis.
    2. As the condition progresses hypotension occurs, with impaired perfusion of the brain, heart, and lungs. This leads to death.

NUTRITIONAL DISEASE (MALNUTRITION)

Protein-Calorie Malnutrition

I. The common type of general malnutrition occurring in the underdeveloped countries of the world; a combination of protein and total calorie deficiencies

II. Manifestations
   A. Growth retardation: assessed as weight and height of a child compared with the norm for the age
   B. Immunologic deficiency: depression of both T and B lymphocyte function, leading to a higher incidence and greater mortality from infections of all kinds
   C. Marasmus
      1. Marasmus represents the compensated phase of malnutrition, in which the protein and calorie deficiency is compensated for by catabolism of the body's "expendable" tissues, notably adipose tissue and skeletal muscle
      2. The calories and amino acids so derived provide for normal cellular metabolism.
      3. The degradation of fat and muscle leads to extreme wasting.
      4. Serum albumin level is maintained and there is no edema.
      5. Marasmic children are alert and will eat ravenously when given food. Since gastrointestinal enzymes are normally secreted, food is absorbed normally. Marasmus is therefore easy to treat (by simply giving food).
   D. Kwashiorkor
      1. Kwashiorkor represents the decompensated phase of malnutrition and commonly follows marasmus.
      2. Amino acids and calories produced by fat and muscle wasting are no longer sufficient for synthesis of enzymes, structural proteins, and serum albumin.
      3. Failure of cellular metabolism in the brain leads to lethargy and somnolence.
      4. Decreased serum albumin is associated with edema.
      5. Gastrointestinal changes include atrophy of villi in the small intestine and deficient enzyme (particularly disaccharidase) secretion, leading to malabsorption.
      6. Abnormal fat metabolism produces fatty liver.
      7. Anemia is caused by a combination of deficient erythropoietin production and decreased intake of iron and folic acid.
      8. Abnormal protein synthesis leads to changes in skin and hair.

Vitamin Deficiency

I. Vitamin A deficiency
   A. Vitamin A is a group of compounds that includes vitamin A_1 (retinol).

B. Being fat soluble, vitamin A is absorbed as micelles and transported in the lymphatics in chylomicrons.
C. It is stored in large amounts in the liver.
D. Vitamin A deficiency occurs as a result of
  1. inadequate dietary intake.
  2. malabsorption of fat.
E. Vitamin A deficiency causes
  1. failure of night vision: retinol is constituent of the retinal rod pigment rhodopsin.
  2. squamous metaplasia and excessive keratinization in
    a) the conjunctival sac: dry eyes (xerophthalmia) and white plaques (Bitot's spots).
    b) the cornea: diminished vision and susceptibility to infection.
    c) the skin: follicular hyperkeratosis.

II. Vitamin D deficiency
A. Vitamin D (cholecalciferol) is derived from
  1. diet: fat soluble.
  2. conversion of 7 dehydro-cholesterol (an endogenous steroid) to cholecalciferol in the skin by the action of sunlight.
B. The active form of the vitamin is 1,25 dihydro-cholecalciferol (1,25 DHCC), which is formed by
  1. hydroxylation of cholecalciferol in liver to 25 hydroxycholecalciferol (25 OH-CC)
  2. hydroxylation of 25 OH-CC in the mitochondria of renal tubular cells to 1,25 DHCC (Fig. 5-5)

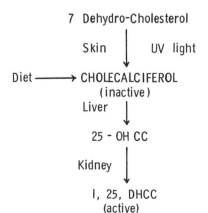

Fig. 5-5. Metabolism of Vitamin D. 25 OHCC = 25 hydroxy cholecalciferol. 1,25 DHCC = 1,25 dihydroxy cholecalciferol.

C. Actions of 1,25 DHCC include the following:
1. Stimulates energy-dependent calcium absorption in the intestine
2. Promotes calcium reabsorption in the renal tubule
3. Stimulates phosphate absorption in the intestine
D. Vitamin D deficiency produces a profound negative calcium balance, leading to a failure of mineralization of bone. This manifests as rickets in children and as osteomalacia in adults.
E. In rickets
1. mineralization of osteoid fails to occur. It affects children.
2. the main feature is a failure of bone growth at the epiphyses, causing growth retardation.
3. uncalcified osteoid accumulates at the epiphysis causing
   a) widening of the wrists and knees.
   b) a double vertical row of bumps on either side of the sternum (the rachitic rosary).
4. the uncalcified bone is much softer than normal, leading to deformities
   a) in bones that bear weight (e.g., bowing of tibiae, deformities in vertebrae and pelvis).
   b) at points of muscle insertion; the respiratory muscles produce forward protrusion of the sternum (pigeon breast) and a trasverse line in the lower rib cage along the diaphragmatic insertion (Harrison's sulcus).
   c) skull bones: softening (craniotabes).
F. In osteomalacia
1. mineralization of osteoid fails to occur. This affects adults.
2. bone is soft with uncalcified, wide osteoid seams.
3. bone pain is often present.
G. Vitamin D deficiency is caused by
1. inadequate dietary intake with insufficient exposure to sunlight.
2. fat malabsorption.
3. chronic renal disease, due to failure of activation of Vitamin D or renal tubular phosphate loss.
III. Vitamin K deficiency
A. The main source of vitamin K is the intestinal bacterial flora.
B. Causes of Vitamin K deficiency include the following:
1. Delay in bacterial colonization of the intestine during the neonatal period.
2. Broad-spectrum antibiotics that alter the gut flora
3. Fat malabsorption
4. Drugs that are Vitamin K antagonists (anticoagulants)

C. Vitamin K is needed for the liver synthesis of prothrombin and factors VII, IX, and X

D. Deficiency causes a bleeding tendency.

IV. Vitamin C deficiency (scurvy)

A. Vitamin C (ascorbic acid) is a water soluble vitamin present in fresh fruit and vegetables. Deficiency is always dietary.

B. It is required for collagen synthesis, the failure of which causes

1. impairment of wound healing and decreased tensile strength in scars.

2. opening up of old scars due to defective collagen turnover.

C. Defective osteoid and ground substance synthesis causes

1. failure of bone growth.

2. disorganization and widening of epiphyseal cartilage.

3. weakening of bone with tendency to fractures.

4. subperiosteal hematomas.

D. Abnormalities develop in teeth and gums. Gums become swollen and inflamed.

V. Vitamin B_1 (thiamine) deficiency

A. Vitamin B_1 deficiency is rare, it occurs most frequently in chronic alcoholics.

B. Thiamine is required

1. as a co-enzyme in the decarboxylation of pyruvate; serum pyruvate levels are increased in thiamine deficiency.

2. in the synthesis of acetylcholine.

C. Thiamine deficiency causes

1. wet beriberi, characterized by congestive cardiac failure due to myocardial fiber degeneration.

2. dry beriberi, characterized by neurological changes, including

a) peripheral neuropathy due to segmental demyelination.

b) neuronal loss in the brain, causing Korsakoff's psychosis.

c) Wernicke's encephalopathy, due to hemorrhage and atrophy of the mamillary bodies and paraventricular brain stem.

VI. Riboflavin (vitamin B_2) deficiency

A. Deficiency is usually due to inadequate dietary intake.

B. Riboflavin deficiency causes

1. cheilosis (inflammation of the lips).

2. glossitis (inflammation of the tongue).

3. eye lesions (vascularization and opacity of the cornea).

VII. Nicotinamide (niacin) deficiency

A. Nicotinamide deficiency is most commonly dietary.

B. It causes pellagra, which is characterized by dermatitis (mainly affecting sun-exposed skin), diarrhea, and dementia.

VIII. Pyridoxine deficiency

  A. Pyridoxine deficiency is most commonly caused by pyridoxine antagonist drugs (isoniazid (INH), oral contraceptives, methyldopa, L-dopa).

  B. The most significant changes caused by deficiency are peripheral neuropathy and sideroblastic anemia.

  C. Deficiency also causes minor changes in mouth, tongue, eyes, skin.

IX. Folic acid (pteroyglutamic acid) and vitamin B_{12} deficiencies

  Folic acid and Vitamin B_{12} deficiencies cause failure of nucleic acid synthesis, manifesting as megaloblastic anemia (see Chapter 7)

Mineral Deficiency

I. Iron deficiency (see Chapter 7: iron deficiency anemia)

II. Other mineral deficiencies: not well established

PHYSICAL AGENTS

Mechanical Trauma

Mechanical trauma is the leading cause of death in children and young adults.

Pressure Injuries (Blast Injuries)

I. Explosives (bombs, grenades, etc.) cause pressure waves that have the maximum effect on gas-filled organs like the lung and the intestine.

II. Compression of the thorax by external pressure waves may lead to rupture of solid viscera like the liver and the spleen.

Temperature Injuries

I. Localized cold injuries

  A. Local changes in a part of the body exposed to cold include vasoconstriction, ischemia, and gangrene.

  B. With exposure to severe cold, these changes occur rapidly (frostbite).

  C. With lesser degrees of cold, long exposure is needed (trenchfoot).

II. Generalized hypothermia
   A. When the whole body is exposed to freezing temperatures, there is reflex vasoconstriction to preserve body heat.
   B. Eventual failure of this protective mechanism causes
      1. a rapid decrease in body core temperature.
      2. peripheral circulatory failure and death.
III. Local heat injury (burns)
   A. Burns are a major cause of death in the United States.
   B. The seriousness of a burn is related to the following factors:
      1. The depth of skin involved: full-thickness (third degree) burns are more serious than partial-thickness burns.
      2. The surface area of the body that is burned.
         a) When more than 20% of the body surface is involved, there is fluid loss sufficient to cause hypovolemia.
         b) When more than 50% of the body surface is burned, there is a high mortality.
IV. Systemic hyperthermia (heat stroke)
   This is a rare condition, defined as an elevation of core body temperature over 40°C.

Electrical Injuries

I. Contact with an electrical source leads to the passage of current through the body between entrance and exit points.
II. Passage of an electrical current through the body causes
   A. paralysis of the cardiac and respiratory centers in the brain stem.
   B. excitation of cardiac muscle, causing ventricular fibrillation.
   C. stimulation of skeletal muscle, causing contractions that may be violent enough to fracture bones.
   D. heat production, mainly causing skin burns. In severe injuries steam production in tissues may cause explosions of tissue.

Ionizing Radiation Injuries

I. Composition of ionizing radiation
   A. Part of the electromagnetic wave spectrum (x-rays, gamma rays)
   B. Certain types of particulate radiation (alpha and beta particles, neutrons, protons and deuterons)
II. Sources of radiation

   A. Nuclear power plants and nuclear weapons

   B. Radioisotopes and x-rays used in medical diagnosis and treatment

III. Mechanism of cell damage by radiation

   A. Direct reaction between the high-energy radiation and vital molecules in the cell (DNA, RNA, proteins, etc.) (target theory)

   B. Indirect effect (indirect action theory): the high-energy radiation causes ionization of water, forming toxic free radicals (such as $H^{.}$, $OH^{.}$, H_2O_2).

IV. Total-body irradiation

   A. Total-body irradiation occurs only as a result of exposure to nuclear fallout from explosion of a nuclear weapon or other nuclear accident.

   B. The effect of total-body irradiation depends on the dosage. Several well-defined syndromes are recognized, depending on the total-body dosage.

     1. Cerebral syndrome (1000+ rads)

       a) Invariably fatal; death instantaneous or in days

       b) Drowsiness, convulsions, and coma preceding death

     2. Gastrointestinal syndrome (300–1000 rads)

       a) Extensive necrosis of the mucosa of the intestine, leading to nausea, vomiting, and diarrhea

       b) Above 500-rad exposure: high mortality from uncontrollable intestinal fluid and electrolyte loss; death occurs in a few days

       c) Recovery of survivors very slow: over many months

     3. Hematopoietic syndrome (200–600 rads)

       a) Commonly occurs in patients with gastrointestinal symptoms who survive for at least a period

       b) First change: lymphopenia and depletion of lymphocytes in lymph nodes and spleen

       c) Subsequent change: bone marrow aplasia

       d) Death in 20–50% of patients

     4. Acute radiation syndrome (50–200 rads)

       a) A nonlethal syndrome characterized by listlessness, fatigue, vomiting, and anorexia for a variable period

       b) Transient reduction in peripheral blood lymphocytes and granulocytes

     5. Survivors of irradiation

       a) Are not "normal," even after low-level exposure

       b) A high incidence of later development of various types of cancer, aplastic anemia, genetic abnormalities in offspring,

cataracts in the eyes, growth and mental retardation
  c) Low limit of "safe" levels of radiation exposure unknown
V. Localized radiation
  A. Localized radiation is used in the therapy of malignant neoplasms.
  B. Prediction of the degree of radiosensitivity of a malignant neoplasm is based on the following factors:
    1. Past experience
    2. Proliferative rate of neoplastic cells
  C. The effect of radiation on normal tissues is predictable on a similar basis.
    1. Past experience of complications observed during radiotherapy
    2. Turnover rate of cells: labile cells (hematopoietic cells, germ cells, and intestinal epithelial cells) extremely sensitive; stable cells (liver and kidney) less susceptible; permanent cells (muscle and nerve) quite resistant

CHEMICAL AGENTS

Ethyl Alcohol Abuse (Alcoholism)

I. Alcoholism is estimated to affect 10% of the population of the United States, directly or indirectly.
II. Acute alcoholic intoxication causes
  A. central nervous system depression.
  B. impairment of fine motor skills and reflexes. Alcohol is implicated in 50% of fatal road traffic accidents.
  C. acute alcoholic liver disease.
  D. hypoglycemia.
  E. death (although rare in acute alcoholism).
III. Chronic alcoholism is associated with
  A. chronic liver disease, leading to cirrhosis.
  B. chronic pancreatitis.
  C. effects on the myocardium, leading to congestive heart failure (alcoholic cardiomyopathy).
  D. malnutrition, particularly deficiencies of folic acid, thiamine, and pyridoxine.

E. nervous system changes: peripheral neuropathy and central pontine myelinolysis.

Psychotropic Drug Abuse

I. Drug abuse is a major problem in the United States.
II. Drugs involved are
  A. stimulants: amphetamines, cocaine
  B. depressants: heroin, barbiturates, diazepam.
  C. hallucinogens: lysergic acid diethylamide (LSD), marijuana, PCP.
III. They may be ingested, inhaled, sniffed, injected into the skin ("skin popping"), or injected intravenously ("mainlining").
IV. Abuse may result in
  A. acute overdosage, which may be fatal.
  B. emotional and physical dependence.
  C. infection: local abscesses, bacteremia, hepatitis B (due to unsterile needles).
  D. foreign-body granulomas either locally (in skin poppers) or systemically in lung and liver.

Heavy Metal Poisoning

I. Lead poisoning causes the following conditions:
  A. Hypochromic anemia
    1. Due to inhibition of hemoglobin synthesis
    2. Characterized by increased free erythrocytic porphyrin level
  B. Nervous system toxicity
    1. Cortical neuronal degeneration (lead encephalopathy)
    2. Demyelination of peripheral motor nerves (lead neuropathy)
    3. Proximal renal tubular dysfunction
    4. Deposition of lead in the gums ("blue line") and epiphyseal region of growing bones in children
II. Mercury poisoning causes the following conditions:
  A. Gastric mucosal inflammation
  B. Acute renal tubular necrosis: occurs in acute poisoning
  C. Glomerular basement membrane thickening with nephrotic syndrome and chronic renal failure: occurs in chronic poisoning

INFECTION

Definition

The entry of a living organism into a tissue and its multiplication or survival therein is known as infection.

Classification of Infectious Agents

I. According to microbiologic group: viruses, rickettsiae, chlamydiae, mycoplasma, bacteria, fungi, protozoa, metazoa
II. According to function: infectious agents are classified according to their capability in terms of multiplying inside or outside cells
   A. Obligate intracellular organisms
      1. Grow and multiply in cells, usually parenchymal cells
      2. Require living cell systems for culture
      3. Viruses, rickettsiae, and chlamydiae
   B. Facultative intracellular organisms
      1. Capable of multiplying extracellularly as well as inside cells; usually macrophages
      2. Organisms belonging to this group
         a) Bacteria: Mycobacteria, *Brucella* spp.; some gram-negative bacilli
         b) Fungi that usually grow as nonmycelial forms in tissues
         c) Protozoa: *Leishmania* spp., *Toxoplasma* spp.
      3. Can be cultured on artificial media (except for *Mycobacterium leprae*)
   C. Extracellular organisms
      1. Organisms that multiply only in the extracellular space
      2. Organisms belonging to this group: those that do not belong in preceding groups
      3. Can be cultured on artificial media (except for the larger parasites)

Tissue Changes in Infection

I. Cellular damage caused by infectious agents
   A. Obligate intracellular organisms
      Viruses, rickettsiae, and chlamydia infect parenchymal cells and multiply causing cellular changes.
      1. Cell necrosis

a) Different agents have affinity for different parenchymal cells (organotropism).

b) In acute viral infections patients die very rapidly (e.g., in viral encephalitis, myocarditis, or massive liver cell necrosis) or recover rapidly.

c) Less frequently, the virus causes chronic or "slow" infections in which continued cell necrosis occurs over months or years (e.g., chronic hepatitis B and slow virus infections of brain).

2. Cellular swelling
   Endothelial cell swelling in Rickettsial infection leads to thrombosis and hemorrhage.

3. Inclusion body formation
   Inclusions are collections of viral products.

   a) Cytomegalovirus infection: cells greatly enlarged and contain huge eosinophilic intranuclear inclusions; also produces multiple, small, basophilic intracytoplasmic inclusions (Fig. 5-6).

   b) Eosinophilic intranuclear inclusions (Cowdry type A) smaller than CMV intranuclear inclusions; occur in
      i) *Herpes simplex* and *Herpes varicella-zoster* infections (Fig. 5-7).
      ii) adenovirus infections.
      iii) measles virus and influenza infections (rare).

   c) Smallpox: multiple, small, eosinophilic cytoplasmic inclusions (Guarnieri bodies)

   d) Rabies virus: multiple, round to oval, eosinophilic cytoplasmic inclusions (Negri bodies)

   e) Chlamydial infections: multiple, irregular cytoplasmic inclusions

   f) Hepatitis B virus: a ground glass appearance of the cytoplasm of infected hepatocytes

4. Giant cell formation
   Multinucleated giant cells occur in
   a) measles: Warthin–Finkeldy cells.
   b) Herpes virus infections (*H. simplex, H. varicella-zoster*), (Fig. 5-7).

5. Neoplastic transformation of cells (viral carcinogenesis)

B. Extracellular organisms

1. Release of locally acting bacterial products, mainly enzymes
   a) Staphylococci: coagulase, hemolysins, staphylokinase
   b) Streptococci: hyaluronidase, streptolysins, streptokinase

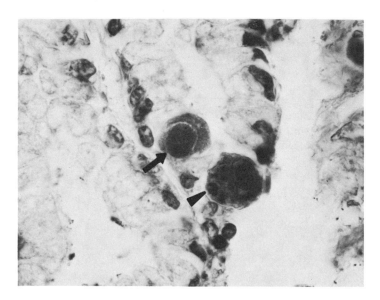

Fig. 5-6. Cytomegalovirus (CMV) in gastric mucosal cells. The infected cells are enlarged and have intranuclear (arrow) and intracytoplasmic (arrowhead) inclusions.

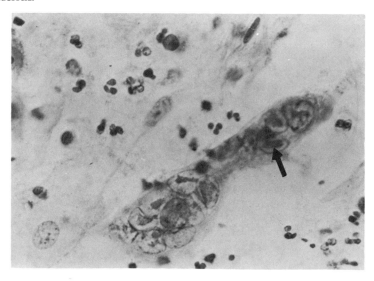

Fig. 5-7. Cervical smear in *Herpes simplex* infection showing multinucleated giant cells and intranuclear inclusions (arrow).

    c) Clostridia (usually *C. perfringens*): collagenases, lecithinases, cytolysins, fibrinolysins, hemolysins, and hyaluronidase (gas gangrene)

    d) *Entamoeba histolytica*: enzymes (amoebic liver abscess)

2. Production of a local vasculitis and ischemic necrosis

    a) Anthrax: plague

    b) Fungi: Aspergillus and Mucor

3. Remote-acting bacterial products

    a) Exotoxins: chemicals secreted by bacteria that act at a site distant to the focus of infection

        (1) *Staphyloccus aureus*: exotoxins that cause

            i) Neonatal bullous impetigo ("scalded skin syndrome") due to an epidermolytic toxin

            ii) Toxic Shock Syndrome

            iii) Food poisoning-enterotoxin

        (2) *Streptococcus pyogenes*: erythrogenic toxin causes scarlet fever

        (3) *Corynebacterium diphtheriae*: exotoxin that causes myocarditis and peripheral neuritis

        (4) *Clostridium tetani* (tetanus): exotoxin that causes convulsions and spasm of muscles

        (5) *Clostridium botulinum* (botulism): exotoxin that, when ingested in contaminated food, causes neuromuscular paralysis

    b) Enterotoxins: special type of exotoxins that are liberated into the lumen of the intestine

        (1) Cause a biochemical defect in mucosal cells, leading to increased secretion of water and electrolytes (severe diarrhea)

        (2) Occur in infections with

            i) *Vibrio cholerae* (cholera)

            ii) *Staphylococcus aureus* food poisoning

        (3) *Clostridium difficile*: toxin that causes necrosis of mucosal epithelial cells (membranous enterocolitis)

    c) Endotoxins

        (1) Lipopolysaccharide cell wall components of gram-negative bacteria

        (2) Cause peripheral circulatory failure and shock (gram-negative shock) when they enter the blood stream

II. Tissue changes due to host response to the agent

  A. The immune and inflammatory reaction to the agent frequently causes tissue injury.

    1. Liquefactive necrosis in suppurative inflammation

2. Caseous necrosis in chronic granulomatous inflammation
B. With many infectious agents, much of the clinical symptomatology is the result of the inflammatory response.

Infection of the Blood Stream

I. The presence of microorganisms in the blood stream (bacteremia, viremia) is always abnormal and is always of clinical significance.
   A. Extreme 1: The microorganisms are present in small numbers, do not actively multiply in the blood and are rapidly removed. Such a mild bacteremia is significant in
      1. immunocompromised patients in whom disseminated infection may occur.
      2. Patients with heart disease who may develop endocarditis.
      3. Normal individuals, where this is a route of infection of internal organs (e.g., viral encephalitis, renal tuberculosis).
   B. Extreme 2: The microorganisms are present in large numbers, multiply actively in the blood, and progressively increase in number. Such severe bacteremia causes high fever, tachycardia, and hypotension, and is sometimes called septicemia or sepsis.

Diagnosis of Infectious Disease

I. The aim of diagnosis is to identify the specific agent.
II. Methods of diagnosis include the following:
   A. Clinical examination: a few agents produce an illness whose clinical characteristics are highly indicative (e.g., herpes zoster, malaria)
   B. Microbiologic examination (culture)
   C. Immunologic techniques
      Antibody titer is a measure of the specific immune response against the infectious agent. A sharp (four-fold) rise in antibody titer indicates acute infection.
   D. Histologic examination of tissues
      1. Larger microorganisms, such as fungi, protozoa, and metazoa, can be identified in histologic sections.
      2. In a few diseases (e.g., leprosy, tuberculosis, actinomycosis, Legionnaire's disease) bacteria can be identified by special stains.
      3. Some viruses are recognizable by changes produced in cells (e.g., giant cells of herpes simplex) and inclusions.

6

Disorders of
Development and Growth

DISORDERS OF FETAL DEVELOPMENT

I. Definitions (Fig. 6-1)
   A. Failure of development of the primitive organ bud (anlage) in the embryo results in complete absence of that organ (agenesis).
   B. Abnormal differentiation of the organ anlage leads to a structurally abnormal organ (dysgenesis).
   C. When the primitive organ anlage differentiates normally but stops growth prematurely, a small organ results (hypoplasia).

II. Causes of abnormal fetal development
   A. Genetic disorders
      1. Structural chromosomal abnormalities
         a) The normal karyotype
            (1) The normal human cell has 46 chromosomes: 22 pairs of autosomes and two sex chromosomes (XX or XY).
            (2) The autosomes are divided into seven groups (A–G) and are numbered 1–22 based on size, position of the centromere, and pattern of banding.
            (3) The sex chromosomes are a pair of X chromosomes in the female or an X and Y chromosome in the male.
            (4) The karyotype is designated as 46,XX (normal female) or 46,XY (normal male).
         b) Mechanisms of chromosomal defects
            (1) Nondisjunction in meiosis
               i) Nondisjunction is the failure of paired homologous chromosomes to separate during meiosis.
               ii) It results in aneuploid (having a number of chromosomes that is not an exact multiple of 23, the haploid number) gametes.
               iii) Union of an aneuploid gamete with a normal gamete leads to an aneuploid cell that either has

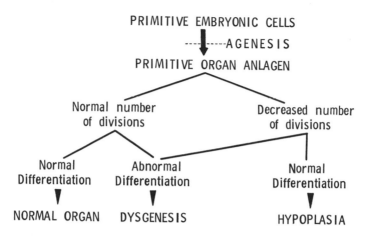

Fig. 6-1. Different ways in which an organ develops abnormally

three of the involved chromosome (trisomy) or only one (monosomy).
(2) Nondisjunction in mitosis
Nondisjunction of the early zygote (diploid cell) during a mitotic division produces two genetically different populations of cells within the embryo (mosaicism).
(3) Deletion: the loss of part of a chromosome after chromosomal breakage
(4) Translocation: the transfer of a broken segment of one chromosome to another chromosome
c) Causes of chromosomal defects
(1) Increasing maternal age: associated with nondisjunction
(2) Ionizing radiation
(3) Drugs, e.g., anticancer agents
d) Common autosomal defects
(1) Down's syndrome (mongolism; trisomy 21)
i) The most common cytogenetic abnormality
ii) Results from the presence in the cell of genetic material of three 21 chromosomes (Fig. 6-2)
iii) Three types of Down's syndrome
(A) Nondisjunction Down's (95% of cases): associated with increasing maternal age; the

child has an extra 21 chromosome (Fig. 6-2)

- (B) Translocation type (3%): part of the long arm of 21 is translocated to 22 or 14; often familial
- (C) Mosaic type (2%): failure of disjunction in embryogenesis: variable mild clinical features

iv) Clinical features

- (A) Mongoloid facial appearance
- (B) Severe mental retardation
- (C) 30% of patients have congenital heart disease, commonly ventricular septal defect
- (D) Increased susceptibility to infections and acute leukemia

(2) Trisomy 18 (Edward's syndrome): severe mental retardation with abnormal hands and feet

(3) Trisomy 13 (Patau's syndrome): abnormal development of the forebrain and midline facial structures. Death in neonatal period

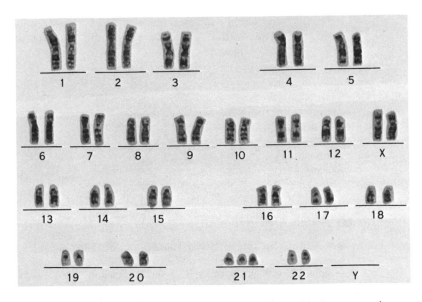

Fig. 6-2. Karyotype of trisomy 21 (Down's syndrome). This karyotype shows banded chromosomes. The patient is female.

(4) Deletion of short arm of chromosome 5 (cri du chat syndrome): severe mental retardation, cardiac anomalies, and a characteristic cat-like cry of the infant

e) Common sex chromosomal defects (Fig. 6-3)

  (1) Klinefelter's syndrome (testicular dysgenesis) (Fig. 6-3)

    i) Common, caused by nondisjunction of the X chromosome (47,XXY).

    ii) Y chromosome dictates development as a male.

    iii) Testes do not develop at puberty; remain small. Seminiferous tubules remain atrophic with absent spermatogenesis.

    iv) Testosterone levels are low, leading to failure of development of male secondary sex characteristics.

    v) Patients are tall and eunuchoid.

    vi) Intelligence is usually normal.

  (2) Turner's syndrome (gonadal dysgenesis; 45,XO)

    i) Common; it is caused by nondisjunction of the X chromosome with loss of an X chromosome (45,XO) (Fig. 6-3); may occur as a mosaic.

    ii) The absence of a Y chromosome leads to development as a female.

    iii) The ovaries fail to develop at puberty (streak ovaries).

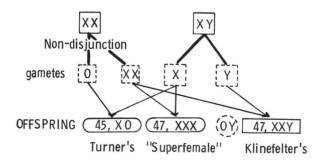

Note: 45, OY is lethal and leads to abortion

Fig. 6-3. Abnormalities of sex chromosome number due to nondisjunction of X chromosomes in the female gametes.

      iv) Patients remain short and infantile with poor breast development, amenorrhea, and infertility.

      v) Lymphedema of the neck is found in infants and webbing of the neck is found in adults.

      vi) Coarctation of the aorta is common.

      vii) Intelligence is usually normal.

2. Single-gene (Mendelian) disorders

  a) Diseases caused by a single abnormal gene are inherited in a predictable manner determined by Mendelian laws.

  b) If one considers a gene that has two alleles A and a

    (1) three genotypes (AA, Aa, aa) are possible.

    (2) the genotypes AA and aa are homozygous; Aa is heterozygous.

    (3) if the genotypes AA and Aa produce an identical phenotype and this is different from aa, the A gene is dominant and the a gene is recessive.

  c) Autosomal dominant traits (Fig. 6-4 and Table 6-1)

    (1) Characterized in the family history by

      i) the presence of the abnormal gene and therefore the disease in every generation.

      ii) affection of males and females equally.

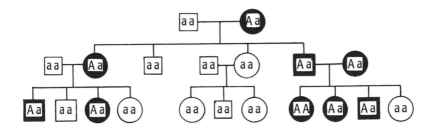

Fig. 6-4. Pedigree of a disease inherited as an autosomal dominant. A = abnormal gene.

Table 6-1. Common Autosomal Disorders

Autosomal Dominant	Autosomal Recessive
Achondroplasia (dwarfism)	Cystic fibrosis (mucoviscidosis)
Marfan's syndrome	Alpha-1-antitrypsin deficiency
Neurofibromatosis	Phenylketonuria
von Willebrand's disease	Wilson's disease
Hereditary hemorrhagic telangiectasia	Tay–Sachs disease
Osteogenesis imperfecta	
Acute intermittent porphyria	
Huntington's chorea	
Hereditary spherocytosis	
Adult renal polycystic disease	
Hereditary angioedema	

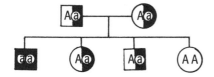

a a – affected male or female

A a – heterozygous carrier

A A – normal female or male

Fig. 6-5. Pedigree of a disease inherited as an autosomal recessive. a = abnormal gene.

  iii) union of an affected heterozygote (Aa) with a
       normal (aa) resulting in offspring that have a 50%
       chance of getting the abnormal gene and
       disease.
  (2) Of the approximately 750 autosomal dominant disorders of man, most are characterized by structural
      abnormalities.
  (3) Variable expression (penetrance) of the abnormal gene
      is common, e.g., in neurofibromatosis.

d) Autosomal recessive traits (Fig. 6-5 and Table 6-1)
   (1) Examination of the family history shows
       i) no disease in the parents.
       ii) expression of the disease in a sibling or a remote family member.
   (2) Both parents of an affected individual must be heterozygous carriers. Siblings have a 25% chance of being affected.
   (3) It is associated with cultures where consanguinous marriage is common.
   (4) Most are characterized by enzyme deficiency leading to "inborn errors of metabolism."
e) Sex-linked traits (Table 6-2)
   All sex-linked traits are linked to the X-chromosome.
   (1) X-Linked recessive traits (Fig. 6-6 and Table 6-2)
       i) These traits are transmitted by female heterozygous carriers of the abnormal gene.
       ii) 50% of male offspring of a union between a carrier and a normal male will be affected.
       iii) Females have disease only when homozygous for abnormal gene: very rare.
   (2) X-Linked dominant traits
       i) Uncommon. The only common disease so inherited is hypophosphatemic rickets.
       ii) Females are more commonly affected than males.
       iii) An affected male transmits the disease to all his daughters.

Table 6-2. Common Sex-Linked Disorders

X-Linked Recessive	X-Linked Dominant	Y-Linked
Hemophilia	Hypophosphatemic rickets	None known
Christmas disease		
Bruton's agammaglobulinemia		
G-6-PD deficiency		
Testicular feminization		
Duchenne muscular dystrophy		
Chronic granulomatous disease		

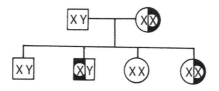

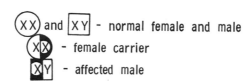

(XX) and [X Y] – normal female and male

(X⊗) – female carrier

[⊗Y] – affected male

Fig. 6-6. Pedigree of a disease inherited as a sex-linked recessive.

3. Polygenic (multiple gene) inheritance

Diseases such as hypertension and diabetes mellitus that tend to "run in families" are believed to be due to the interaction of several genes as well as to environmental factors.

B. Abnormal fetal development due to external agents (teratogens) resulting in other congenital abnormalities (Table 6-3)

1. Ionizing radiation

The minimum safe radiation dosage in early pregnancy is not known.

Table 6-3. Common Congenital Anomalies

Congenital heart disease
Neural tube defects (meningomyelocele)
Cleft lip and palate
Congenital pyloric stenosis
Intestinal atresia
Tracheoesophageal fistula
Imperforate anus
Clubfoot (talipes equinovarus)
Congenital dislocation of hip

2. Infections
   a) Rubella
      (1) Rubella is the best known teratogenic virus.
      (2) The risk is greatest (up to 70%) in the first 8 weeks.
      (3) Rubella virus interferes with protein synthesis.
      (4) "Rubella syndrome" refers to the triad of congenital heart disease, deafness, and cataracts.
      (5) Other defects include microcephaly with mental retardation, and microphthalmia.
   b) Other viruses in early pregnancy: uncertain
   c) Infections of the developed fetus
      (1) Cytomegalovirus and *Toxoplasm gondii* produce necrosis and calcification in the brain. This causes microcephaly and mental retardation.
      (2) *Treponema pallidum*, crosses the placenta and infects the fetus (congenital syphilis).
3. Drugs
   a) Thalidomide
      (1) A mild sedative drug that was commonly used in Europe in the 1960's
      (2) Shown to cause failure of the limbs with the hands appearing as short stumps off the trunk: phocomelia
   b) Diethylstilbestrol (DES)
      (1) Was used in 1950–1960 in the treatment of threatened abortion
      (2) Associated with abnormal development of the vaginal epithelium (vaginal adenosis) and an increased risk of vaginal cancer (clear cell carcinoma) in childhood

POSTNATAL DEVELOPMENT

I. The newborn infant is structurally fully formed and, apart from minor developmental changes, merely grows into an adult.
II. Abnormalities in psychosocial development cause psychiatric illness. The pathological basis of these diseases is unknown.
III. Aging is the final phase of postnatal development.
   A. Defined as the sum total of changes that occur with the passage of time. "Old" is impossible to define.
   B. Man has a finite life span of 90–110 years.
   C. Morphologic changes of aging
      1. Organ and tissue atrophy
      2. Decreased T-lymphocyte function and increased incidence of autoantibodies

  3. DNA changes due to defective repair mechanisms contributing to cell loss
  4. Accumulation of lipofuscin in brain and myocardial cells
  5. Changes in the extracellular connective tissue
    a) Decreased elasticity of the skin, elastic arteries and lungs (senile emphysema)
    b) Deposition of amyloid ("senile amyloidosis")
    c) Changes in ground substance in the lens (cataract), joint cartilages (osteoarthritis)
    d) Bone loss (osteoporosis)
    e) Medial calcification of muscular arteries (Monckeberg's sclerosis)
  D. The cause of aging is unknown. Theories include the following:
    1. Programmed aging
      a) The aging process is programmed into the genome.
      b) *Progeria*, where there is a greatly accelerated aging process, is believed to be due to faulty programming.
    2. Changes in DNA
      Decreased replication of DNA and decreased efficiency of DNA repair occur increasingly with age.
    3. Immune theory of aging
      The decline of the immune system functions that occur with increasing age contributes to aging of all tissues.

DISORDERS OF CELLULAR GROWTH AND MATURATION

  I. Atrophy, hypertrophy, and hyperplasia
  A. Definitions (Fig. 6-7)
    1. Atrophy: a decrease in the size of a tissue after it has developed due to a decrease in size of individual cells or a decrease in their number
    2. Hypertrophy: an increase in size of a tissue due to an increase in size of its component cells
    3. Hyperplasia: an increase in the size of a tissue or organ due to an increase in the number of component cells
    4. Not uncommonly, an increase in size is due to a combination of both hypertrophy and hyperplasia.

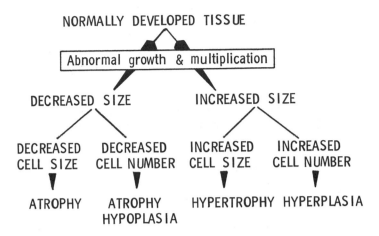

Fig. 6-7. Different types of abnormal growth in tissues.

B. Causes of atrophy
   1. Disuse atrophy, e.g., in skeletal muscle and bone during immobilization
   2. Denervation atrophy of skeletal muscle due to damage to the lower motor neurone
   3. Atrophy due to loss of trophic hormones
      a) Withdrawal of female sex hormones at menopause leads to atrophic changes in the endometrium, vaginal mucosa, and breast.
      b) Withdrawal of pituitary trophic hormones leads to atrophy of all target organs: thyroid, adrenal cortex, gonads.
      c) High-dose adrenocortical steroid therapy suppresses pituitary ACTH, leading to adrenal cortical atrophy.
   4. Atrophy caused by nutrient lack
      a) Malnutrition (marasmus) due to utilization of body tissues such as skeletal muscle as an energy and protein source
      b) Ischemia: chronic ischemia causes progressive cell loss and atrophy.
   5. Senile atrophy
      Cell loss is one of the morphologic changes of the aging process.
   6. Pressure atrophy
      Prolonged compression of a tissue causes atrophy.

C. Causes of hypertrophy and hyperplasia
1. Increased functional demand leads to various combinations of physiologic hypertrophy and hyperplasia.
   a) Skeletal and cardiac muscle hypertrophy with increased load.
   b) Hypertrophy of the smooth muscle wall of the bladder or intestine occurs proximal to an obstruction.
   c) Hyperplasia occurs in labile and stable cells in response to demand.
      (1) In hemolytic processes, there is erythroid hyperplasia in bone marrow.
      (2) Pregnancy and lactation are associated with hyperplasia and hypertrophy of uterine muscle and breast parenchyma.
2. Pathologic hypertrophy and hyperplasia
   An increase in size of a tissue without there being an increased demand
   a) Myocardial hypertrophy sometimes occurs without any recognizable cause (hypertrophic cardiomyopathy).
   b) Endometrial hyperplasia is associated with excessive bleeding, and predisposes to cancer of the endometrium.
   c) Prostatic hyperplasia, a very common disease in older men, is characterized by hyperplasia of both the glandular and stromal elements.
II. Metaplasia
   A. The replacement of one type of adult tissue with another different type of adult tissue that is abnormal for that site
   B. Epithelial metaplasia
      1. Squamous metaplasia is the most common type and occurs in
         a) the columnar epithelia of the endocervix, endometrium, and respiratory tract.
         b) the transitional epithelium of the bladder.
      2. Glandular metaplasia occurs in
         a) the squamous epithelium of the lower esophagus (Barrett's esophagus).
         b) intestinal metaplasia of the gastric mucosa in chronic gastritis.
      3. Most epithelial metaplasias occur as a result of chronic irritation.
      4. The metaplastic epithelium matures normally and does not carry an increased risk of neoplasia.

C. Mesenchymal metaplasia
   1. Rare
   2. Osseous metaplasia sometimes occurs in fibroblastic proliferations in soft tissue.
   3. Of little clinical significance
III. Dysplasia
   A. The term *dysplasia* should be reserved for a specific abnormality in maturation of dividing epithelial cells. Dysplasia is recognized by the following:
      1. Nuclear abnormalities, including
         a) increase in size of nucleus relative to the amount of cytoplasm (increased nuclear: cytolasmic ratio).
         b) hyperchromasia: increased amount of chromatin.
         c) abnormal chromatin: thicker than normal and tending to form coarse clumps
         d) irregularity, wrinkling and thickening of the nuclear membrane.
      2. Increased rate of multiplication of cells, leading to
         a) disorderly maturation.
         b) the presence of mitoses at all levels in the epithelium.
      3. Failure of development of cytoplasmic features such as keratinization (squamous epithelium) and mucin (columnar epithelium).
   B. So defined, dysplasia is associated with an increased risk of developing into a neoplastic disease.
   C. The term *intraepithelial neoplasia* is synonymous with severe dysplasia.
   D. The time frame in which dysplasia progresses to invasive cancer is variable depending on site.
   E. Dysplasia is usually graded into mild, moderate, severe, and carcinoma-in-situ; the latter is a misleading term that is used for the most severe form of dysplasia.
   F. The risk of developing cancer increases with increasing grades of dysplasia.
   G. Dysplasia and carcinoma-in-situ differ from cancer.
      1. There is no invasion in dysplasia or carcinoma-in-situ.
         a) Because the epithelium contains no lymphatics or blood vessels, metastasis does not occur.
         b) Complete removal of the area of dysplasia is 100% curative.
      2. Dysplasia, particularly the milder grades, appears to be reversible, unlike neoplasia.

H. Diagnosis of dysplasia

    (1) Dysplasias, including carcinoma-in-situ, are often asymptomatic.

    (2) As a rule, diagnosis is made by examining cells in scrapings (exfoliative cytology) or biopsies.

    (3) Routine cytologic screening of cervical smears ("Pap smears") has permitted recognition and early treatment of cervical dysplasia. This has contributed to a striking decline in the incidence of invasive cervical cancer in the past two decades.

IV. Neoplasia

  A. Definition

    1. Neoplasia is an abnormality of cellular growth that:

      a) is characterized by excessive cellular proliferation.

      b) is uncoordinated with the growth of surrounding normal cells and occurs without any apparent purpose and without the controls that govern normal cellular growth.

      c) persists in the same excessive manner after removal of the stimulus that evoked the change.

    2. The above definition indicates how poorly the process of neoplasia is understood (Fig. 6-8).

      a) Neoplasia cannot be defined by its causative agents because these are largely unknown.

      b) Neoplasia cannot be defined by a fundamental change in the cell because this is unknown.

      c) Neoplasia is therefore defined by its characteristic growth abnormality.

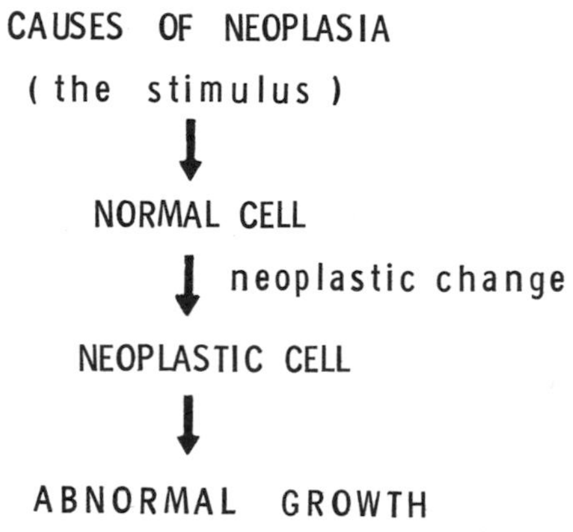

CAUSES OF NEOPLASIA

(the stimulus)

NORMAL CELL

 neoplastic change

NEOPLASTIC CELL

ABNORMAL GROWTH

Fig. 6-8. The process of neoplasia.

B. The neoplastic change: theories of oncogenesis
   Normal cellular growth is under the control of regulator genes
   that act through growth regulating proteins. The abnormal
   growth of neoplasia may result from the following:
   1. Somatic mutation involving regulator genes
      Acquired chromosomal abnormalities are associated with
      neoplasia in
      a) Bloom's syndrome (rare), which is characterized by in-
         stability of chromosomes and increased incidence of skin
         cancer.
      b) leukemias (particularly chronic granulocytic leukemia),
         lymphomas and many other neoplasms.
   2. Abnormal DNA repair mechanisms involving regulator
      genes
      a) DNA alterations occur frequently in normal cells, which
         have active repair mechanisms.
      b) In the elderly, DNA repair mechanisms are frequently
         defective. The incidence of neoplasia progressively in-
         creases with age.
      c) Xeroderma pigmentosum
         (1) An autosomal recessive inherited disease characterized
             by deficiency of an important DNA-repairing en-
             zyme.
         (2) DNA dimers produced in skin by exposure to ultra-
             violet (sun) light persist as mutations.
         (3) These patients have a very high incidence of skin
             cancer and are extremely sensitive to sunlight.
   3. The virogene–oncogene theory
      a) Suggest that viral genetic material introduced many
         generations ago may have integrated into the genome
         ("endogenous viruses," cellular oncogenes).
      b) These cause neoplastic transformation after appropriate
         derepression by various carcinogens.
      c) A number of oncogenic viral nucleotide sequences (viral
         oncogenes) have been identified in cells of experimental
         animals (cellular oncogenes) and man.
      d) For some oncogenes the gene product is a protein kinase-
         tyrosine phosphorylase which appears to play a role in cell
         growth regulation.
   4. Abnormalities of growth regulating proteins (epigenetic
      theory)
      a) Many stimuli that cause neoplasia, such as chemical
         agents, do not produce DNA changes.
      b) Some of these agents bind cellular proteins as the major

biochemical action. If such binding involves regulator proteins, neoplasia may result.
5. Neoplasia as a failure of immune surveillance
  a) Neoplastic changes in cells result in new antigens that are recognized and destroyed by the immune system.
  b) Neoplasia results only if the immune system fails to recognize and destroy the altered cell.
  c) States of immune deficiency in which neoplasms occur with increased frequency include:
    (1) congenital immunodeficiency syndromes.
    (2) acquired immunodeficiency syndrome (AIDS).
    (3) old age.
C. Causes of neoplasia (carcinogens, oncogens)
  A cause of neoplasia (a carcinogen) is a stimulus that produces the basic neoplastic change in a cell. While a large number of carcinogens have been identified the causes of most types of human neoplasms remain unknown.
1. Chemical carcinogens
  a) Polycyclic hydrocarbons: benzpyrene, dibenzanthracene
    Soot containing hydrocarbons was the first chemical to be recognized as a carcinogen (Percival Pott, 1775, in chimney sweeps).
  b) CIGARETTE SMOKING
    (1) Is associated with cancer of the lung, bladder and oral cavity
    (2) Is believed to be due to the polycyclic hydrocarbon ("tar") content of cigarettes
    (3) Probably causes more cases of cancer than all other known carcinogens combined
  c) Cyclamates and saccharin
    Used as artificial sweeteners; cause bladder cancer in experimental animals
  d) Nitrosamines
    (1) Carcinogenic in experimental animals in very small doses
    (2) Produced in the human stomach from nitrites which are extensively used as meat preservatives
    (3) Role in human carcinogenesis uncertain
  e) Azo-dyes
    Used as food coloring agents in the past ("butter yellow"), induce liver cell cancer in experimental animals
  f) Aflatoxin
    (1) A metabolite of the fungus *Aspergillus flavus*, which

grows on improperly stored ground nuts and grain
- (2) High levels of aflatoxin in the diet in parts of Africa associated with a high incidence of liver cell cancer
- g) Betel leaf and areca nut chewing in India and Sri Lanka is associated with a high incidence of oral cavity cancer.
- h) Asbestos has been clearly shown to cause
  - (1) mesothelioma of the pleura, pericardium and peritoeum.
  - (2) bronchogenic carcinoma ("lung cancer").
- i) Heavy metals like arsenic (skin and lung cancer), nickel (lung), chromium (lung), and cadmium (lung).
- j) Polyvinyl chloride (PVC), is a widely used synthetic plastic, causes angiosarcoma of the liver.
- k) Unknown environmental carcinogens
  - (1) 70–90% of all cancers may be due to unknown environmental carcinogenic agents.
  - (2) The marked geographic variation of different cancers is probably due to environmental agents.
2. Radiation carcinogenesis
  - a) Ultraviolet radiation of sunlight
    - (1) Associated with skin cancers (basal cell carcinoma, squamous cell carcinoma, and malignant melanoma)
    - (2) Common in fair-skinned races. The melanin pigment of dark-skinned individuals is protective against ultraviolet light.
  - b) X-rays
    - (1) Early radiologists had an increased incidence of skin cancer and leukemia.
    - (2) Neck radiation for respiratory obstruction in infants in 1950–60 led to a high incidence of thyroid cancer 15–25 years later.
  - c) Radioisotopes
    - (1) Exposure to radioactive minerals in mines of Central Europe and Western United States caused lung cancer.
    - (2) An epidemic of bone cancer (osteosarcoma) occurred in a watch factory among radium watch-dial painters who sharpened their brushes with their lips.
    - (3) Thorotrast, a radio-active thorium-containing dye that was used in radiography, is deposited in liver and causes angiosarcoma, liver cell cancer, and bile duct cancer.
  - d) Nuclear fall-out

(1) The Hiroshima–Nagasaki survivors have an increased incidence of leukemia, breast, lung, and thyroid cancer.

(2) The accidental exposure of Marshall Islanders during nuclear device testing produced benign and malignant thyroid neoplasms.

3. Viral carcinogenesis

a) Mechanisms (see Virogene–Oncogene Theory)

b) Oncogenic RNA viruses

(1) In animals, RNA viruses have been proven to cause

   i) leukemia and lymphomas in mice, cats and birds.

   ii) sarcomas in birds (Rous sarcoma virus) and primates.

   iii) breast carcinoma in mice (the Bittner milk virus, mouse mammary tumor virus—MMTV).

(2) No definite proof is available for RNA viruses causing any human neoplasm. HTLV-I, associated with human T-cell leukemia, and HTLV-III, the so-called AIDS virus, are RNA retroviruses.

c) Oncogenic DNA viruses

DNA viruses are strongly incriminated in human oncogenesis.

(1) Papova viruses

The papilloma virus group causes benign squamous epithelial neoplasms in skin and mucous membranes (verruca vulgaris, condyloma acuminatum, laryngeal papillomatosis).

(2) Pox viruses: *Molluscum contagiosum* virus produces a wart-like benign neoplasm in the skin.

(3) Adenoviruses: role in human oncogenesis is unknown

(4) Herpes viruses

   i) Epstein Barr Virus (EBV) in African Burkitt's lymphoma. EBV selectively infects B lymphocytes.

   ii) EBV is also believed to be associated with nasopharyngeal carcinoma in the Far East.

   iii) Herpes simplex type II virus may be associated with carcinoma of the uterine cervix.

4. Nutritional oncogenic factors

a) In Japan a relationship exists between gastric cancer and a high intake of fish. Smoked fish has a high hydrocarbon content.

    b) A high fiber content in the diet is postulated to decrease colon cancer risk.
    c) A high fat diet has been associated with colon cancer.
  5. Hormones and neoplasia
    a) Hormone induction of neoplasms
      (1) Diethylstilbestrol (DES) administration in pregnancy has been shown to cause vaginal clear cell adenocarcinoma in female offspring.
      (2) Oral contraceptives have been associated with liver cell adenomas.
      (3) Unopposed estrogen effect of the endometrium causes endometrial hyperplasia and cancer.
    b) Hormone dependence of neoplasms
      (1) Prostate carcinoma is dependent on androgens.
      (2) Breast carcinoma
        i) Frequently dependent on estrogens; more rarely on progesterone.
        ii) Hormone dependence correlates well with the presence of estrogen and progesterone receptors on the cancer cell membrane.
      (3) Well differentiated thyroid cancer is dependent on TSH.
  6. Inherited neoplasms
    a) Single gene inheritance of neoplasms
      (1) Retinoblastoma
        i) Occurs in both inherited (40%) and noninherited (60%) forms
        ii) Inherited form has bilateral neoplasms.
        iii) Chromosome analysis shows a deletion of the long arm of chromosome number 13.
      (2) Other autosomal dominant single-gene inherited diseases characterized by the occurrence of neoplasms are
        i) neurofibromatosis.
        ii) familial multiple endocrine adenomatosis (MEA).
        iii) familial polyposis coli.
        iv) multiple nevoid basal cell carcinoma syndrome.
    b) Familial tendency (? polygenic) of neoplasms
      Breast carcinoma has an increased incidence in families.
D. The neoplastic cell (morphologic and biochemical alterations)
  1. Lag period
    a) A constant feature of all known carcinogens is a time

interval between exposure and development of the neoplasm.

b) This lag period is the main reason why it has been difficult to identify carcinogenic agents for common neoplasms.

c) The lag period also suggests that more than one process is involved in the production of a neoplasm (so-called 2-hit theory).

 (1) Initiation is the actual neoplastic change produced by the carcinogen (initiator).

 (2) Promotion is the action of a second agent (co-carcinogen or promotor) that causes the neoplastic cell to express its growth abnormality.

d) In the lag period, the neoplastic cells resemble normal cells, or are so few as to be undetectable.

2. Monoclonal (single cell) origin vs. field origin

a) It is probable that neoplasms arise in two separate ways:

 (1) From a single cell (monoclonal origin).

 (2) From several cells in multiple foci that undergo neoplastic transformation simultaneously (field origin).

b) Monoclonality has been proven in the following cases:

 (1) Immunoglobulin-producing neoplasms (B-cell lymphomas and plasma cell neoplasms): the presence of only one light chain and/or one heavy chain indicates monoclonality.

 (2) The presence of only one of the two isoenzymes of glucose-6-dehydrogenase in the cells of a neoplasm indicates monoclonality.

c) Multifocal (field effect) neoplasms are seen in the liver, urothelium, skin, breast, and colon. In all of these sites the occurrence of one neoplasm increases the risk of another.

3. Preneoplastic (or precancerous) changes

a) In most cases the neoplastic cell, after a lag period, transforms directly by cellular proliferation into the neoplasm.

b) In a few instances there is an intermediate nonneoplastic lesion (preneoplastic change).

c) Preneoplastic lesions are important because their recognition and removal may prevent the occurrence of the neoplasm.

d) Preneoplastic lesions include

 (1) dysplasia of cervix, skin, respiratory epithelium, bladder, stomach, and colon.

(2) hyperplasia of the endometrium and liver.
(3) some types of metaplasia: Barrett's esophagus.
(4) chronic inflammatory conditions: ulcerative colitis, chronic atrophic gastritis (in pernicious anemia).
(5) benign neoplasms: colonic adenoma, neurofibroma.
4. Biochemical, immunologic, and karyotypic changes
   a) Surface membrane alterations
      (1) Include changes in enzymes, microfilaments, glycoprotein and fibronectin content and electrical charge
      (2) Are associated with loss of contact inhibition
      (3) May contribute to the ability of malignant cells to invade and metastasize
   b) Appearance of new "tumor-specific" antigens
      (1) With viral-induced neoplasms the new antigen is a function of the virus. All neoplasms caused by one virus will show the same new antigen.
      (2) Chemically induced neoplasms manifest surface antigens that vary with each different neoplasm induced by the chemical. More often neoplasms lose antigens.
      (3) Tumor-specific antigens evoke a cellular immune response. In malignant melanoma, Hodgkin's disease, and breast carcinoma the magnitude of this lymphocytic response correlates with the behavior of the neoplasm.
      (4) Very rarely, spontaneous regression of neoplasms occurs; this is believed due to immune destruction.
   c) Karyotype abnormalities
      The following neoplasms and karyotypic abnormalities are associated:
      (1) The Philadelphia chromosome (Ph^1) (a small 22 chromosome resulting from translocation of part of chromosome 22 to chromosome 9): chronic granulocytic leukemia (90% of cases)
      (2) Acute promyelocytic leukemia: 15, 17 translocation
      (3) Burkitt lymphoma: 8, 14 and 8, 22 translocation
      (4) Retinoblastoma: deletion of 13
      (5) Wilms' tumor (nephroblastoma): deletion of 11
   d) Production of abnormal molecules (tumor markers)
      (1) Oncofetal antigens
         i) These are antigens that are usually only expressed in fetal life.
         ii) CEA (carcinoembryonic antigen) is elevated in most cases of colon and pancreatic carcinoma

and in some cases of gastric, breast, and lung cancer.

iii) AFP (alpha feto-protein) is elevated in most patients with liver cell carcinoma and with primitive gonadal germ cell neoplasms.

(2) Enzymes
   i) Elevation of prostatic acid phosphatase in prostate cancer
   ii) Regan iso-enzyme of alkaline phosphatase in pancreatic carcinoma

(3) Excessive secretion of normal substances
   Neoplasms of cells that synthesize molecules frequently secrete excessively, e.g., endocrine neoplasms, choriocarcinoma (human chorionic gonadotropin), plasma cell myeloma (immunoglobulin).

(4) "Ectopic" hormones (paraneoplastic syndromes)
   Many malignant neoplasms of cells that do not normally secrete hormones produce "ectopic" hormones.
   i) Human chorionic gonadotrophin: testicular germ cell neoplasms
   ii) Parathormone: squamous carcinoma of lung, renal adenocarcinoma, breast carcinoma
   iii) ACTH: oat cell carcinoma of lung, islet cell carcinoma of pancreas
   iv) Anti-diuretic hormone: oat cell carcinoma of lung
   v) Erythropoietin: renal adenocarcinoma, cerebellar hemangioblastoma

(5) Other paraneoplastic syndromes: occur in malignant neoplasms; no known cause
   i) Neuromyopathic syndromes: myasthenic (Eaton–Lambert) syndrome, cerebellar degeneration
   ii) A variety of skin lesions
   iii) Clubbing of fingers: lung cancer
   iv) Migratory superficial thrombophlebitis—leg: pancreatic, gastric, and lung cancer

E. Changes in cell growth pattern of neoplasms
   1. Excessive cellular proliferation
      a) Often produces a mass of neoplastic cells (a tumor).
      b) Rate of proliferation of neoplastic cells is extremely variable.

    c) As a general rule the degree of malignancy of a neoplasm increases with increasing rate of growth.

    d) Rate of growth is assessed by

      (1) mitotic rate: frequency with which mitotic figures are seen.

      (2) cellularity: rapidly growing neoplasms tend to be more cellular.

    e) Clinically the time taken for the neoplasm to double its size (doubling time). This varies from a few days in Burkitt's lymphoma to many months in most malignant epithelial neoplasms (carcinomas).

2. Anaplasia, differentiation

    a) As the neoplastic cell proliferates it may differentiate normally to resemble the cell of origin, e.g., a lipoma looks like fat; it is said to be well differentiated.

    b) With increasing degrees of malignancy, the degree of differentiation becomes less.

    c) When the examination of the neoplasm does not permit recognition of the cell of origin, the neoplasm is said to be undifferentiated or anaplastic (Fig. 6-9).

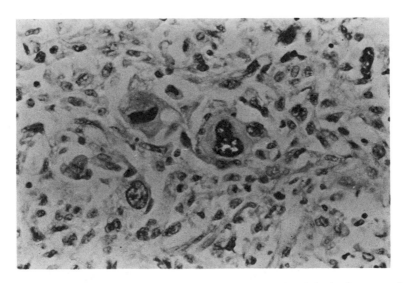

Fig. 6-9. Malignant neoplasm showing anaplasia and cytologic features of malignancy.

    d) On occasion, the neoplastic cell differentiates in directions abnormal for the cell of origin, e.g., squamous differentiation in an endometrial adenocarcinoma.

3. Infiltration (invasion)
   a) Benign neoplasms tend to expand by pushing and compressing surrounding tissue, forming fibrous capsules.
   b) Malignant neoplasms extend out on all sides as tongues of cells.
   c) Infiltration or invasion destroys tissues and may result in entry of tumor cells into blood vessels and lymphatics.
   d) Infiltration is a poorly understood process. Surface membrane abnormalities are believed to be important.

4. Metastasis
   a) Defined as an established second neoplastic mass at a site that is physically separate from the primary neoplasm.
   b) Occurs only with malignant neoplasms.
   c) Lymphatic metastasis
      (1) Occurs early in malignant epithelial neoplasms (carcinomas) and melanoma.
      (2) The cells are carried by lymphatics as emboli to the regional nodes.
   d) Blood stream metastasis
      (1) Establishment of neoplastic cells that are transported in the blood stream to remote sites is a complex process.
      (2) Most cancer cells that enter the blood are destroyed by the immune system.
      (3) Entrapped neoplastic cells must obtain a vascular supply if they are to survive. The production of a tumor angiogenesis factor (TAF) by neoplastic cells has been demonstrated.
      (4) The site of metastasis is most commonly the first capillary bed into which veins from the primary site drain: the lungs for the systemic venous drainage, and the liver for a tumor draining to the portal system.
      (5) Some sites are favored for metastasis, e.g., bone (thyroid and prostate cancer), adrenals (lung cancer).
      (6) Vascular dissemination occurs early in malignant mesenchymal neoplasms (sarcomas).
   e) Metastases in body cavity fluids
      Entry of neoplastic cells into the cerebrospinal fluid or celomic cavities may lead to dissemination.

Table 6-4. Differences between benign and Malignant Neoplasms

Benign	Malignant
Well differentiated	Poorly differentiated
Grow with compression (capsule)	Infiltrative growth
Slow growth	Rapid growth
Few mitoses (appear normal)	Many mitoses (often abnormal)
Nuclei appear normal	Nuclei hyperchromatic, "primitive"
Nucleoli rarely prominent	Nucleoli often prominent
Cells regular—"normal appearing"	Pleomorphic
Well-formed blood vessels	Rudimentary blood channels
No invasion	Invasion
No metastases	Metastases
Not fatal (unless in critical site)	Usually fatal (unless treated early)

F. Classification of neoplasms
   1. According to biologic behavior (benign vs. malignant) (Table 6-4)
      a) Neoplasms are classified as benign or malignant.
      b) Though broadly similar, the terms benign or malignant differ for different neoplasms; there are no universal criteria.
      c) Criteria used for differentiating benign from malignant neoplasms
         (1) Rate of growth
            Malignant neoplasms grow rapidly and benign neoplasms slowly.
         (2) Degree of differentiation
            Benign neoplasms resemble normal tissue. Anaplastic or poorly differentiated neoplasms are malignant. In between are many gradations.
         (3) Cellularity is greater and number of mitoses is higher in malignant neoplasms.
         (4) Cytologic features of malignancy (Fig. 6-9) include:
            i) pleomorphism: variation in size and appearance.
            ii) increased nuclear size and high nuclear: cytoplasmic ratio.
            iii) hyperchromatism, abnormal chromatin pattern, chromatin clumping.

        iv) wrinkling and thickening of nuclear membrane.

        v) lack of cohesion leading to separation of cells.

        vi) large nucleoli.

        vii) abnormal mitotic figures.

(5) Infiltration

    i) Benign neoplasms are generally surrounded by a capsule.

    ii) Some benign neoplasms have infiltrating borders and are not encapsulated (e.g., benign fibrous histiocytoma of skin).

    iii) Generally, infiltration is a reliable sign of malignancy.

    iv) In cancer of the uterine cervix, colon, stomach, and melanoma, the depth of invasion bears a close relationship to prognosis.

(6) Metastasis

    The occurrence of metastases represents absolute evidence that a given neoplasm is malignant.

2. According to cell of origin (Figs. 6-10, 6-11)

    a) A neoplasm arises from a cell in the body that has undergone neoplastic transformation. Neoplasms are classified and named according to the cell of origin.

    b) Neoplasms of totipotent cells (germ cells)

        (1) Capable of differentiating into any tissue, including trophoblast (choriocarcinoma) and yolk sac (yolk sac carcinoma).

        (2) Teratoma is a tumor arising in totipotent cells that differentiates into somatic tissues derived from all three germ layers: ectoderm, mesoderm, and endoderm.

    c) Neoplasms of pluripotent cells

        (1) The cell of origin has differentiated partially, but is still capable of differentiating into multiple cell types.

        (2) Neoplasms of such cells are known as embryomas or blastomas, (nephroblastoma, neuroblastoma).

        (3) They usually occur in young children.

        (4) They are composed of primitive, highly malignant, small, round cells with hyperchromatic nuclei, which may show differentiation into a variety of tissues.

    d) Neoplasms of unipotential cells (Fig. 6-11)

        (1) These are "adult"-type cells that comprise differenti-

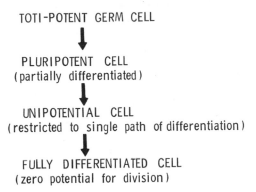

Fig. 6-10. Classes of cells from which neoplasms are derived based on their differentiating potential.

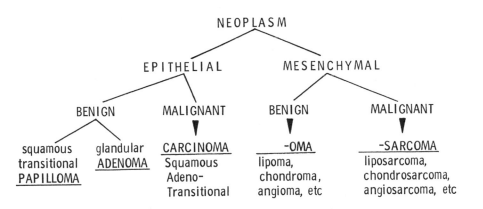

Fig. 6-11. Classification and terminology of neoplasms arising from unipotential cells.

ated organs; they differentiate into one cell type only; the majority of human neoplasms.

(2) Classification and naming of these neoplasms depend on

   i) whether they are epithelial or mesenchymal.

   ii) whether they are benign or malignant.

(3) A benign epithelial neoplasm is termed

   i) adenoma, if it arises in glandular epithelium (e.g., thyroid adenoma, colonic adenoma).

   ii) papilloma, if it arises in squamous (squamous papilloma) or transitional (transitional cell papilloma) epithelium.

(4) Malignant epithelial neoplasms are carcinomas.

(5) Benign mesenchymal neoplasms are named by the cell of origin to which is attached the suffix "oma," e.g., lipoma (fat).

(6) Malignant mesenchymal neoplasms are named according to the cell origin to which is attached the suffix, "sarcoma."

(7) Many neoplasms are named specifically by adding "oma," e.g., lymphoma, melanoma, glioma, mesothelioma, plasmacytoma (many of these are malignant in spite of the "oma" suffix).

(8) Neoplasms of hematopoietic tissue include the leukemias.

(9) The term *cancer* is used for any malignant neoplasm.

e) Mixed tumors

(1) These have more than one cellular component, with both components usually considered as neoplastic.

(2) Malignant mixed neoplasms may have

   i) two types of epithelia: adenosquamous carcinoma.

   ii) mesenchymal and epithelial elements: carcinosarcoma.

   iii) multiple mesenchymal elements: mesenchymoma.

f) Eponymous neoplasms

Neoplasms of uncertain origin are given the name of the person that described them: Ewing's sarcoma, Brenner tumor.

g) Hamartoma and choristoma

(1) These are developmental anomalies that produce abnormal, proliferating masses of tissue.

(2) A hamartoma is composed of tissues normally present in the tissue in which it is found (e.g., a hamartoma of the lung is composed of a disorderly mass of cartilage and bronchial epithelium).

(3) A choristoma is similar except that it contains tissues not normally present in that site (e.g., a disorderly mass of pancreatic acini, smooth muscle, and ducts in the wall of the stomach).

G. Incidence and distribution of human cancers

   1. Cancer is the second leading cause of death in the United States (after ischemic heart disease), being responsible for 375,000 deaths per year, or 25% of all deaths. The rate is increasing; approximately 1 in 4 of you, the readers, will die of cancer.

   2. Of fatal cancers in males, lung cancer dominates.

   3. In females, deaths due to breast and lung cancer dominate. Most recent figures indicate equal number of deaths due to breast and lung cancer.

   4. Carcinoma of the lung and colon are the leading fatal cancers when both sexes are considered together.

   5. In children, central nervous system malignancies, plus leukemia, neuroblastoma, and nephroblastoma dominate.

   6. In adolescence, lymphomas represent the common neoplasm.

   7. Geographic variations in cancer incidence is often marked.

H. Diagnosis of neoplasms

   1. Clinical detection

     a) Routine examination in asymptomatic patients. Routine annual cervical Pap smears and physical examination including sigmoidoscopy

     b) Self-examination of breasts monthly to detect lumps

     c) Hemorrhage, either acute (hematuria, rectal bleeding, etc) or chronic (manifesting as blood loss anemia)

     d) Compressive and obstructive symptoms

     e) Pain: a late feature of neoplasia

     f) Paraneoplastic syndromes

     g) Cachexia: a combination of weight loss, loss of appetite, weakness and anemia that occurs in advanced malignant neoplasms

   2. Cytologic diagnosis

    a) Examination of cells for evidence of malignant changes.

    b) Samples include

        (1) sputum, body fluids, cerebrospinal fluid, gastric and colonic lavage, and urine (exofoliative cytology).

        (2) brushing or scraping a lesion that has been visualized by endoscopy.

        (3) fine needle aspiration, directed by ultrasound or CT scan, if necessary

3. Histologic diagnosis

    a) This is considered the ultimate test.

    b) The diagnosis may be made on examination of

        (1) the entire neoplasm (excisional biopsy).

        (2) an incision or needle biopsy of the specimen.

    c) Histologic diagnosis of excised tissue may be made

        (1) immediately at the time of surgery by examination of sections made of frozen material.

        (2) after tissue processing and paraffin-embedding, which takes 12–24 hours; such "permanent" sections provide optimal material for microscopic examination.

    d) The histologic diagnosis will generally provide

        (1) the name of the neoplasm.

        (2) whether it is benign or malignant.

        (3) where relevant, a histologic grading, which is a scheme of grading the degree of differentiation of the neoplasm.

        (4) where relevant, the degree of invasion and spread. This information provides the basis of the pathologic staging, which is an expression of the extent of spread and generally correlates well with survival.

Part II

Systemic Pathology

7

Blood

STRUCTURE AND FUNCTION

Peripheral Blood Cells (Table 7-1)

I. Erythrocytes (red blood cells)
   A. In the first 2 days after release from the marrow, red cells are larger and show cytoplasmic basophilia (reticulocytes).
   B. Erythrocytes have a life span of 120 days.
II. Granulocytes (polymorphonuclear leukocytes)
   A. Granulocytes are classified as neutrophils, eosinophils, or basophils according to their cytoplasmic granules.
   B. Young granulocytes have a bandlike nucleus (band form) before nuclear lobation occurs.
III. Lymphocytes: part of the immune defense of the host
IV. Monocytes: part of the macrophage system
 V. Platelets: very small, anucleate, cytoplasmic fragments of megakaryocytes

Bone Marrow

I. Sole site of production of erythrocytes, granulocytes, monocytes, and platelets after birth
II. Methods of obtaining bone marrow specimens
   A. Aspiration
   B. Needle biopsy using a special needle capable of extracting a core of bone with marrow inside for histologic sections
III. Structure of bone marrow
   A. Cellularity
      1. The ratio of area occupied by hematopoietic cells to the total area of the bone marrow
      2. Varies with age and site; in childhood, the marrow is highly cellular in almost all bones
   B. Cell types (Fig. 7-1)
      1. Cells of the granulocyte (=myeloid) series exceed erythroid cells by a ratio of 3–4:1.

Table 7-1. Normal Blood Cell Counts

Red cells (million/ml)	4.2–6 (man)	4.2–5.4 (woman)

White cells/ml (both sexes)		% of total
Total	4,000–11,000	100
Lymphocytes	1,500–3,500	20–40
Monocytes	100–1000	4–8
Neutrophils	2,000–7,500	40–60
Eosinophils	40–400	1–3
Basophils	0–100	0–1
Platelets/ml	200,000–400,000	

2. More mature elements outnumber the early precursors (blasts) in all series.

IV. Hypercellularity of the marrow

A. Hypercellularity is recognized as an increased cellularity, taking the site of biopsy and age of patient into consideration.

B. It represents either hyperplasia or neoplasia.

C. Hyperplasia of the marrow occurs when there is an increased demand for hematopoietic cells.

1. In conditions of increased red cell need (chronic anoxia) or red cell destruction (hemolytic anemia) there is erythroid hyperplasia.

2. In severe acute inflammation there is hyperplasia of the neutrophil series.

3. In peripheral destruction of platelets there is megakaryocyte hyperplasia.

D. Neoplasms of bone marrow cells include leukemias, myeloproliferative diseases, malignant lymphoma, and plasma cell myeloma.

E. Hypercellularity may also be seen when the marrow is infiltrated by malignant neoplasms.

V. Hypocellularity of the marrow: hypoplastic or aplastic anemia

A. Hypocellularity is caused by failure, suppression, or destruction of stem cells.

B. It results in decreased production of one or all cell lines (pancytopenia).

C. In severe cases, death results from infections, bleeding, and the effects of anemia.

D. The etiology of hypocellularity is as follows:

1. Drugs: most common cause

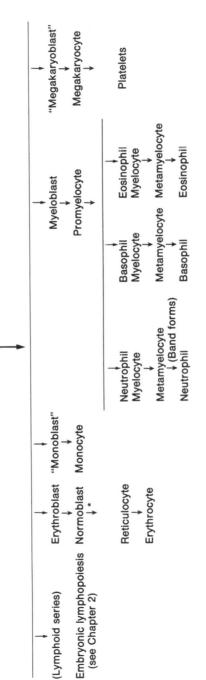

Fig. 7-1. Production of blood cells from stem cells in the bone marrow.

a) Expected (dose-related): high doses of chloramphenicol, anti-cancer drugs
b) Unexpected (hypersensitivity): chloramphenicol, phenylbutazone, phenothiazines, etc.
2. Radiation
3. Infections: viral hepatitis, miliary tuberculosis
4. Chemical agents: benzene, insecticides
5. Idiopathic: in about 50% of cases of aplastic anemia, cause is not found; course unpredictable and often fatal.

DISORDERS OF RED CELLS

Decreased Number of Red Cells (Anemia)

I. Introduction
   A. Anemia is defined as a reduction in the hemoglobin concentration of the blood.
   B. Anemia may result from (etiologic classification)
      1. blood loss: either acute or chronic.
      2. hemolysis: increased rate of destruction of red cells.
      3. decreased production: either due to bone marrow failure or deficiency of essential nutrients.
   C. Morphological classification of anemia depends on the changes in erythrocyte size (mean corpuscular volume (MCV) and hemoglobin content (mean corpuscular hemoglobin concentration (MCHC).
      1. Normocytic, normochromic anemias (normal MCV and MCHC)
      2. Macrocytic anemias (increased MCV)
      3. Microcytic, hypochromic anemias (decreased MCV and MCHC)
II. Anemias of diminished erythropoiesis (Table 7-2)
   A. Pure red cell aplasia: very rare
   B. Megaloblastic anemias: due to abnormal DNA synthesis
      1. Etiology of abnormal DNA synthesis
         a) Vitamin B_{12} deficiency: causes:
            (1) Inadequate dietary intake: very rare; only in strict vegetarians
            (2) Failure of absorption due to intrinsic factor deficiency: pernicious anemia, total and subtotal gastrectomy
            (3) Disease affecting the terminal ileum, the site of absorption of the vitamin B_{12}-intrinsic factor complex

Table 7-2. Anemia Due to Insufficient Erythropoiesis

Replacement of bone marrow
  Malignant neoplasms: leukemias, myeloma, lymphoma, metastatic carcinoma
  Myelofibrosis
Inadequate erythropoietin stimulation
  Chronic renal disease
Erythroid stem cell failure
  Aplastic anemia
  Pure red cell aplasia
Defective DNA synthesis (megaloblastic anemia)
  Folic acid deficiency and folate antagonist drugs
  Vitamin B_{12} deficiency
Defective hemoglobin synthesis
  Iron deficiency
  Anemia of chronic disease
  Sideroblastic anemia

(4) Competition for vitamin B_{12} by intestinal microorganisms: the fish tapeworm (*Diphylobothrium latum*); vitamin B_{12}-utilizing bacterial overgrowth
  b) Folic acid deficiency: causes:
    (1) Inadequate intake: most common cause of megaloblastic anemia, due to malnutrition, chronic alcoholism
    (2) Failure of absorption: all malabsorptive states but especially tropical sprue
    (3) Increased demand: pregnancy, infancy
    (4) Folic acid antagonistic drugs: anticancer agents (e.g., methotrexate), and anticonvulsants (dilantin)
2. Effect of abnormal DNA synthesis
  a) In megaloblastic erythropoiesis, megaloblasts differ from normoblasts in that
    (1) they are larger at all stages.
    (2) while cytoplasmic hemoglobinization occurs normally, there is marked delay in nuclear maturation.
  b) Megaloblasts show a decrease in the normal rate of maturation, causing
    (1) decreased output of erythrocytes.
    (2) increased numbers of early megaloblasts in the marrow with appearance of hyperplasia.

    c) They undergo intramedullary hemolysis (ineffective erythropoiesis).

    d) The peripheral blood shows a macrocytic anemia.

    e) Neutrophils are hypersegmented; neutrophil precursors in the marrow show enlargement (giant metamyelocytes).

3. Diagnosis of the etiology of megaloblastic anemia
   a) Folate vs vitamin B_{12} deficiency
      (1) Determination of serum vitamin B_{12} and folic acid; red cell folate
      (2) Occurrence of subacute combined degeneration of the spinal cord: only in vitamin B_{12} deficiency
   b) Pernicious anemia: a specific disease characterized by the following:
      (1) Megaloblastic anemia due to vitamin B_{12} deficiency
      (2) Chronic atrophic gastritis with achlorhydria and failure of production of intrinsic factor
      (3) Failure to absorb radiolabelled vitamin B_{12} (Schilling's test)
      (4) Presence in the serum of antibody against gastric parietal cells (in 95% of patients)
      (5) Presence of antibody against intrinsic factor (in 75% of patients); specific for pernicious anemia

C. Iron-deficiency anemia
   1. Causes of iron deficiency (Fig. 7-2)
      a) Dietary: common
      b) Malabsorption of iron: rare
      c) Blood loss, acute or chronic: common
      d) Increased demand: pregnancy
   2. Effects of iron deficiency
      a) Depletion of iron stores in bone marrow
      b) Decreased serum iron and decreased saturation of iron-binding capacity
      c) Decreased hemoglobin production causing
         (1) anemia: decrease in hemoglobin and red cell count
         (2) microcytosis: decrease in mean corpuscular volume (MCV)
         (3) hypochromia: decrease in mean corpuscular hemoglobin concentration (MCHC)
         (4) increased amounts of free protoporphyrin in the erythrocytes
      d) Variable normoblastic hyperplasia in the bone marrow
      e) Atrophic changes in mucous membranes of tongue, pharynx, esophagus, and stomach

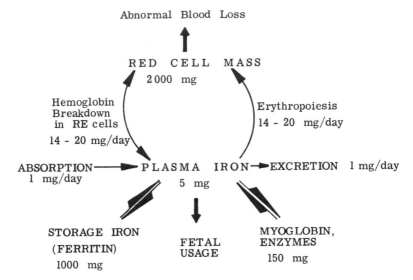

Fig. 7-2. Iron metabolism.

      f) Koilonychia (split, concave fingernails). Iron deficiency anemia, glossitis, dysphagia, and koilonychia is called Plummer–Vinson syndrome
 D. Anemia of chronic disease
   1. Anemia of chronic disease occurs in longstanding disorders such as chronic infections, rheumatoid arthritis, and neoplasia.
   2. It is caused by failure of transport of storage iron into plasma and developing erythrocytes, leading to
     a) normocytic and normochromic anemia.
     b) increased iron stores in the reticuloendothelial system.
     c) decreased serum iron.
 E. Anemia of chronic renal disease: caused by deficient erythropoietin secretion by the kidney; the anemia is normochromic, normocytic
 F. Sideroblastic anemia: rare
III. Anemias due to red cell destruction: hemolytic anemia
 A. Definition and effects
    Hemolytic anemias are characterized by a shortened survival of red blood cells in the circulation.

1. Extravascular hemolysis occurs in the reticuloendothelial system and has the following characteristics:
   a) Increased levels of indirect unconjugated bilirubin, which does not appear in urine (acholuric jaundice)
   b) Formation of pigment stones in the gall bladder
   c) Increased urobilinogen in the urine and feces
   d) Compensatory erythroid hyperplasia of the bone marrow
   e) Increased numbers of reticulocytes in the blood
   f) Increased serum lactate dehydrogenase from lysed erythrocytes
2. Intravascular hemolysis is characterized by additional features:
   a) Decreased level of serum haptoglobin, which binds free hemoglobin
   b) Free hemoglobin in the plasma (hemoglobinemia)
   c) Free hemoglobin in the urine (hemoglobinuria)
   d) Binding to albumin of oxidized heme groups leading to the formation of methemalbumin
B. Classification of hemolytic anemias
   1. Congenital abnormalities
      a) Enzyme deficiency in erythrocyte
         (1) Glucose-6-phosphate dehydrogenase deficiency
         (2) Pyruvate kinase deficiency
         (3) Others
      b) Membrane defects: hereditary spherocytosis
      c) Abnormal hemoglobin synthesis
         (1) Sickle cell disease and its variants
         (2) Unstable hemoglobins
         (3) Thalassemias
   2. Acquired abnormalities
      a) Immune hemolytic anemia
         (1) Autoimmune (with autoantibodies)
            i) Associated with "warm" antibodies
            ii) Associated with "cold" antibodies
         (2) Isoimmune (blood group antigens: commonly ABO, Rh)
            i) Hemolytic blood transfusion reactions
            ii) Hemolytic disease of the newborn
         (3) Drug-(hapten-) induced immune reactions
      b) Membrane defects: Paraxysmal nocturnal hemoglobinuria
      c) Directly acting external agents
         (1) Infections: malaria

      (2) Snake venom

      (3) Physical trauma

         i) Microangiopathic hemolytic anemia

         ii) Hypersplenism

C. Hemolytic diseases due to membrane defects

  1. Hereditary spherocytosis

    a) This is an autosomal dominant inherited disease with variable penetrance

    b) It is caused by structural abnormality involving the contractile membrane protein spectrin that causes the cell to become spherocytic

    c) Spherocytes have a shortened life span and are abnormally permeable to sodium, showing

      (1) increased osmotic fragility in vitro.

      (2) autohemolysis when incubated at 37°C for 24–48 hours.

    d) Spherocytes are destroyed in the spleen, which is enlarged. Removal of the spleen is effective treatment.

  2. Paroxysmal nocturnal hemoglobinuria (PNH)

    a) PNH is a rare acquired disease of red cells characterized by an increased sensitivity of the membrane to complement.

    b) Activation of complement causes intravascular hemolysis.

    c) It is associated with aplastic anemia.

    d) Complement activation occurs through the alternate pathway and is precipitated by

      (1) decreased pH: Ham's (acidified serum) test is positive.

      (2) Sucrose: the sucrose lysis test.

D. Hemolysis due to erythrocyte enzyme deficiency

  1. G-6-PD deficiency: the most common

    a) Several variants exist; the most common (X-linked) occurs predominantly in blacks.

    b) Red cells are hemolysed by oxidants (mainly oxidant drugs like primaquine).

    c) Clinically, patients

      (1) may be asymptomatic (common).

      (2) develop acute hemolytic episodes (common).

      (3) develop chronic hemolytic anemia (rare).

  2. Pyruvate kinase deficiency

    a) Less common than G-6-PD deficiency but more often produces clinical effects

b) Autosomal recessive
3. Other enzyme deficiencies: rare

E. Structure of hemoglobin (Hb)
1. All hemoglobin types have four polypeptide chains. Each chain is linked with one heme group. ʼ
2. The different kinds of Hb have different polypeptide chains.
   a) HbA ($\alpha_2\beta_2$): comprises 95-97% of normal adult hemoglobin
   b) HbF (fetal hemoglobin) ($\alpha_2\gamma_2$)
      (1) Predominant hemoglobin in fetal life
      (2) Progressive switch from gamma chain production to beta chain production at about the 20th week of fetal life
      (3) Rapid fall in HbF levels after birth; less than 1% by age 6 months.
   c) HbA$_2$ ($\alpha_2\delta_2$): accounts for 1.5-3.5% of normal adult hemoglobin

F. Qualitatively abnormal hemoglobin syndromes (hemoglobinopathies)
1. The common hemoglobinopathies involve abnormalities in the beta chain (beta hemoglobinopathies).
2. These are inherited single gene diseases.
3. Sickle cell anemia (HbSS) has the following characteristics:
   a) This is a common disorder in Africa and India, affects 0.1-0.2% of black people in the United States
   b) Homozygous (SS) individuals synthesize an abnormal beta chain that has valine at position 6 instead of glutamic acid.
   c) This substitution results in polymerization of hemoglobin with the production of semisolid, crystalline structures known as tactoids.
   d) Tactoid formation occurs under states of decreased oxygen tension and causes
      (1) decreased solubility of the hemoglobin.
      (2) "sickling," due to surface membrane alterations consequent on interaction between the tactoids and the spectrin–actin cytoskeleton.
      (3) decreased deformability of the erythrocyte causing hemolysis.
   e) Clinical characteristics include the following:

(1) Severe anemia in childhood, growth retardation, cardiac enlargement, and cardiac failure
(2) Extreme normoblastic erythroid hyperplasia in the bone marrow
(3) Chronic leg ulcers
    f) Complications include the following:
(1) Aplastic crisis: a sudden failure of the marrow, precipitated by infections, drugs, etc.
(2) Hemolytic crisis: a sudden acceleration of hemolysis
(3) Positive iron balance in the body (secondary hemochromatosis or hemosiderosis)
(4) Vaso-occlusive crisis: due to plugging of the microcirculation by aggregates of sickle cells
(5) Splenic changes: repeated infarcts leading to decrease in spleen size (autosplenectomy)
(6) Predisposition to infections with encapsulated bacteria (Pneumococci, Salmonella) due to asplenic state
    g) Diagnosis is confirmed by
(1) presence of sickle cells in peripheral blood.
(2) hemoglobin electrophoresis: over 80% HbS and absence of HbA.
4. Sickle cell trait (HbAS) has the following characteristics:
    a) Heterozygous for the abnormal gene
    b) Very common; present in 9% of American blacks
    c) Usually asymptomatic and without hematologic abnormalities
    d) Diagnosis by a positive metabisulfite sickle preparation: hemoglobin electrophoresis shows moderate amounts of HbS (30–35%)
5. Other abnormal hemoglobins are associated with the following:
    a) Milder forms of hemolytic anemia: diagnosed by Hb electrophoresis
(1) Hemoglobin C disease (HbCC) and trait (HbAC)
(2) Hemoglobin D disease (HbDD) and trait (HbAD)
(3) Hemoglobin SC disease and Hemoglobin SD disease
    b) Methemoglobinemia (HbM): cyanosis
    c) Increased affinity for oxygen (Hb Chesapeake), causing tissue hypoxia, erythropoietin secretion, and polycythemia
    d) Decreased affinity for oxygen (Hb Kansas), causing anemia and cyanosis
    e) Unstable hemoglobins (Hb Hammersmith); the hemoglobin precipitates in the erythrocyte as Heinz bodies

G. Quantitative hemoglobin abnormalities (thalassemias)
  1. Decreased rate of synthesis of structurally normal hemoglobin chains
  2. Beta thalassemia (common): beta chain production decreased
  3. Common in persons of Mediterranean, African, and Asian ancestry
  4. Homozygous beta thalassemia (major thalassemia; Cooley's anemia)
     a) Severe deficiency of beta chain production; marked decrease in $\alpha_2\beta_2$ (HbA)
     b) Persistence of compensatory gamma chain production into adult life, leading to high HbF ($\alpha_2\gamma_2$) levels
     c) Increased delta chain production; elevated HbA$_2$ ($\alpha_2\delta_2$) levels
     d) Clinical manifestations in early childhood
        (1) Severe anemia, jaundice, splenomegaly
        (2) Extreme erythroid hyperplasia of the bone marrow
        (3) Growth retardation, delayed puberty
        (4) Positive iron balance due to stimulated iron absorption and multiple blood transfusions (secondary hemochromatosis)
     e) Diagnosis
        (1) Hypochromic microcytic anemia with many target cells
        (2) Hemoglobin electrophoresis: markedly decreased HbA with elevated HbF and HbA$_2$
  5. Heterozygous beta thalassemia (minor thalassemia; Cooley's trait)
     a) One normal gene, one abnormal
     b) Often asymptomatic
     c) May have mild hemolytic anemia
     d) Hemoglobin electrophoresis shows slight elevation of HbA$_2$ (4–7%) and HbF (2–6%)
  6. Sickle cell–beta thalassemia
     a) Heterozygous for both the sickle cell gene and thalassemia gene
     b) Causes a clinical syndrome that is intermediate in severity between sickle cell disease and sickle cell trait
H. Autoimmune hemolytic anemias (AIHA)
  1. Classification
     a) Associated with warm antibodies (70%)
        (1) Idiopathic (40%)

      (2) With lymphoma (13%)
      (3) With systemic lupus erythematosus (5%)
      (4) Others (12%)
    b) Associated with cold antibodies (30%)
      (1) Idiopathic cold hemagglutinin disease (13%)
      (2) With mycoplasma pneumonia (8%)
      (3) With infectious mononucleosis (1%)
      (4) With lymphoma (2%)
      (5) With paroxysmal cold hemoglobinuria (1%)
  2. Autoantibodies
    a) Warm antibodies are those that have maximum binding to
       the red cell membrane at 37°C (body temperature); cold
       antibodies bind maximally at 4°C.
    b) The antibodies have specificity against red cell membrane
       antigens.
    c) Autoantibodies may be IgG, IgM, or rarely, IgA.
    d) They cause hemolysis by inducing immune adherence to
       phagocytes (extravascular hemolysis) or activating com-
       plement (intravascular hemolysis).
  3. Idiopathic AIHA
    a) Idiopathic AIHA presents as hemolysis (anemia and mild
       jaundice) of variable severity in the over-40-year age
       group.
    b) The diagnosis is made by demonstrating antibodies
       against the patient's own erythrocytes. This is done by the
       antiglobulin test (Coombs' test).
      (1) Direct Coombs' test: detects the presence of red cells
          coated with IgG
      (2) Indirect Coombs' test: detects the presence of free
          antierythrocyte antibodies in the patient's serum
  4. Idiopathic cold hemaglutinin disease
    a) Older patients (50 plus), especially females
    b) Cold-induced hemolysis
    c) Caused by an IgM autoantibody that acts by complement
       fixation
I. Isoimmune hemolytic anemia: due to an immune reaction between
  red cells of one individual and antibodies of another that occurs in
  the following:
  1. Hemolytic blood transfusion reactions: follows transfusion of
     incompatible blood; transfused red cells are hemolysed by
     antibody in recipient's serum
  2. Hemolytic disease of the newborn
    a) This is commonly due to Rh incompatibility.

     b) Anti-Rh antibodies (IgG) in an Rh-negative mother cross the placenta and hemolyse red cells of an Rh positive fetus.

     c) Rh-negative individuals develop anti-Rh antibodies when exposed to Rh-positive red cells in blood transfusion or during pregnancy.

J. Drug-induced immune hemolysis

  1. A large number of drugs are known to cause immune hemolysis and a positive Coombs' Test.

  2. Mechanisms include the following:

     a) Induction of autoantibody (methyldopa)

     b) Hapten effect: the drug combines with an erythrocyte membrane protein (penicillin, cephalosporins).

     c) Immune complex mechanism: the drug plus antibody immune complexes adsorb to erythrocyte membrane (quinidine, phenacetin, para-amino salicylic acid)

     d) Alteration of erythrocyte membrane (cephalosporins)

K. Hemolysis due to infectious agents

  1. Malaria

     a) Caused by four species of Plasmodium

     b) Intravascular and extravascular hemolysis due to infection of red blood cells

     c) Hemolysis most severe with *P. falciparum* (malignant tertian malaria), where hemoglobinuria (blackwater fever) may occur

  2. *Mycoplasma pneumoniae*, by inducing cold antibodies

L. Microangiopathic hemolytic anemia

  1. Hemolysis caused by the traumatic disruption of red cells as they traverse an abnormal circulation

  2. Causes

     a) Many diseases, including vasculitis, malignant hypertension, prosthetic heart valves, disseminated intravascular coagulation, vascular neoplasms

     b) Hemolytic uremic syndrome: a disorder (cause unknown) of young children characterized by renal failure and microangiopathic hemolytic anemia

     c) Thrombotic thrombocytopenic purpura: a serious disease (cause unknown) of young adults characterized by microangiopathic hemolytic anemia, fever, marked central nervous system changes, and renal failure

  3. Diagnosis

     a) Features of intravascular hemolysis

     b) Presence of fragmented abnormally shaped erythrocytes (schistocytes) in the peripheral blood smear.

Increased Number of Red Cells (Polycythemia)

I. Polycythemia: an increased number of erythrocytes in the blood
   A. Absolute polycythemia is an increase in the total red cell mass in the body.
   B. Relative polycythemia is an increased red cell count in the blood due to a decreased plasma volume.
II. Secondary polycythemia
   A. Polycythemia secondary to hypoxia: via increased erythropoietin
   B. Seen in chronic pulmonary disease, cyanotic congenital heart disease, cigarette smokers (high CO level), and persons living at high altitudes
III. Inappropriate erythropoietin secretion
   A. By neoplasms (e.g., by renal carcinoma, cerebellar hemangioblastoma, hepatoma)
   B. By renal cysts, hydronephrosis
IV. Polycythemia rubra vera (primary polycythemia)
   A. A myeloproliferative disorder predominantly affecting the erythroid series; neutorphils and platelets also commonly increased
   B. Diagnosis: demonstrating increased red cell mass in the absence of hypoxemia

DISORDERS OF WHITE CELLS

Abnormalities in White Cell Count (Nonneoplastic)

I. Neutrophilia (neutrophil leukocytosis)
   A. An increase in the number of neutrophils usually signifying the presence of an acute inflammation in the body
   B. Leukemoid reaction
      1. A very severe reactive neutrophilia in which the neutrophil count may exceed 50,000/mm^3 with the presence of metamyelocytes (early forms) in the peripheral blood.
      2. Distinguished from leukemia by an elevated neutrophil (leukocytic) alkaline phosphatase (NAP) level
II. Neutropenia (agranulocytosis)
   A. A decrease in the neutrophil count below normal
   B. Results in an inability to defend against bacterial infection (when the count is below 1,000/mm^3)

  C. Causes
    1. Inherited: rare
    2. Drug-induced
       a) The most common cause of neutropenia in adults
       b) Variety of actions
          (1) Direct suppression of bone marrow
          (2) Immune destruction of peripheral neutrophils
III. Eosinophilia: increased number of eosinophils
  A. Causes
    1. Type I hypersensitivity states
    2. Other immunologically mediated diseases, such as polyarteritis nodosa, Wegener's granulomatosis, and pemphigus vulgaris
    3. Parasitic infections of all kinds

Neutrophil Dysfunction Syndromes

  I. Defects of movement of neutrophils (rare)
  A. Chediak–Higashi syndrome
  B. Lazy leukocyte syndrome: extremely rare
 II. Defects of microbial killing (rare)
  A. Chronic granulomatous disease (CGD) of childhood: X-linked recessive disease characterized by failure to produce microbicidal hydrogen peroxide in neutrophils
  B. Myeloperoxidase deficiency
III. Effect of corticosteroid therapy: decreased neutrophil migration and phagocytic activity

Neoplasms of Hematopoietic Cells (Leukemias)

  I. Definition: malignant neoplastic proliferations of hematopoietic cells in the bone marrow
 II. Classification
  A. According to onset and clinical course
    1. Acute leukemia
    2. Chronic leukemia
  B. According to cell type
    1. Lymphocytic leukemia
    2. Granulocytic (=myelocytic) leukemia
    3. Monocytic leukemia
    4. Other cell types (rare)
  C. According to the peripheral blood picture

    1. Leukemic: white count elevated; abnormal cells present.
    2. Subleukemic: total white count normal; abnormal cells present
    3. Aleukemic: no abnormal cells detectable in peripheral blood

III. Etiology
    A. Etiology unknown
    B. Viruses: cause animal leukemias; are highly suspect in man.
    C. Radiation

IV. Incidence
    A. Number of new cases per year is 20,000–25,000 (United States); number of deaths is 10,000–15,000/year.
    B. Acute leukemias account for 50–60% of cases.
    C. ALL occurs in young children (peak 3–4 years); AGL occurs at any age, but especially in young adults (peak 15–20 years).
    D. Chronic granulocytic leukemia (CGL) occurs in the 30–50-year age group and chronic lymphocytic leukemia (CLL) in the over-60-year group.

V. Acute leukemias
    A. Clinical characteristics
        1. Sudden onset; rapid progression
        2. Rapidly developing anemia
        3. A decrease in mature functioning granulocytes, with fever and mucous membrane ulceration
        4. Thrombocytopenia with purpura
    B. Diagnosis
        1. The total white count is usually increased. Abnormal primitive (blast) cells are present in the peripheral blood in most cases (exception: aleukemic leukemia).
        2. The diagnosis is confirmed by examination of the bone marrow, which shows
            a) extreme hypercellularity.
            b) infiltration with primitive "blasts."
        3. Morphologic features must be supplemented by a battery of special staining techniques to identify the type of acute leukemia (Table 7-3).
    C. Acute lymphocytic leukemia (ALL)
        1. Acute leukemia characterized by lymphoblast proliferation in bone marrow and lymphoid tissue
        2. Lymph node enlargement common
        3. Classification (French–American–British (FAB): based on morphologic features
            a) L1: this is the usual type of childhood leukemia (Fig. 7-3).

Table 7-3. Identification of Acute Leukemia by Morphology and Histochemical Staining Reactions

	Sudan Black & Peroxidase	Chloroacetate Esterase (CAE)	Nonspecific Esterase (NSE)	PAS	Morphology
Lymphocytic	−	−	−	+	Single nucleolus
Granulocytic	+	+	−	−	Multiple nucleoli; Auer rods
Monocytic	−	−	+	−	
Unclassified	−	−	−	−	

The lymphocytes do not mark either as T or B cells (hence null cells). This type has the best prognosis.
  b) L2: this is less common in children; it is the usual type in adults. The cells frequently mark as T cells and have convoluted nuclei. This type is frequently associated with mediastinal mass and has a bad prognosis.
  c) L3: Burkitt type; cells frequently mark as B cells; bad prognosis
4. "Immunologic" classification depends on the presence of common ALL antigens (CALLA). Many "null" cells of ALL (L1 type) show CALLA positivity and early T- and B-lymphocyte markers (Fig. 7-4).
D. Acute granulocytic leukemia (AGL)
  1. Acute leukemia characterized by myeloblast proliferation
  2. Classification (FAB): based on morphologic and cytochemical features
    a) M1: myeloblasts without maturation
    b) M2: myeloblasts with some maturation into more differentiated granulocytic cells
    c) M3: promyelocytic leukemia
    d) M4: myelomonocytic leukemia
    e) M5: monocytic leukemia
    f) M6: erythroleukemia (Di Guglielmo's syndrome)
  3. Features peculiar to AGL variants
    a) Auer rods are characteristic rod-shaped purple-staining

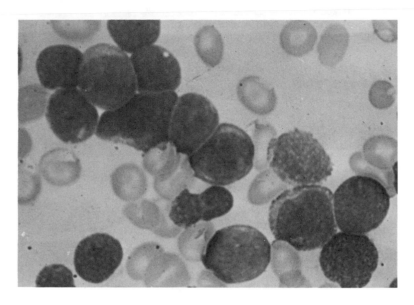

Fig. 7-3. Peripheral blood smear in acute lymphocytic leukemia of childhood (L1) showing increased number of lymphoblasts.

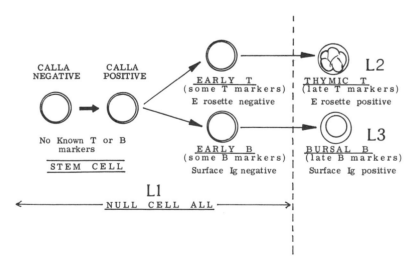

Fig. 7-4. Immunologic classification of acute lymphocytic leukemia (see text).

cytoplasmic inclusions in myeloblasts and promyelocytes.

b) Promyelocytic leukemia (M3). Granules in promyelocytes have coagulant material that causes disseminated intravascular coagulation.

c) Myelomonocytic leukemia (M4) is diagnosed when the blasts stain as myeloblasts (CAE+) and monoblasts (NSE+).

d) Erythroleukemia (M6) is characterized by proliferation of erythroid as well as myeloid precursors.

VI. Chronic leukemias

A. Chronic lymphocytic leukemia (CLL)

1. CLL is a disease of older (over 60 years) individuals having an insidious onset and slow progression.

2. Lymph node, spleen, and liver enlargement is common.

3. The peripheral blood shows increase in the absolute lymphocyte count, often in excess of 100,000/mm^3. The lymphocytes are "mature" B lymphocytes, (95%) or T lymphocytes (5%).

4. Anemia and thrombocytopenia due to bone marrow infiltration are later features.

5. The bone marrow is infiltrated by small lymphocytes (Fig. 7-5).

6. Involved lymph nodes and spleen are enlarged and firm. They are microscopically indistinguishable from lymphocytic lymphoma (well differentiated).

7. Diffuse leukemic infiltration is common in other organs (skin, liver, heart, kidneys, etc.).

8. Average survival is 4 years after diagnosis.

B. Chronic granulocytic (myeloid) leukemia (CGL; CML)

1. This occurs most often in the 30–50 year age group.

2. It presents with anemia, weight loss, and effects of splenic enlargement.

3. Peripheral blood shows marked increase in granulocytes (all types). Primitive forms such as metamyelocytes are common. Blasts account for less than 5% of cells in the periphery.

4. The platelet count is elevated initially, but later falls.

5. CGL is differentiated from other causes of neutrophilia by the markedly decreased neutrophil alkaline phosphatase (NAP) level.

6. Philadelphia chromosome (a small 22 chromosome due to translocation of part of 22 to 9) is present in over 90% of cases.

7. Bone marrow shows marked hypercellularity with increased

numbers of granulocytes, normoblasts and megakaryocytes (myeloproliferative disease)
   8. The spleen is massively enlarged. Splenic infarction due to vascular occlusion by aggregates of granulocytes is common.
   9. The accelerated phase of CGL
      a) occurs after a median time of about 3–4 years of onset.
      b) is characterized by an increased number of blast cells in the bone marrow and peripheral blood (acute blast crisis). The median survival after blast crisis is 2 months.
      c) can be predicted by the appearance of new karyotype abnormalities.
VII. Myeloproliferative disorders
   A. This is a group of diseases in which there is proliferation of erythroid, granulocytic, and megakaryocytic cell lines in the bone marrow.
   B. The cause is unknown.
   C. Peripheral blood shows an increase in all cell lines. Usually, one cell line dominates:

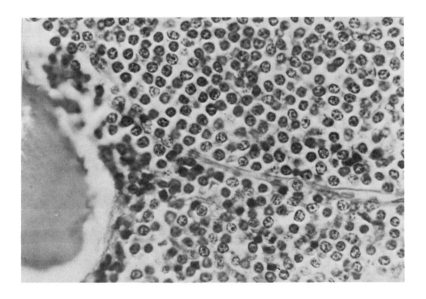

Fig. 7-5. Bone marrow in chronic lymphocytic leukemia. A monomorphous population of mature small lymphocytes has infiltrated the marrow.

1. Chronic granulocytic leukemia (granulocytes).
2. Polycythemia rubra vera (erythrocytes).
3. Idiopathic thrombocythemia (platelets).
D. Tends to cause progressive fibrosis of the marrow (myelofibrosis).

DISORDERS OF PLATELETS

Decreased Blood Platelets (Thrombocytopenia)

I. Causes
   A. Decreased production in the marrow
      1. Aplastic anemia
      2. Infiltration of the marrow in leukemia, carcinoma, infections
      3. Folate and vitamin B_{12} deficiency
   B. Pooling (sequestration) of platelets in an enlarged spleen
   C. Increased peripheral destruction
      1. Immune destruction
         a) Idiopathic thrombocytopenic purpura
         b) Systemic lupus erythematosus
         c) Drug- (hapten-) induced thrombocytopenia
         d) Neonatal thrombocytopenia due to transfer of maternal IgG antibodies with activity against fetal platelets
      2. Platelet consumption
         a) Disseminated intravascular coagulation
         b) Thrombotic thrombocytopenic purpura
II. Idiopathic thrombocytopenic purpura
   A. Rare disease of young adults
   B. Caused by autoimmune reaction (antibody) against platelets
   C. Splenectomy (spleen is the site of platelet destruction) effective in treatment
   D. Bone marrow: frequently shows megakaryocytic hyperplasia
III. Effects of thrombocytopenia
   A. Clinically significant bleeding occurs only with a marked decrease in the platelet count (less than 40,000/ml).
   B. Bleeding most commonly occurs into the skin (purpura) and mucous membranes (menorrhagia, melena, hematuria).

Abnormal Platelet Function

I. Characterized by symptoms and signs of platelet deficiency with a normal platelet count
II. Platelet function tests like clot retraction, bleeding time, platelet adhesion, and aggregation in vitro abnormal
III. Associated diseases
    A. Bernard–Soulier disease: abnormal giant platelets in blood
    B. Storage pool disease: decreased stored ADP granules
    C. Glanzmann's disease (thrombasthenia)

DISORDERS OF BLOOD COAGULATION

Normal blood coagulation is depicted in Fig. 7-6.

Abnormal Blood Coagulation

I. This occurs due to
    A. deficiency of one or more coagulation factors.
    B. the presence of anticoagulants, which may be drugs, antibodies, or natural anticoagulants.
II. It is characterized by increased bleeding after minor trauma. The bleeding is usually slow.
III. Coagulation tests are abnormal:
    A. Clotting time is abnormal only in very severe defects.
    B. Prothrombin time is abnormal in defects of the extrinsic pathway.
    C. Partial thromboplastin time (PTT) is abnormal in defects of the intrinsic pathway.
    D. Defects of the final common pathway cause abnormalities in both prothrombin and partial thromboplastin times.

Hemophilia A (Classical Hemophilia)

I. Coagulation Factor VIII is a complex molecule composed of (Fig. 7-7):
    A. Factor VIII coagulant portion. This is inherited as a sex-linked factor and is deficient in Hemophilia A.
    B. Factor VIII related antigen. This is inherited as an autosomal dominant factor. It is present in normal amounts in Hemophilia A.
    C. Factor VIII -von Willebrand's factor.

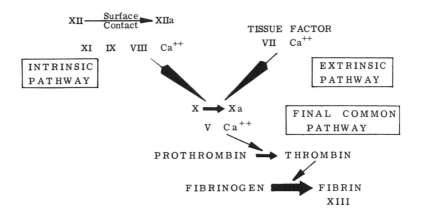

Fig. 7-6. Coagulation of blood.

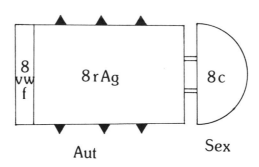

Fig. 7-7. The factor VIII molecule. 8rAg = VIII related antigen, 8vwf = VIII von Willebrand's factor, and 8c = VIII coagulant factor.

II. Hemophilia A is an X-linked recessive disease, predominantly affecting males and carried by females.

III. Severe cases have less than 1% Factor VIII coagulant activity and have "spontaneous" bleeding.

IV. Carrier females can be identified by a decreased Factor VIII coagulant activity: Factor VIII related antigen ratio.

V. It can be treated effectively with Factor VIII concentrates (cryoprecipitate of plasma). Recently, transmission of acquired immunodeficiency syndrome (AIDS) has occurred through these blood products.

Von Willebrand's Disease

I. This is inherited as an autosomal dominant trait.

II. It is characterized by deficiency of all three parts of the Factor VIII molecule to the same extent.

III. Deficiency of Factor VIII-von Willebrand's factor is detected by abnormal platelet aggregation with the antibiotic ristocetin.

IV. The Factor VIII coagulant activity: Factor VIII related antigen ratio is 1 (normal).

Hemophilia B (Christmas Disease)

I. This is inherited as an X-linked recessive trait and is very similar in its clinical features to Hemophilia A.

II. It is caused by deficiency of Factor IX.

8

The Lymphoid System

LYMPH NODES

I. Normal structure (see Chapter 2)

II. Infections of lymph nodes

A. Acute pyogenic bacterial infection (acute lymphadenitis): spread of bacteria from a regional focus of infection producing an acute inflammation with neutrophils in the lymph node

B. Viral lymphadenitis

1. Characterized by a marked T-cell proliferation expanding the deep paracortical T-cell zone

2. Specific features in viral infections

a) Measles: large multinucleated (Warthin–Finkeldy) giant cells

b) Infectious mononucleosis (Epstein–Barr virus)

(1) This is an acute illness of young adults with fever, sore throat, lymph node enlargement, and hepatosplenomegaly.

(2) B lymphocytes have surface receptors for E–B virus and are specifically infected.

(3) There is an atypical T-lymphocytic hyperplasia. These large atypical cells (Downey–McKinley cells) are seen in peripheral blood and lymph nodes.

(4) The diagnosis is confirmed serologically by finding

i) increased antibody against E–B virus (specific).

ii) heterophile antibodies (Paul Bunnell test; mono spot test).

C. Toxoplasmosis (*Toxoplasma gondii*)

1. Acquired toxoplasmosis presents most commonly as an acute illness with fever and lymph node enlargement.

2. The following histologic changes in the lymph node are characteristic:

a) Marked follicular hyperplasia.

b) Collections of histiocytes in the paracortical zone and in reactive follicles.

    c) Sickle-shaped *Toxoplasma gondii* trophozoites are almost never seen. Rarely a toxoplasma pseudocyst is seen.

    d) Immunoperoxidase techniques with toxoplasma antibodies show the presence of organisms in the node.

D. Infective granulomatous lymphadenitis

  1. This is a common condition.

  2. It is characterized by the presence of multiple epithelioid cell granulomas. Caseation necrosis, often extensive, is characteristic.

  3. Its causes include

    a) tuberculosis: common in cervical and mediastinal areas.

    b) atypical mycobacteria: cervical and mediastinal.

    c) histoplasmosis.

    d) coccidioidomycosis.

  4. The lymphadenitis may be

    a) secondary to an obvious focus of infection elsewhere in the body.

    b) the only manifestation of the disease, the result of reactivation of a dormant focus in the lymph node.

  5. Diagnosis is made by

    a) identification of the agent by histologic examination, using acid-fast stains for mycobacteria and methenamine silver or PAS for fungi.

    b) Culture: the most reliable method.

E. Suppurative (stellate) granulomas

  1. These are epithelioid cell granulomas in which the central necrotic area is infiltrated by neutrophils. In the fully formed state, these have a stellate (star) shape.

  2. Causes of suppurative granulomas are numerous.

    a) Lymphogranuloma venereum (LGV): a chlamydial infection

    b) Cat-scratch disease: caused by a bacterium that stains positively with a Dieterle (silver) stain

    c) Tularemia: *Pasteurella tularensis*

    d) Brucellosis

    e) Glanders and melioidosis: rare diseases caused by *Pseudomonas mallei* and *pseudomallei*.

    f) Mesenteric lymphadenitis: a relatively common disease in young children caused by *Yersinia enterocolitica* and *Y. pseudotuberculosis*

III. Reactive hyperplasia

A. Histologically nonspecific hyperplasia is characterized by

  1. reactive lymphoid follicular hyperplasia (B lymphocyte).

2. expansion of the paracortex (T lymphocytes).
3. sinus histiocytosis (macrophages).
B. Histologically characteristic types of reactive hyperplasia
   1. Dermatopathic lymphadenitis
      a) A lymph node hyperplasia occurring in nodes draining chronic skin diseases
      b) Characterized by
         (1) follicular hyperplasia and sinus histiocytosis
         (2) many histiocytes which contain brown melanin pigment
   2. Angioimmunoblastic lymphadenopathy
      a) This is a disease that occurs in older individuals (around 50 years); it presents with fever, weight loss, skin rashes, generalized lymph node enlargement, and hepatosplenomegaly.
      b) Polyclonal elevation of serum immunoglobulins is common.
      c) The lymph node shows
         (1) loss of normal architecture with obliteration of lymphoid follicles.
         (2) a large number of immunoblasts (B and T).
         (3) proliferation of vascular endothelial cells in postcapillary venules.
         (4) amorphous, eosinophilic, PAS-positive material between the cells which causes an appearance of hypocellularity.
      d) This is a serious disease.
         (1) It results in susceptibility to infections.
         (2) About 15% develop immunoblastic sarcoma.
      e) Overall as many as 50% die within 2 years.
   3. Giant lymph node hyperplasia, plasma cell variant (Castleman–Iverson disease, plasma cell type)
      a) A disease characterized by low grade fever, anemia, hyperglobulinemia and the presence of a large mass of matted lymph nodes, commonly in the mediastinum
      b) Characterized by marked follicular hyperplasia with large numbers of plasma cells in the paracortical and medullary areas
      c) Usually resolves when the mass is excised; may be progressive
   4. Giant lymph node hyperplasia, angiofollicular or hyaline-vascular type (Castleman–Iverson disease, hyaline-vascular type)

     a) Massive lymph node enlargement in mediastinum, retroperitoneum, cervical, or axillary region

     b) Lymph nodes show

        (1) distortion of normal architecture

        (2) numerous abnormal lymphoid follicles

        (3) extensive vascularization

        (4) deposition of fibrohyaline material around vessels

     c) A benign, nonprogressive disorder

  5. Sinus histiocytosis with massive lymphadenopathy

     a) This is a specific benign disease most commonly seen in black children.

     b) It is characterized by fever, and massive bilateral cervical lymph node enlargement.

     c) Involved lymph nodes show

        (1) dilated medullary sinuses packed with histiocytes.

        (2) lymphocytes in cytoplasm of histiocytes.

        (3) numerous plasma cells in medullary cords.

  6. Persistent generalized lymphadenopathy

     a) This occurs in those at risk for Acquired Immunodeficiency Syndrome (AIDS), mainly homosexual males.

     b) It is characterized by marked follicular hyperplasia with expanded germinal centers, disruption of mantle zones, and immunoblastic proliferation.

     c) Its significance is uncertain.

IV. Histiocytic proliferations

  A. Noninfectious epithelioid cell granulomas

    1. These are usually noncaseating.

    2. They are caused by

     a) sarcoidosis, which commonly affects mediastinal and cervical nodes.

     b) Crohn's disease, which affects mesenteric nodes, usually associated with intestinal disease.

     c) berylliosis: the mineral can be identified in the lymph node.

  B. Lipidoses: Gaucher's disease, Niemann–Pick disease

  C. Whipple's disease

  D. Foreign body reactions: following lymphangiography, in "skin popping" drug addicts

  E. Histiocytosis X: an overall rare group of diseases including

    1. Hand–Schuller Christian disease (more chronic; systemic)

    2. Letterer–Siwe disease (more acute; systemic)

    3. eosinophilic granuloma (localized):

a) The most common variant; in children and young adults
b) Composed of infiltrate composed of a distinctive histiocytes (Langerhan's cell), giant cells and eosinophils
c) Commonly associated with bone lesions
V. Metastatic neoplasms
  A. Are a common cause of enlarged lymph nodes
  B. Can be very difficult to differentiate from large cell malignant lymphomas
VI. Malignant neoplasms arising from lymphocytes (malignant lymphomas)
  Several different classifications (Table 8-1):
  A. Morphologic classification (Rappaport)
    1. This is based on the features of malignant lymphoma as seen on histologic examination of excised lymph nodes.
    2. It is still widely accepted and used in the United States.
    3. Nodular lymphomas are those which are composed of large, defined nodules of neoplastic lymphocytes. Diffuse lymphomas are composed of a diffuse proliferation of neoplastic lymphocytes.
    4. Four cellular patterns are recognized (Table 8-1):
      a) Well differentiated lymphocytic.
      b) Poorly differentiated lymphocytic
      c) Mixed lymphocytic: "histiocytic"
      d) "Histiocytic": most cases classified as "histiocytic" lymphomas are composed of large transformed lymphocytes.
  B. Immunologic classification (Lukes/Collins)
    1. B-cell lymphomas
      a) Normal transformation of B cells (Fig. 8-1; see Chapter 2)
      b) Types of B-cell lymphoma
        (1) B-cell small lymphocytic lymphoma (part of a spectrum with chronic lymphocytic leukemia)
        (2) Follicular center cell (FCC) lymphomas, which are composed of neoplastic cells that resemble one of the normal cell types in the transformation sequence:
          i) Small cleaved
          ii) Large cleaved
          iii) Small noncleaved (including Burkitt and Burkitt-like lymphomas)
          iv) Large noncleaved
        The neoplastic cells may adopt a follicular or diffuse pattern of involvement of the lymph node.

Table 8-1. Classification of Malignant Lymphoma

Immunological (Lukes/Collins)	Morphological (Rappaport)
Small lymphocytic ⟨ T / B	Well differentiated lymphocytic
FCC[a]—small cleaved ⟨ diffuse / follicular	Poorly differentiated lymphocytic ⟨ diffuse / nodular
FCC[a]—small noncleaved ⟨ diffuse / follicular	Poorly differentiated lymphocytic ⟨ diffuse / nodular
Burkitt type	(Burkitt lymphoma)
FCC[a]—large cleaved ⟨ diffuse / follicular	
	Mixed or histiocytic[b] ⟨ diffuse / nodular
FCC[a]—large noncleaved ⟨ diffuse / follicular	
Immunoblastic sarcoma ⟨ T / B	Histiocytic[b]
Plasmacytoid lymphocytic (B cell)	Well differentiated lymphocytic
Histiocytic (true histiocyte)	Histiocytic

[a]Note all FCC (follicular center cell) lymphomas are B cell by definition.

[b]Note that almost all lymphomas designated as "histiocytic" are in fact composed of large transformed lymphocytes; this is because the Rappaport scheme was developed prior to recognition that this large cell represents a transformed lymphocyte.

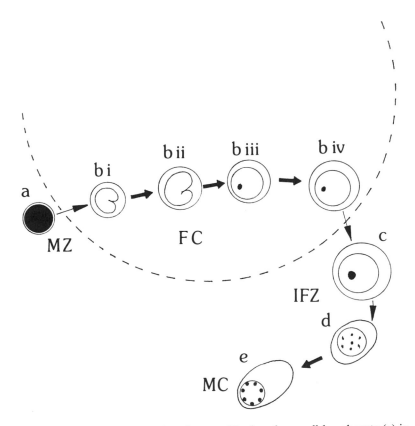

Fig. 8-1 Transformation of B lymphocytes. The inactive small lymphocyte (a) in the mantle zone (MZ) moves into the follicular (germinal) center (FC), transforming through small cleaved (bi), large cleaved (bii), small noncleaved (biii), large noncleaved (biv) lymphocytes, B-immunoblast (c), intermediate plasmacytoid lymphocyte (d), and finally the plasma cell (e). The transformed lymphocytes move out of the follicle center into the interfollicular zone (IFZ) and medullary cords (MC).

a   b   c

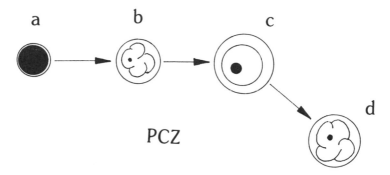

PCZ

            d

Fig. 8-2 Transformation of T lymphocytes in the paracortical zone (PCZ). The inactive small lymphocyte (a) transforms into a lymphoblast (b), T-immunoblast (c) and a group of effector T cells (d). Note that T cells tend to have convoluted nuclei.

   (3) B-immunoblastic sarcoma (B-IBS)
   (4) Plasmacytoid lymphocytic lymphoma (=Waldenstrom's macroglobulinemia)
   (5) Plasma cell myeloma
 2. T-cell lymphomas
  a) Normal transformation of T cells (Fig. 8-2)
  b) Types of T-cell lymphoma
   (1) T-cell small lymphocytic lymphoma (=T-cell chronic lymphocytic leukemia)
   (2) Convoluted T-cell lymphoma (=type L2 acute lymphocytic leukemia)
   (3) T-immunoblastic sarcoma
   (4) Mycosis fungoides, Sezary's syndrome
 3. Immunologic diagnosis
  a) Diagnosis requires special processing of lymph nodes removed for biopsy.
  b) The presence of surface or cytoplasmic immunoglobulin identifies B cells. A "monoclonal" (i.e., stains exclusively for either kappa or lambda light chain) pattern of staining is strong evidence for a neoplastic process.
  c) T-cell lymphomas are identified by the use of monoclonal anti-T cell antibodies.
 C. Translation of immune/morphologic classifications
The types of lymphomas of the Lukes/Collins and Rappaport schemes can be compared (Table 8-1).

D. Specific types of malignant lymphoma
1. Small (well-differentiated) lymphocytic lymphoma (WDLL)
    a) Lymph node equivalent of chronic lymphocytic leukemia, with bone marrow and peripheral blood involvement occurring in almost 100%
    b) A B-cell process; less than 5% are T cell (except in Japan)
2. Follicular center cell lymphomas
    a) Neoplasms of follicular center B lymphocytes; the most common type of lymphoma
    b) Frequently nodular; slowly progressive; median survival of 7 years or more. Small noncleaved and large cell types more aggressive (see Burkitt's lymphoma, below)
    c) Involvement of bone marrow and peripheral blood common
    d) Commonly affects adults, presenting with lymph node enlargement, either regional or generalized
3. T-lymphoblastic (convoluted) lymphoma
    a) Composed of T lymphocytes that have a convoluted nucleus, delicate chromatin and small nucleoli; bear early T or thymic markers (see Chapter 2)
    b) Presents a diffuse proliferation with a high mitotic rate and frequently have a "starry-sky" appearance due to the presence of interspersed macrophages
    c) Typically presents as a mediastinal mass and rapidly progresses to an acute lymphocytic leukemia (L2 type; see Chapter 7)
    d) Has a poor prognosis
4. "Histiocytic" lymphoma/immunoblastic sarcoma (IBS)
    a) As defined by Rappaport, is extremely heterogeneous (5 types); composed of large follicular center cell lymphomas (cleaved and noncleaved types), B-IBS, T-IBS, and true histiocytic lymphoma
    b) Diffuse, composed of large cells, and may have a high mitotic rate
    c) Immunoblastic sarcomas, large cell lymphomas have aggressive course and poor prognosis
5. Burkitt's lymphoma (Fig. 8-3)
    a) A B-cell lymphoma of intermediate-sized lymphocytes having an extremely aggressive course, rapid growth, and poor prognosis
    b) Cells have a moderate amount of vacolated, lipid-con-

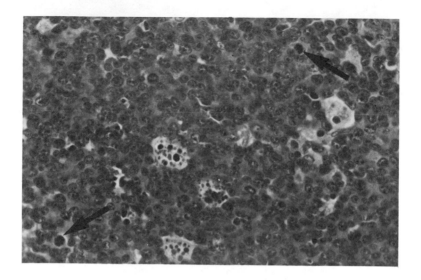

Fig. 8-3 Burkitt's lymphoma, microscopic.

taining cytoplasm, a primitive noncleaved nucleus with multiple small nucleoli, and a very high mitotic rate
  c) A "starry-sky" pattern due to the presence of macrophages among the diffuse lymphocytic proliferation
  d) Common neoplasm in African children, where it has been etiologically related to Epstein–Barr virus
  e) A similar neoplasm occurs among children and young adults in the United States
  f) Characterized clinically by extranodal (jaw in African cases; gastrointestinal tract elsewhere) involvement.
6. Mycosis fungoides and Sezary's syndrome
  a) T-cell neoplasm composed of cells having characteristic cerebriform (complex lobulations like brain) nuclei
  b) Mycosis fungoides: involves the skin, appearing as plaques and nodules, and eventually becomes disseminated
  c) Sezary's syndrome: characterized by generalized erythrodema and early involvement of the peripheral blood
  d) Neoplastic cells frequently express T-helper cell markers (see Chapter 2)
7. Plasma cell myeloma (multiple myeloma)
  a) A common disease affecting older (over 50 years) individuals

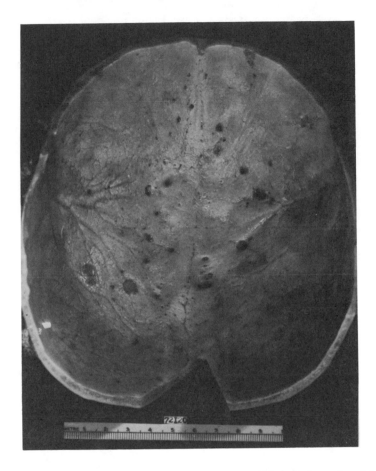

Fig. 8-4 Inner surface of skull showing multiple small lytic lesions of multiple myeloma.

b) A multifocal, progressive neoplastic proliferation of a single clone of plasma cells in the bone marrow; lymph node involvement usually minimal
c) Causes multiple lytic lesions in bones (Fig. 8-4)
d) Produces excessive amounts of a single clone of immunoglobulin, usually IgG or free light chains (light chain myeloma)

   e) This immunoglobulin causes a sharp spike on protein electrophoresis because it is monoclonal

   f) When free light chains are produced, they are excreted in the urine as Bence–Jones protein

   g) Renal dysfunction more common in cases where free light chains are secreted

   h) Hypercalcemia often present due to lytic lesions in bone

   i) Prognosis is poor; median survival is about 3 years after diagnosis

  8. Plasmacytoid lymphocytic lymphoma (clinical syndrome of Waldenstrom's macroglobulinemia)

   a) An uncommon disease affecting older individuals

   b) Characterized by proliferation of small lymphocytes and cells with plasmacytoid features

   c) Neoplastic cells secrete a monoclonal immunoglobulin of the IgM class (macroglobulin): produces hyperviscosity

  9. Heavy chain diseases: rare; alpha, gamma and mu chain diseases

VII. Malignant neoplasms of histiocytes

 A. True histiocytic lymphomas

  1. Tumor cells mark with histiocyte markers such as muramidase, or monoclonal anti-monocyte/histiocyte antibodies

  2. Extremely rare (less than 1% of lymph node neoplasms)

 B. Malignant histiocytosis ("histiocytic medullary reticulosis")

  1. A highly malignant disease characterized by proliferation of histiocytes having marked nuclear atypia, hyperchromatism and pleomorphism

  2. Phagocytosis of erythrocytes and leukocytes by the malignant histiocytes characteristic

VIII. Hodgkin's lymphoma

 A. A malignant lymphoma characterized by the presence of Reed-Sternberg cells. The classical Reed–Sternberg cell is a large cell which has two nuclei, each having a large inclusion-like nucleus.

 B. Four histologic subclasses are recognized:

  1. Lymphocyte-predominant Hodgkin's disease

   a) There is a complete obliteration of lymph node architecture by a proliferation of lymphocytes and histiocytes; may be nodular or diffuse.

   b) Typical Reed–Sternberg cells are rare.

   c) A variant of Reed–Sternberg cells typical for the disease is the polyploid cell, a highly irregular, multi-lobulated, polyploid cell ("popcorn" cell).

   d) It is a slowly progressive disease with a long survival.

2. Nodular sclerosing Hodgkin's disease
   a) Comprising 40% of cases of Hodgkin's disease; it is the most common type in most series.
   b) It is characterized histologically by
      (1) nodules of lymphoid tissue containing lymphocytes, plasma cells, histiocytes, eosinophils, and Reed–Sternberg cell variants.
      (2) broad bands of collagen which encircle the nodules.
      (3) rare finding of classic Reed–Sternberg cells.
      (4) the "lacunar cell": a variant Reed–Sternberg cell that characterizes this type. This is a cell that has a central lobulated nucleus with abundant pale cytoplasm.
   c) Clinically tends to occur more frequently in young females and commonly presents as a mediastinal mass
   d) Slowly progressive disease often with long survival
3. Mixed cellularity Hodgkin's disease
   a) 25% of all cases of Hodgkin's lymphoma
   b) Characterized by obliteration of the lymph node by a diffuse proliferation of lymphocytes, histiocytes, plasma cells, eosinophils, and typical Reed–Sternberg cells
   c) Necrosis and disorderly fibrosis may be present
   d) Prognosis worse than lymphocyte-predominant Hodgkin's disease
4. Lymphocyte-depleted Hodgkin's disease
   a) 15-20% of Hodgkin's lymphoma
   b) A rapidly progressive systemic disease characterized by acute fever, pancytopenia, and lymphadenopathy
   c) Characteristics of affected lymph nodes
      (1) Obliteration of normal architecture
      (2) Marked depletion of lymphocytes
      (3) Large number of Reed–Sternberg cells, often showing marked pleomorphism
      (4) Diffuse fibrosis of the lymph node common
   d) Bone marrow involvement common
C. Clinical features
   1. Hodgkin's disease usually presents with lymph node enlargement, either of a single group of nodes or generalized lymphadenopathy.
   2. Spleen and liver enlargement occur in advanced disease.
   3. It occurs from childhood to old age. The greatest frequency is between 15 and 30 years.
   4. Systemic symptoms include fever, pruritus, weight loss, and anemia.

D. Clinical staging
1. Using skeletal radiographic scans, bone marrow biopsy, lymphangiography, laparotomy with splenectomy, and liver biopsy
2. Important in planning appropriate treatment, which can be very successful and has improved survival dramatically
3. Four clinical stages
   a) Stage I: disease limited to lymph nodes in one anatomic region (or two contiguous regions)
   b) Stage II: disease involves two or more noncontiguous regions on one side of the diaphragm
   c) Stage III: disease is present on both sides of the diaphragm but is limited to lymphoid tissue (including spleen)
   d) Stage IV: involvement of nonlymphoid organs, including bone marrow and liver, lung, etc.
4. All stages are subdivided into A if systemic symptoms are absent, or B if systemic symptoms are present.
E. Etiology of Hodgkin's disease
1. Unknown; viral cause suspected but not proven
2. Origin of the neoplastic Reed–Sternberg cell uncertain

THYMUS

I. Normal structure and function
A. The thymus is composed of
1. epithelial cells, which are present diffusely and form aggregates of concentric keratinized cells known as Hassall's corpuscles.
2. T lymphocytes.
3. myoid cells, which contain cross-striations.
B. Involution and atrophy occur after childhood, and in the adult the gland is difficult to identify in the mediastinal fat pad.
II. Thymic hypoplasia (see Chapter 2), in DiGeorge's syndrome, Nezelof's syndrome, and Swiss-type combined immunodeficiency, is associated with defective T cell function.
III. Thymic hyperplasia
A. The appearance of lymphoid follicles containing germinal centers in an involuted adult thymus
B. Most commonly associated with myasthenia gravis; 70% of patients with myasthenia have thymic hyperplasia
C. Also occurs in a variety of other autoimmune diseases (Graves' disease, Addison's disease, systemic lupus erythematosus, rheumatoid arthritis, scleroderma, etc.)

IV. Neoplasms of the thymus
  A. Thymoma
    1. One of the most common neoplasms of the anterior mediastinum; usually occurs in adults within an age range of 30–80 years
    2. Gross characteristics
      a) The majority of thymomas are encapsulated. Infiltration of adjacent structures is evidence of malignancy.
      b) They may be large (up to 20 cm), and characteristically are divided into lobules by fibrous septa.
      c) Cystic change is common.
    3. Histologic characteristics
      a) Thymomas may be predominantly epithelial with few lymphocytes.
      b) They may be predominantly lymphocytic with the neoplastic epithelial cells obscured and difficult to identify.
      c) Thymomas that are mixed epithelial and lymphocytic are the most common type.
      d) The neoplastic cell is the thymic epithelial cell.
    4. Biologic behavior
      a) 80–90% of thymomas are benign and slow growing.
      b) 10–20% are malignant; but still are slow growing.
      c) Even thymomas that are locally invasive rarely metastasize.
    5. Clinical characteristics
      a) The majority of patients present with an anterior mediastinal mass, detected at chest x-ray, or because of local compressive effects.
      b) Associated diseases occur in about one-third of patients with thymoma.
        (1) Myasthenia gravis is most common.
        (2) Patients may have hematologic abnormalities, notably pure red cell aplasia and pancytopenia.
        (3) Malignant neoplasms elsewhere in the body.
        (4) Hypogammaglobulinemia.
        (5) Autoimmune disease.
    6. Good prognosis: less than 5% of patients die of their disease.
  B. Germ cell tumors of the thymus
    1. Rare
    2. May be seminoma (germinoma), embryonal carcinoma, choriocarcinoma, yolk sac carcinoma, or teratoma
  C. Carcinoid tumor: rare

SPLEEN

I. Congenital anomalies
   A. Absence of spleen (asplenia): very rare
   B. Accessory spleens (splenunculi)
      1. Common, present in 10% of people, usually in the hilum of the spleen or tail of pancreas
      2. A cause of treatment failure in patients who have splenectomy as part of their treatment (e.g., in hereditary spherocytosis)
II. Rupture of the spleen
   A. Traumatic
      1. Trauma resulting in rupture of the splenic capsule causes acute, often massive, intraperitoneal hemorrhage.
      2. When the capsule is intact bleeding occurs in the spleen (subcapsular hematoma) and the capsule may rupture at a later time, often several days after the trauma.
   B. "Spontaneous" rupture of a diseased spleen
      1. An enlarged spleen from any cause is more susceptible to rupture with minimal trauma ("spontaneous") than a normal spleen.
      2. Rupture is particularly common in infections such as infectious mononucleosis, typhoid, and malaria.
III. Vascular lesions
   A. Passive venous congestion: in portal hypertension
   B. Infarction
      1. Causes
         a) Embolism: in infective endocarditis
         b) Splenic artery disease: atherosclerosis, polyarteritis nodosa
         c) Leukocyte plugging of arteries in chronic granulocytic leukemia
         d) Sickle cell anemia: "autosplenectomy"
IV. Splenomegaly
   A. Venous congestion (congestive splenomegaly)
   B. Infections
      1. Bacterial: bacteremia, typhoid, infective endocarditis
      2. Viral–rickettsial: infectious mononucleosis, typhus
      3. Protozoal: malaria, visceral leishmaniasis (kala-azar)
   C. Immunologic: Felty's syndrome
   D. Splenomegaly due to accumulation of abnormal substances
      1. Amyloidosis
      2. Lipid, glycogen, and mucopolysaccharide storage diseases
   E. Increased phagocytic activity: chronic hemolytic anemia, idiopathic thrombocytopenia

F. Hematopoiesis in spleen (myeloid metaplasia), e.g., in myelofibrosis
G. Benign neoplasms, hamartomas, and cysts
H. Malignant neoplasms
   1. Myeloproliferative disorders
   2. Leukemias and lymphomas
   3. Metastatic cancer
V. Infections of the spleen
   A. Acute bacteremia
      1. Acute bacteremia is characterized by mild splenomegaly, marked congestion, and neutrophil infiltration in pyogenic bacterial infections.
      2. The spleen is purple and very soft, and becomes almost semisolid.
   B. Chronic infections are associated with marked hyperplasia of phagocytic cells, often causing massive enlargement of the organ. Identification of malarial pigment or specific etiologic agents (e.g., Leishmania) may permit diagnosis.
VI. Neoplasms of the spleen
   A. Hamartoma: rare; composed of a nodular mass of disorganized splenic tissue
   B. Leukemia and lymphoma
      1. Leukemia and lymphoma commonly involve the spleen.
      2. There may be a diffuse infiltration of the spleen by neoplastic cells or involvement of only the Malpighian follicles (white pulp).
      3. Involvement of the spleen by lymphoma may be present in a spleen of normal size and detected only by microscopic examination.
   C. Primary malignant neoplasms: almost never occur
   D. Metastatic cancer: rare

9

The Circulatory System

HEART

Manifestations of Cardiac Disease

I. Cardiac pain
   A. Ischemic pain ("angina")
      1. Caused by contraction of myocardial fibers under hypoxic conditions
      2. Retrosternal and usually described as tightening
   B. Pericardial pain: caused by irritation of the lower third of the parietal pericardium, which is pain sensitive
II. Cardiac hypertrophy
   A. Produces no symptoms
   B. Recognized clinically by enlargement of the heart and by electrocardiography
III. Cardiac failure
   A. The inability to maintain a normal cardiac output despite a normal venous return
   B. Left-sided heart failure
      1. Sudden death follows cessation of left ventricular contraction due to asystole or ventricular fibrillation.
      2. Cardiogenic shock follows severely impaired contraction.
      3. Pulmonary edema follows less severely impaired contraction and causes severe dyspnea and cough with pink, frothy sputum.
      4. Chronic left-sided heart failure
         a) Causes fibrous thickening of alveolar septa
         b) Manifests as exertional and nocturnal dyspnea
         c) Alveoli contain hemosiderin-laden macrophages (brown induration of lung)
   C. Right-sided heart failure
      1. Acute right heart failure occurs as a result of massive pulmonary embolism and may cause sudden death.
      2. Chronic right heart failure causes

a) elevated jugular venous pressure.
b) enlargement of the liver due to centrilobular congestion.
c) peripheral edema.

D. In both left- and right-sided chronic heart failure: sodium and water retention occurs due to secondary aldosteronism

Ischemic Heart Disease (IHD)

I. Incidence
  A. Very common; responsible for 500,000 deaths per year in the United States
  B. The leading single cause of death in most affluent countries
II. Causes of coronary artery narrowing
  A. Atherosclerosis: accounts for 98% of cases
  B. Coronary artery spasm
  C. Coronary artery embolism, most commonly in infective endocarditis
  D. Coronary ostial narrowing in syphilitic aortitis
  E. Dissecting aneurysm of the aorta
  F. Various types of arteritis: polyarteritis nodosa, giant cell arteritis, Buerger's disease
III. Effects of coronary artery disease
  A. Myocardial infarction (MI) (Fig. 9-1)
    1. Incidence: over 1¼ million cases each every year (in the United States); about 40% fatal
    2. Etiology
      a) Atherosclerosis of one or more coronary arteries
      b) Fresh thrombosis overlying an atherosclerosis plaque: found in 40–90% of cases
    3. Distribution of infarcts
      a) Anterior descending artery occlusion produces infarction of the anterior left ventricle and anterior interventricular septum.
      b) Occlusion of the right coronary produces infarction of the posterior left ventricle and posterior septum and frequently involves the conducting system.
      c) Left circumflex thrombosis leads to lateral left ventricle infarction.
      d) Infarction may be
        (1) transmural: involving the entire wall thickness.
        (2) subendocardial.
    4. Clinical characteristics
      a) Pain: sudden onset, severe; may rarely be absent
      b) Autonomic changes: sweating, changes in heart rate

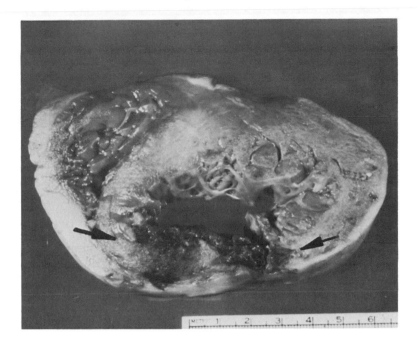

Fig. 9-1. Transverse section of the ventricles showing a transmural infarct (arrows) in the left ventricle (LV). The infarcted area is hemorrhagic.

    c) Electrocardiographic abnormalities: deviation of the S-T segment (acute injury), Q wave, T wave inversion

    d) Serum enzyme changes: elevation of creatine kinase (MB isoenzyme), lactate dehydrogenase (isoenzyme I), asparate aminotransferase (GOT)

5. Sequence of pathologic changes

    a) At 4–6 hours changes appear only at electron microscopic level.

    b) Light microscopic changes appear at 4–6 hours but become obvious only after 12–24 hours.

    c) Gross changes are absent in the first 12 hours.

        (1) After 18–24 hours the area appears soft, flabby, and pale. Fibers show eosinophilia and loss of myofibrils.

        (2) After 2–4 days necrotic cells begin to disintegrate and neutrophil infiltration becomes prominent. The infarct is now yellow with a hyperemic border.

        (3) After the 4th day healing begins with ingrowth of

granulation tissue; deposition of collagen begins in about 10 days.
d) The time taken for healing depends on the size of the infarct: 4–6 weeks.
6. Complications of myocardial infarction
   a) Cardiac arrhythmias: common. Caused by
      (1) ectopic electrical foci: ventricular tachycardia, fibrillation
      (2) involvement of conducting system: heart block
      (3) autonomic stimulation: sinus bradycardia, tachycardia
   b) Left ventricular failure: cardiogenic pulmonary edema
   c) Pericarditis: either fibrinous or hemorrhagic
   d) Systemic emboli: derived from mural thrombi that form over areas of injured ventricular endocardium
   e) Rupture: results from excessive softening of the infarcted muscle (myomalacia cordis)
      (1) Free wall rupture: hemopericardium
      (2) Septal rupture: acute ventricular septal defect
      (3) Papillary muscle rupture: acute mitral regurgitation
   f) Ventricular aneurysm: may result from transmural infarcts healing by fibrosis
B. Angina pectoris: ischemic cardiac pain of short duration, not associated with myocardial infarction; usually precipitated by effort
C. Chronic left ventricular failure: with or without a history of angina or myocardial infarction; the heart shows diffuse myocardial fibrosis.
D. Sudden death: probably due to an arrhythmia

Rheumatic Heart Disease

I. Acute rheumatic fever
A. Etiology
   1. Immunological hypersensitivity reaction to antigens associated with group A beta hemolytic streptococci
   2. Latent period of about 14 days between streptococcal pharyngitis and rheumatic fever
   3. Elevated serum titer of antistreptolysin O
   4. Immunologic mechanism unknown
      a) Antibodies to streptococcal antigens cross-react with myocardial antigens

   b) Alteration of myocardial antigens by the streptococcus leads to "autoimmunity."

B. Incidence
 1. Occurs between 5 and 15 years
 2. Common in underdeveloped "third-world" countries; rare in the United States, and Western Europe

C. Clinical manifestations
 1. Affects multiple tissues, producing a characteristic clinical illness
 2. Sudden onset with fever and either or both of the following:
  a) Acute onset with migratory polyarthritis affecting large joints, fever, chorea (involuntary movements), and skin lesions (rashes, subcutaneous nodules)
  b) Carditis, which occurs in about 30% of patients with a first attack of rheumatic fever
 3. Chorea (Sydenham's), skin rashes (erythema marginatum and nodosum).

D. Pathologic characteristics
 1. Cardiac involvement: affects all the layers (pancarditis)
  a) Endocarditis: particularly the valves (valvulitis)
   (1) Inflammatory edema
   (2) Formation of platelet–fibrin thrombi (vegetations) on traumatized endocardium; these are small, firmly attached and occur along the line of valve apposition
  b) Myocarditis: acute myocardial failure; rare
  c) Pericarditis: of dry fibrinous type
 2. Aschoff bodies
  a) Diagnostic of acute rheumatic fever
  b) Occur in the connective tissue of the heart commonly perivascular
  c) Central area of fibrinoid necrosis surrounded by histiocytes and Aschoff giant cells; heal by fibrosis

E. Sequelae of rheumatic fever
 1. Complete recovery the rule; a few die from severe myocarditis
 2. Susceptibility to recurrence; prevented by penicillin prophylaxis
 3. Chronic rheumatic heart disease

II. Chronic rheumatic heart disease
 A. Follows acute rheumatic fever after a long latent interval
 B. An endocardial disease affecting cardiac valves primarily
 C. Fibrosis, with fusion of the commissures, leads to a rigid valve with a narrowed orifice: stenosis

D. More severe involvement of the valvular apparatus leads to an incompetent valve
E. Valves affected: mitral valve only (50%); combined mitral and aortic; others rare
F. Nonvalvular endocardial fibrosis in left atrium: McCallum's patch

Acquired Diseases of Cardiac Valves

I. Mitral stenosis (Fig. 9-2)
   A. Etiology: almost always the result of chronic rheumatic heart disease
   B. Effects
      1. Obstruction to flow of blood through the open valve in diastole, with turbulence (diastolic murmur).
      2. Prolonged left atrial emptying causing a loud first heart sound
      3. Left atrial muscular hypertrophy and dilatation

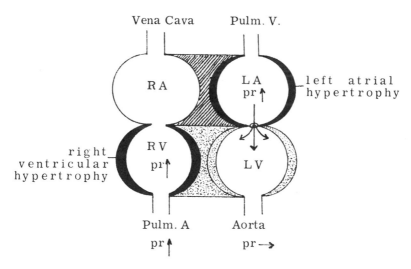

Fig. 9-2. Mitral stenosis. Obstruction to blood flow at the narrowed mitral valve increases pressure in the left atrium, causing left atrial hypertrophy and dilatation. Pulmonary hypertension and right ventricular hypertrophy follows (solid = hypertrophy).

4. Stagnation of blood causing thrombosis in left atrium, leading to
   a) systemic embolism
   b) obstruction of mitral valve orifice ("ball-valve thrombus")
5. Increase in pulmonary venous pressure, with changes of left heart failure
6. Right ventricular hypertrophy and failure

II. Mitral regurgitation
   A. Etiology
      1. Rheumatic heart disease: the most common cause
      2. Mitral valve prolapse syndrome ("floppy valve syndrome"): associated with myxomatous degeneration of the valve
      3. Rupture of chordae tendineae: in infective endocarditis or trauma
      4. Rupture or dysfunction of papillary muscles: in ischemic heart disease
   B. Effects
      1. Regurgitation of blood into the atrium throughout systole, producing a pan-systolic murmur
      2. Left ventricular dilatation and hypertrophy
      3. Left atrial dilatation and hypertrophy
      4. Pulmonary hypertension and right ventricular hypertrophy and failure

III. Aortic stenosis
   A. Etiology
      1. Rheumatic heart disease
      2. Congenital bicuspid aortic valve with progressive fibrous thickening and calcification
      3. Valve calcification in the elderly
   B. Effects
      1. Decreased aortic flow and pressure, leading to hypotension and syncopal attacks
      2. Soft aortic valve closure (second heart) sound
      3. Turbulent flow across the narrowed valve in systole producing a rough mid systolic murmur
      4. Left ventricular hypertrophy
      5. Angina pectoris caused by decreased coronary blood flow and increased left ventricular oxygen demand

IV. Aortic regurgitation
   A. Etiology
      1. Rheumatic heart disease
      2. Syphilis, with aortic scarring and valve ring dilatation

   3. Ankylosing spondylitis
   4. Traumatic rupture of aortic valve cusps
   5. Infective endocarditis, which may lead to valve cusp perforation
   6. Myxomatous degeneration and Marfan's syndrome
 B. Effects
   1. Regurgitation of blood across the incompetent aortic valve causing an early diastolic murmur
   2. Leakage of blood back from the aorta leading to an increased pulse pressure (collapsing pulse)
   3. Left ventricular dilatation and hypertrophy often massive
V. Stenosis of right-sided valves: very rare
 A. Congenital pulmonic stenosis
 B. Carcinoid syndrome

Congenital Heart Disease

I. Etiology
 A. Chromosomal abnormalities
   1. Down's syndrome (trisomy 21): endocardial cushion defects affecting mitral and tricuspid valves and ventricular septum

Table 9-1. Congenital Cardiac Disease

Acyanotic: with left-to-right shunt
  Atrial septal defect
  Ventricular septal defect
  Patent ductus arteriosus
Acyanotic: no shunt
  Coarctation of the aorta
  Pulmonic stenosis
  Ebstein's anomaly of the tricuspid valve
Cyanotic heart disease
  Tetralogy of Fallot
  Transposition of great vessels
  Total anomalous pulmonary venous return
  Tricuspid atresia
  Truncus arteriosus
  (Note: The five "T"s causing congenital cyanotic heart disease)

---

      2. Trisomy 18: right ventricular origin of both great arteries

      3. Turner's syndrome (45,XO): coarctation of the aorta

   B. Rubella: during the first trimester of pregnancy

II. Classification (Table 9-1)

III. Common congenital cardiac diseases

   A. Atrial septal defect (ASD)

      1. The atrial septum develops from two membranes, the septum primum and the septum secundum.

      2. Septum secundum defects are the common type of ASD: mild disease; often asymptomatic

      3. Septum primum defects rare, but more severe and frequently associated with mitral valve lesions

      4. Effects of large defects in the atrial septum

         a) Left-to-right atrial shunt

         b) Right ventricular dilatation and hypertrophy

         c) Increased flow through pulmonary circulation

   B. Ventricular septal defect (VSD) (Fig. 9-3)

      1. The most common congenital cardiac defect

      2. Occurs in the membranous part of the interventricular septum just below the semilunar valve rings

      3. Small VSD: with a small shunt produces a pan-systolic

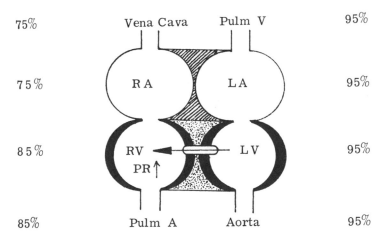

Fig. 9-3. Ventricular septal defect. The shunt increases oxygen saturation of right side blood at ventricle level (75% to 85%). Both ventricles handle increased volumes causing biventricular hypertrophy (solid). Numbers are percent oxygen saturation.

murmur; may be asymptomatic; cardiac catheterization shows entry of oxygenated blood into the right ventricle
4. Large VSD
   a) A serious defect, commonly manifesting in early life
   b) Results in
      (1) biventricular hypertrophy
      (2) increased pulmonary blood flow with pulmonary hypertension
   c) Right ventricular hypertension may lead to shunt reversal (Eisenmenger's complex) and cyanosis.
C. Tetralogy of Fallot (Fig. 9-4)
   1. This is the most common congenital cyanotic heart disease.
   2. It is characterized by four features (hence tetralogy).
      a) a large ventricular septal defect
      b) stenosis of the pulmonary outflow tract
      c) dextroposition of the aorta which over-rides the right ventricle
      d) right ventricular hypertrophy
   3. Pulmonary stenosis raises right ventricular pressure so that

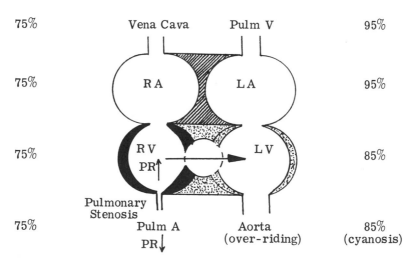

Fig. 9-4. Tetralogy of Fallot. The stenosis of the pulmonic valve produces a right-to-left shunt through the ventricular septal defect. The oxygen saturation of left ventricular blood drops (95% to 85%) leading to cyanosis. The right ventricle undergoes hypertrophy. Numbers are percent oxygen saturation.

the shunt across the VSD is a right-to-left shunt with cyanosis.
4. It presents at birth with severe central cyanosis ("blue baby").
5. The prognosis is poor without treatment. With corrective surgery normal survival is the rule.

Infections of the Heart

I. Infective endocarditis
  A. Classification
    1. Acute endocarditis
      a) Caused by virulent organisms, most commonly *Staphylococcus aureus*
      b) Can occur in previously healthy endocardium
    2. Subacute endocarditis
      a) Caused by organisms that are less virulent; e.g., *Streptococcus viridans, Streptococcus faecalis*
      b) Usually occurs in a previously abnormal valve
    3. Important to identify the agent causing infective endocarditis to select therapy
  B. Pathogenesis
    1. Endocardial injury
      a) Causes
        (1) Jet effects of blood
        (2) Turbulent flow
      b) Predisposing endocardial diseases
        (1) Chronic rheumatic heart disease, especially mitral regurgitation and aortic valve disease
        (2) Congenital heart disease, most commonly a small VSD or bicuspid aortic valve
        (3) Prosthetic heart valves
    2. Causes of bacteremia
      a) oral and dental procedures: *Streptococcus viridans*
      b) Urologic procedures: *Streptococcus faecalis* and gram-negative bacilli
      c) "Mainlining" by drug addicts: *Staphylococcus aureus*
      d) severe infection anywhere in the body
  C. Pathological characteristics (Figs. 9-5, 9-6)
    1. Vegetations: friable masses of fibrin and platelets in which are colonies of multiplying organisms.
    2. Vegetations are often multiple and are bulkier in acute endocarditis than subacute.

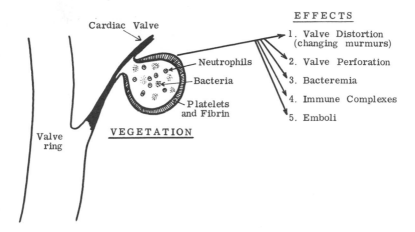

Fig. 9-5. Diagrammatic representation of a vegetation on a cardiac valve, its composition and its effects.

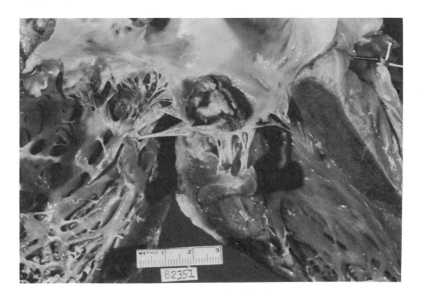

Fig. 9-6. Gross appearance of a large vegetation on the mitral valve in infective endocarditis.

3. Vegetations occur principally on the valves, particularly mitral and aortic.
4. Right-sided endocarditis: rare; occurs in
   a) drug addicts (tricuspid)
   b) patients with catheters extending into the right atrium
   c) gonococcal endocarditis
   d) VSD

D. Clinical characteristics
   1. Caused by bacteremia: entry of bacteria into blood from the vegetations
      a) Blood culture positive in over 95% of cases
      b) Low-grade and persistent fever in subacute endocarditis; high fever with rigors in acute endocarditis
      c) Splenomegaly
      d) Petechial hemorrhages in the skin, retina, nails
      e) In acute endocarditis with pyogenic organisms, miliary abscesses produced in all organs
   2. Caused by immune complexes (antibody + bacterial antigen): focal and diffuse proliferative glomerulonephritis
   3. Valvular vegetations
      a) Cause cardiac murmurs
      b) Destroy the valve; perforations; with acute incompetence
   4. Embolism by detached vegetations
      a) When vegetations are left-sided: embolism is systemic (cerebral, coronary, renal, mesenteric)
      b) In right-sided endocarditis: emboli are pulmonary

E. Other causes of cardiac vegetations
   1. Acute rheumatic fever
   2. Systemic lupus erythematosus (Libman–Sacks endocarditis)
   3. Non-bacterial thrombotic endocarditis
      a) Occurs in ill patients, commonly in advanced cancer
      b) Vegetations on the mitral and aortic valves; usually small but may be large enough to produce murmurs and emboli; sterile

II. Myocarditis
   A. Causes of myocarditis
      1. Viral myocarditis: most common
         a) Usually caused by Coxsackie B virus
         b) Focal necrosis of myocardial fibers, interstitial edema, and lymphocytic infiltrate
      2. Diphtheritic myocarditis
         a) Caused by diphtheritic exotoxin

      b) Myocardial fiber necrosis, interstitial edema, and lymphocytic infiltration

   3. Parasitic myocarditis

      a) *Trypanosoma cruzi* (Chagas' disease): the parasite is seen as pseudocysts in myocardial fibers; common in South America; acute and chronic myocardial disease

      b) *Trichinella spiralis* (Trichinosis): severe myocarditis is unusual

      c) Toxoplasmosis rarely causes acute myocarditis

B. Effects of myocarditis

   1. Cardiac failure with a dilated, flabby heart

   2. Arrhythmias and conduction defects

   3. Elevation of cardiac enzymes in serum; electrocardiographic changes

Cardiomyopathy

  I. Definition: Rare primary myocardial diseases of unknown etiology; sometimes familial

 II. Classification

   A. Congestive cardiomyopathy: characterized by greatly dilated ventricles and heart failure

   B. Hypertrophic cardiomyopathy: characterized by marked ventricular hypertrophy; involvement of the ventricular septum may obstruct left ventricular outflow (hypertrophic obstructive cardiomyopathy: subvalvular aortic stenosis)

   C. Restrictive cardiomyopathy: characterized by failure of the ventricle to dilate in diastole to accomodate the venous return

Neoplasms of the Heart

Neoplasms of the heart are rare; the commonest is cardiac myxoma, which occurs mainly in the left atrium.

Pericardial Diseases

  I. Acute pericarditis

   A. Causes

     1. Idiopathic pericarditis: common in young adults, frequently following a viral infection; mild, self-limited

     2. Viral: Coxsackie B virus most common

     3. Myocardial infarction

      a) In the acute phase: common

b) Rarely, delayed pericarditis occurs during the recovery phase
4. Tuberculous pericarditis: due to extension from a mediastinal node; an acute hemorrhagic pericarditis with effusion
5. Connective tissue diseases: systemic lupus erythematosus, rheumatoid arthritis
6. Acute rheumatic fever
7. Pyogenic bacterial infection: rare
8. Chronic renal failure (uremia)

B. Effects of acute pericarditis
1. Pathologic effects
   a) Fibrin and the inflammatory exudate produces a rough, yellowish appearance ("bread and butter" appearance).
   b) Exudation of fluid may be minimal ("dry" pericarditis) or it may cause an effusion.
2. Clinical effects
   a) "Dry" fibrinous pericarditis causes pericardial pain and a pericardial rub.
   b) When a significant effusion is present, cardiac tamponade occurs (see below).

II. Chronic pericarditis
A. Adhesive pericarditis: clinically insignificant
B. Constrictive pericarditis
1. Etiology
   a) Unknown in many cases
   b) Complicates tuberculous and pyogenic pericarditis
2. Pathological characteristics
   a) Marked thickening of the pericardium by fibrosis or calcification
   b) Prevention of expansion of the heart to accomodate the systemic venous return (restrictive)

III. Pericardial effusion
A. Hydropericardium (serous fluid)
1. Transudate occurring in any condition of generalized edema
2. Exudate in acute pericarditis
B. Hemopericardium (blood)
1. Acute penetrating injuries of the heart
2. Rupture of the heart in myocardial infarction
3. Rupture of the root of the aorta, most commonly by a dissecting aneurysm of the aorta
C. Clinical effects
1. The effusion causes enlargement of the heart, dullness, and muffled heart sounds.

2. Increased intrapericardial pressure impairs diastolic venous filling and decreased cardiac output (cardiac tamponade).

DISEASES OF THE VASCULAR SYSTEM

Degenerative Diseases

I. Atherosclerosis (Fig. 9-7)
   A. Definition: a disease of large and medium-sized arteries characterized by the deposition of lipid in the intima leading to the formation of plaques
   B. Incidence
      1. The major primary cause of death (causing ischemic heart and ischemic cerebral disease) in developed countries
      2. Decline in mortality from atherosclerotic vascular disease since 1975
   C. Distribution of lesions
      1. Involvement of the aorta in most cases; maximal in the abdominal aorta.
      2. Large muscular arteries: coronary, carotids, vertebrobasilar, mesenteric, renal, iliofemoral
   D. Risk factors for atherosclerosis
      1. Age: increases progressively after age 30 years
      2. Sex
         a) More frequent in males up to age 50 years
         b) Increases in females after menopause and becomes equal to male incidence at age 75 years
      3. Hypertension: particularly diastolic hypertension; is the strongest risk factor in patients over age 45 years.
      4. Hyperlipidemia
         a) The strongest risk factor in patients under age 45 years.
         b) Risk increased with
            (1) hypercholesterolemia: low-density lipoprotein on electrophoresis (LDL)
            (2) hypertriglyceridemia: very low density lipoprotein (VLDL)
            (3) low levels of high-density lipoprotein (HDL)
         c) Causes of hyperlipidemia
            (1) Familial: especially familial hypercholesterolemia
            (2) Diet
               i) A high intake of fatty acids (animal fat) and cholesterol; increases serum cholesterol

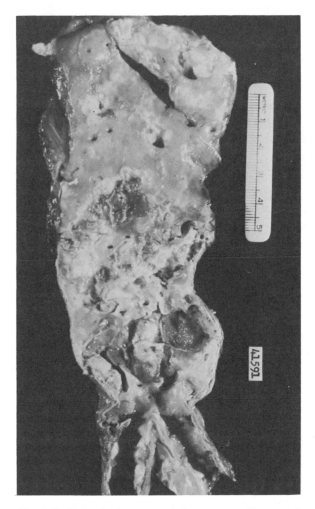

Fig. 9-7. Abdominal aorta and the common iliac arteries showing severe atheromatous disease with ulceration of plaques and formation of thrombi in ulcerated areas.

           ii) High intake of polyunsaturated fats (vegetable oils): decreases serum cholesterol

           iii) High intake of calories, refined sugar and alcohol: increases serum triglyceride levels

        (3) Other diseases associated with hypercholesterolemia

           i) Hypothyroidism

           ii) Nephrotic syndrome

           iii) Obstructive jaundice

  5. Cigarette smoking: smoking over a pack per day increases the risk 2–3 fold

  6. Diabetes mellitus: high risk

  7. Other less significant factors

    a) Obesity

    b) Lack of physical activity

    c) Type A personality (aggressively competitive, ambitious)

E. Pathological characteristics

  1. Development of the atheromatous plaque

    a) Proliferation of smooth muscle cells in the intima

    b) Accumulation of lipid intracellularly in the cytoplasm of the smooth muscle cells

    c) Disruption of lipid-laden cells leading to the extracellular accumulation of lipid in the intima

    d) Vascularization and collagen deposition

  2. Appearance of plaques (Fig. 9-7)

    a) An endothelialized fibrous surface with a central mass of yellow, semi-solid material

    b) When there is less lipid, the plaque is firm and white (fibromuscular plaques)

  3. Effects and complications of atheromatous plaques

    a) Progressive narrowing of affected vessels

    b) Calcification: of very little significance

    c) Ulceration: an endothelial injury which favors thrombosis

    d) Cholesterol embolization

    e) Hemorrhage into a plaque: rare cause of sudden occlusion

    f) Occurrence of thrombosis, which causes obstruction

      (1) due to slowing and turbulence of blood in the narrowed arteries

      (2) when ulceration occurs

      (3) when hemorrhage occurs into the plaque

II. Hypertension

A. Definition

     1. A sustained elevated arterial blood pressure
     2. Controversy over exact levels that constitute hypertension
  B. Etiology
     1. "Essential" hypertension: hypertension occurring as a primary phenomenon without a known disease
       a) Is the most common form of hypertension
       b) Has a strong familial tendency
       c) Usually occurs after the age of 40 years
       d) Basic mechanism causing elevation of blood pressure unknown
     2. Secondary hypertension: hypertension as part of a disease process elsewhere in the body
       a) Renal hypertension
         (1) Chronic renal disease: chronic glomerulonephritis, chronic pyelonephritis, polycystic disease, renal artery stenosis
         (2) Hypertension in acute glomerulonephritis transient
         (3) Renal hypertension caused by sodium retention due to
           i) decreased glomerular filtration
           ii) increased renin: in renal artery stenosis, malignant hypertension
       b) Mineralocorticoid excess
         (1) Primary aldosteronism (Conn's syndrome)
         (2) Hypercortisolism (Cushing's syndrome)
         (3) Congenital adrenal hyperplasia due to 11-hydroxylase deficiency
       c) Catecholamine excess: pheochromocytoma
       d) Hypertension in pregnancy (preeclampsia)
       e) Coarctation of the aorta
  C. Effects of hypertension
     1. Hypertensive heart disease: left ventricular hypertrophy and failure
     2. Increased risk of atherosclerotic vascular disease (ischemic heart disease, cerebral thrombosis)
     3. Changes in peripheral arterioles: mainly renal and retinal
       a) "Benign" hypertension
         (1) Characterized by hyaline arteriolosclerosis: medial hypertrophy and replacement of muscle by hyalinized collagen
         (2) Formation of micro-aneurysms which may rupture: (cerebral hemorrhage)
       b) "Malignant" or accelerated hypertension

(1) Occurs with very high pressures: diastolic over 110 mm/Hg
(2) Arterioles show fibrinoid necrosis, thrombosis, and intimal fibrosis leading to luminal narrowing
(3) These changes produce microinfarction, hemorrhages, and marked edema (retinal hemorrhages, papilledema)
(4) In the kidney, acute renal failure may result (malignant nephrosclerosis)
  4. Hypertensive encephalopathy
    a) An acute and transient dysfunction of the brain that occurs with very high blood pressures
    b) The result of spasm of cerebral arterioles
III. Medial calcification (Monckeberg's sclerosis)
  A. An unimportant but very common degenerative disease affecting large muscular arteries (femoral, radial, tibial, uterine, splenic, etc.)
  B. Characterized by extensive calcification of the media, often in a concentric manner, causing hardening and elongation of the arteries with increased tortuosity
  C. No luminal narrowing, or any predisposition to endothelial damage and thrombosis, so that medial calcification produces no clinical effects
  D. Cause unknown: deterioration associated with aging

Congenital Diseases of the Aorta

  I. Coarctation of the aorta: narrowing usually near site of fetal ductus arteriosus
 II. Marfan's syndrome
  A. An autosomal-dominant disease characterized by defective formation of connective tissue
  B. Occurrence of myxomatous degeneration of aortic wall (dissecting aneurysm, rupture), aortic valve (aortic incompetence), and mitral valve (prolapse, incompetence)

Inflammatory Diseases of Blood Vessels

  I. Syphilitic aortitis
  A. Rare; occurs in the late (tertiary) stage; thoracic aorta maximally involved
  B. Media shows lymphocytic infiltration around vasa vasorum with muscle degeneration and fibrosis
  C. Scarring caused by intimal fibrosis ("tree-bark" appearance)

D. Dilatation caused by weakening of wall (aortic aneurysm)
E. Clinical effects of syphilitic aortitis
    1. Aortic valve incompetence due to aortic root dilatation
    2. Coronary artery stenosis due to intimal fibrosis at the ostia
    3. Aortic aneurysms
II. Takayasu's disease (aortic arch syndrome)
    A. Uncommon in the United States; common in Japan
    B. Panaortitis of the aortic arch with extensive fibrosis constricting openings of arteries arising from the aorta ("pulseless disease")
III. Giant-cell arteritis
    A. An inflammatory disease affecting medium-sized muscular arteries
    B. Occurs almost exclusively in the elderly (over 50 years)
    C. Etiology is uncertain, probably immunological
    D. The lesion commonly affects
        1. Temporal arteries: severe headache, thickening and tenderness of the superficial temporal artery, (temporal arteritis).
        2. Intracranial arteries: cranial nerve palsies and sudden blindness due to retinal artery involvement
        3. Parascapular arteries: muscle pain, fever (polymyalgia rheumatica)
    E. Pathologic effects
        1. Granulomatous inflammation of the media with numerous giant cells around fragmented elastic fibers
        2. Irregular fibrosis
IV. Polyarteritis nodosa
    A. Uncommon; occurs in young adults; more common in males
    B. Etiology: unknown; hepatitis B surface antigen, antibody, and immune complexes present in 30–40% of patients
    C. Pathologic characteristics
        1. Small arteries maximally involved
        2. Segmental nodular reddish swellings with microaneurysms and hemorrhages
        3. Microscopic features
            a) Fibrinoid necrosis of the media
            b) Acute inflammation with neutrophils and eosinophils involving all layers of the artery
            c) Microaneurysm formation and hemorrhage
            d) Thrombosis
        4. In the chronic phase: artery shows concentric fibrosis
    D. Clinical characteristics
        1. A chronic disease with remission and exacerbations
        2. Presents with fever and variable organ involvement

    3. Renal: hematuria, proteinuria, oliguria, and hypertension
    4. Gastrointestinal: abdominal pain and bleeding (melena)
    5. Involvement of joints, skeletal muscle and peripheral nerves common
    6. Peripheral blood commonly shows eosinophilia
V. Thromboangitis obliterans (Buerger's disease)
  A. Predominantly involves peripheral vessels of the lower extremity
  B. Occurs almost exclusively in males aged 20–30 years
  C. Has a strong relationship to cigarette smoking
  D. Pathologic characteristics
    1. Segmental involvement of small and medium-sized arteries, frequently involving adjacent veins and nerves
    2. In the acute phase: marked swelling and neutrophilic infiltration of the neurovascular bundle; thrombosis common
    3. Production of occluded, cord-like vessels due to healing by fibrosis
  E. Clinical characteristics
    1. Calf pain on exercise (intermittent claudication) produced by ischemia of skeletal muscle
    2. Pain at rest, trophic changes, and dry gangrene produced by ischemia of the skin

Aneurysms

  I. Definition: a localized dilatation of an artery
 II. Types of aneurysm
  A. Saccular: a balloon-like bulge of one side
  B. Fusiform: a circumferential dilatation
  C. Dissecting: an intimal tear permits blood to dissect between layers of medial smooth muscle
III. Causes of aneurysms
  A. Congenital: commonly in cerebral Circle of Willis (Berry aneurysm)
  B. Atherosclerotic: commonest cause; occurs in low abdominal aorta
  C. Syphilis: rare; occurs in thoracic aorta
  D. Trauma: rare; blunt chest trauma; common site is at the insertion of the ligamentum arteriosum
  E. Mycotic (infectious) aneurysm: the result of an infected embolus, usually in infective endocarditis
  F. Dissecting aneurysm of the aorta

1. Associated with myxomatous degeneration (common in Marfan's syndrome)
2. Intimal tear commonly present, usually just above the aortic valve
3. Entrance of blood in the media at the site of intimal injury and dissection between layers of smooth muscle
4. Effects of a dissecting aneurysm
   a) Compression of blood vessels taking origin from the aorta
   b) Rupture through the outer wall producing massive hemorrhage
   c) Rupture back into the aortic lumen at a distal site producing a "double-barrelled" aorta
   d) Rupture into pericardial cavity: hemopericardium

IV. Clinical effects of fusiform and saccular aneurysms
   A. A pulsatile swelling; may compress adjacent structures
   B. Compression of vessels taking origin from the aorta
   C. Rupture causing massive hemorrhage
   D. Rupture into adjacent veins: arteriovenous fistulae
   E. Thrombosis in the wall of an aneurysm possibly leading to distal embolism

10

The Respiratory System

STRUCTURE AND FUNCTION

I. Structure of the respiratory system
   A. Air passages
      1. the upper respiratory tract: nasal cavity, pharynx, larynx
      2. the lower respiratory tract: trachea, bronchi, bronchioles
   B. Lung parenchyma (Fig. 10-1)
      1. The pulmonary lobule: structures derived from a small bronchiole. These include 3–5 terminal bronchioles.
      2. The pulmonary acinus: structures arising from a single terminal bronchiole, consisting of respiratory bronchioles, alveolar ducts, and alveoli. The acinus is the functional unit of lung parenchyma.
   C. Pleura: the mesothelial lining of the cavity in which each lung is situated
II. Function of the lung: is gas exchange. Normal PaO_2 is 95 mm Hg and normal $PaCO_2$ is 40 mm Hg. Gas exchange involves the following:
   A. Ventilation: supplies oxygen-rich air to the alveoli
      1. Abnormalities in ventilation may be caused by diseases that are
         a) restrictive: lung expansion does not occur normally due to brain stem, nerve, muscle disease or due to intrinsic lung disease that prevents expansion (e.g., pulmonary fibrosis).
         b) obstructive: ventilation of the lung does not occur because of obstruction of the air passages.
      2. Abnormal alveolar ventilation leads to changes in blood gases:
         a) Decreased alveolar ventilation leads to hypoxemia (decreased PO_2) and hypercapnia (increased PCO_2) in arterial blood.
         b) Increased alveolar ventilation washes out carbon dioxide and causes hypocapnia. If the individual is breathing air, the PO_2 does not increase with hyperventilation.

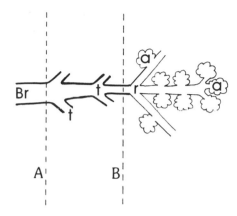

Fig. 10-1. Normal lung parenchyma. Pulmonary lobule includes structures distal to line A. Br = small bronchiole. Acinus includes structures distal to line B. t and r = terminal and respiratory bronchiole. a = alveolus.

B. Perfusion: supplies blood to alveolar capillaries.
C. For proper gas exchange, ventilation and perfusion must be balanced. Mismatching of perfusion and ventilation results in the following:
   1. Increased physiologic dead space if ventilated alveoli are not perfused.
   2. Right-to-left shunting of blood if perfused alveoli are not ventilated.
   3. Both these imbalances lead to hypoxemia.
D. Diffusion: transfer of gases between alveolar air and blood.
   1. Diffusion occurs across the alveolar diffusion membrane (Fig. 10-2).
   2. Abnormal diffusion causes hypoxemia. Carbon dioxide, being much more diffusible than oxygen, is not affected. Stimulation of respiration by hypoxemia causes hyperventilation and hypocapnia.

INFECTIONS OF THE RESPIRATORY SYSTEM

I. Infections of the air passages
   A. Coryza (the common cold): A common acute self-limited infection caused by many different viruses, most commonly Rhinoviruses
   B. Acute pharyngotonsillitis ("sore throat")
      1. This is very common.

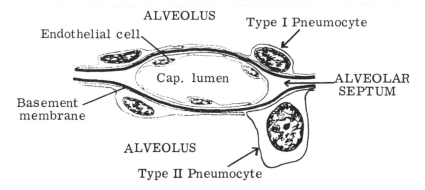

Fig. 10-2. Gas exchange occurs between alveoli and capillary across the diffusion membrane, which is composed of endothelial cell, basement membrane, and alveolar epithelial cell (pneumocyte).

   2. Its Etiology includes the following:
      a) Influenza, parainfluenza, myxoviruses, adenoviruses: 90%
      b) Beta-hemolytic streptococci (Landsteiner group A): 5%
      c) Epstein–Barr virus (infectious mononucleosis) and Cytomegalovirus: produce a systemic illness with pharyngitis
      d) Other bacteria such as gonococci and diphtheria bacilli
   3. Clinically, all of these present with sore throat and fever.
   4. The diagnosis is made by throat culture.
  C. Diphtheria
   1. Caused by *Corynebacterium diphtheriae*
   2. Has become rare in the United States because of routine active immunization against the disease (the D in the triple DPT vaccine)
   3. Is now as commonly seen in adults as it is in children.
   4. Characterized by
      a) local acute inflammation and mucosal necrosis. The necrotic mucosa appears as an adherent membrane on the surface. The sites maximally affected are the fauces, larynx and nasal cavity.
      b) high fever and marked cervical lymph node enlargement ("bull-neck"). There is no bacteremia.
   5. Complications
      a) Locally, respiratory obstruction due to the acute laryngeal inflammation or aspiration of a detached membrane

b) Systemic complications due to exotoxin produced by the bacillus and absorbed into the blood stream, including
   (1) toxic myocarditis with acute cardiac failure
   (2) peripheral nerve dysfunction
D. Acute epiglottitis ("croup")
   1. This is caused by
      a) *Haemophilus influenzae*, mainly in children under 5 years old.
      b) viruses, notably influenza and para-influenza.
   2. Acute inflammation of the epiglottis, larynx, and trachea causes severe edema and may obstruct the narrow respiratory passages.
E. Pertussis ("whooping cough")
   1. Caused by *Bordetella pertussis*
   2. Another childhood communicable disease that has been controlled by active immunization (the P in the DPT vaccine)
   3. Causes mucosal acute inflammation in the larynx, trachea, and bronchi; associated edema stimulates the cough reflex, producing paroxysms of coughing that are followed by a high-pitched inspiration (the whoop)
F. Acute bronchiolitis
   1. Caused by viruses, most commonly respiratory syncytial virus
   2. A common disease in children under 2 years of age
   3. Acute inflammation of the bronchiole with edema, exudation, and mucus production leading to bronchiolar obstruction and wheezing
   4. In severe cases, a serious ventilatory defect causing respiratory failure and death
G. Fungal infections of the air passages
   1. Candidiasis
      a) An opportunistic infection caused by *Candida albicans*, a yeast
      b) Occurs in debilitated states associated with immuno-deficiency
         (1) Neonates
         (2) Diabetes mellitus
         (3) Immunodeficient patients, particularly those with the acquired immunodeficiency syndrome (AIDS) and those undergoing cancer therapy
         (4) Patients undergoing broad-spectrum antibiotic therapy, in whom suppression of normal flora favors the overgrowth of the yeast

c) Causes white plaques on the surface of the mucosa of the oral cavity, esophagus, and large air passages that are composed of masses of budding yeasts
d) Diagnosis made by a scraping, biopsy, or culture; budding yeasts forming pseudohyphae (Fig. 10-3) typical
e) The yeast may enter the blood stream (fungemia); this is of considerable significance in
   (1) patients with cardiac valve prostheses where candida produces endocarditis
   (2) in immunocompromised patients where a severe dis-

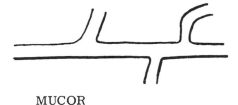

MUCOR
Broad hyphae; non-septate
Perpendicular branching

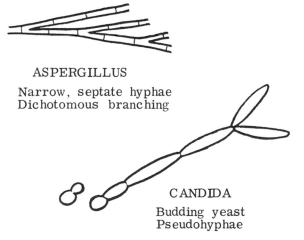

ASPERGILLUS
Narrow, septate hyphae
Dichotomous branching

CANDIDA
Budding yeast
Pseudohyphae

Fig. 10-3. Candida, Mucor, and Aspergillus: differential features.

seminated infection occurs with abscesses in virtually all organs.

2. Mucormycosis (phycomycosis)
   a) An opportunistic infection of the nasal cavity and paranasal sinuses by mycelial fungi belonging to the family Phycomycetes: Mucor, Rhizopus, or Absidia
   b) Occurs in
      (1) diabetes mellitus with ketoacidosis
      (2) severely immunosuppressed patients, commonly in terminal cancer
   c) Causes a severe necrotizing inflammation due to invasion of blood vessels by the fungus; extension to bone and brain occurs in severe infections, where mortality is high
   d) Diagnosed by finding the characteristic large, perpendicular branching, nonseptate hyphae (Fig 10-3) in tissue and culture

3. Aspergillosis
   a) An opportunistic infection caused by mycelial fungi of the genus Aspergillus (Fig 10-3)
   b) Three types of disease in the respiratory tract
      (1) Aspergilloma ("fungus ball"): a mass of fungus growing in a cavity such as a tuberculous or bronchiectatic cavity
      (2) Invasive pulmonary aspergillosis: occurs in immunosuppressed patients; fungal dissemination commonly occurs
      (3) Allergic aspergillosis: a hypersensitivity reaction to spores of *Aspergillus* species, causing bronchospasm and wheezing

II. Infections of the lung parenchyma
   A. Lobar and bronchopneumonia
      1. Multiplication of extracellular organisms in the alveoli leads to hyperemia of septal capillaries, exudation, and neutrophil emigration into the alveolar spaces (consolidation of alveoli).
      2. It may be classified by distribution of lesions into
         a) lobar pneumonia, characterized by involvement of an entire lobe or bronchopulmonary segment.
         b) bronchopneumonia, in which there is a patchy, often bilateral involvement. The areas of consolidation are usually smaller and tend to occur around inflamed bronchioles.

3. It may be classified according to pathogenetic mechanism into
   a) primary pneumonias, which occur in previously healthy individuals and are caused by virulent organisms.
   b) secondary pneumonias.
      (1) Occur when there is an underlying cause such as
         i) following a viral respiratory infection
         ii) bronchial obstruction with stagnant secretions
         iii) chronic lung disease such as emphysema, bronchiectasis
         iv) aspiration of pharyngeal secretions in comatose states
      (2) Caused by virulent as well as less virulent organism such as *Haemophilus influenzae.*
4. The classification that is of greatest importance is the etiologic classification.
5. Pneumococcal pneumonia
   a) Pneumococci cause 90% of lobar and many cases of bronchopneumonia
   b) The disease falls into four clinicopathologic stages
      (1) Acute congestion
         i) The pneumococci are actively multiplying in the alveoli.
         ii) Microscopically there is active dilatation of alveolar capillaries and early fluid exudation into the alveoli.
         iii) Clinically, there is high fever, bacteremia (positive blood culture), and a cough productive of purulent, blood-tinged (rusty) sputum.
      (2) Red hepatization
         i) Exudation and neutrophil emigration cause the alveoli to become consolidated and look like liver ("hepatization").
         ii) Physical signs of consolidation are present.
      (3) Gray hepatization
         i) The early recovery phase. The organism has been controlled and the patient has recovered clinically.
         ii) The hyperemia has disappeared, but the alveoli still contain the exudate. Physical signs of consolidation are still present.

(4) Resolution

    i) The process by which the alveolar exudate is removed and the lung returns to normal.

    ii) It may take several weeks, during which radiologic abnormalities persist despite return of the clinical state to normal.

c) The above natural history of pneumonia is rarely seen today because of antibiotic therapy.

6. Type 3 pneumococcal pneumonia

    a) Type 3 pneumococcus has a thick mucoid capsule that gives it considerable antiphagocytic capability.

    b) It causes a severe pneumonia with a high incidence of suppuration, bacteremia, and death.

7. Staphylococcal pneumonia

    a) *Staphylococcus aureus* affects the extremes of life, complicating emphysema and influenza in the elderly and viral infections and cystic fibrosis in the very young.

    b) It causes a severe pneumonia with suppuration and bacteremia. This is a common "hospital" infection.

8. Klebsiella pneumonia

    a) Occurs in alcoholics and debilitated individuals; a similar pneumonia is caused by other coliform gram-negative bacilli

    b) Severe suppurative pneumonia with much tissue necrosis

9. Legionnaire's disease (*Legionella pneumophilia*)

    a) Produces epidemics (like that at the Legionnaire's convention in Philadelphia from which it got its name), as well as sporadic cases, particularly in immunocompromised hosts

    b) Contamination of air-conditioners, ventilation systems, shower-heads with the gram-negative bacillus represent important sources of infection

    c) Causes a severe necrotizing pneumonia with high mortality

    d) Diagnosis by demonstrating the organism in the alveolar exudate (sputum, bronchial washings, lung biopsy)

10. *Pneumocystis carinii* pneumonia

    a) *Pneumocystis carinii* is a protozoan parasite that is a commensal in the pharynx of normal individuals.

    b) It is an organism of very low virulence that causes infection only in immunocompromised hosts. It appears most commonly in patients with acquired immunodeficiency syndrome (AIDS).

c) The organism multiplies in the alveoli, filling them. On routine sections, the alveoli are filled with a pink, frothy mass that is seen to be a mass of organisms on special stains (methenamine silver stain). The organism has a typical cup or crescent shape and measures about 2 μm.

d) The inflammatory response is a plasma cell and lymphocytic response in the alveolar septa.

e) Pneumocystic pneumonia is a severe disease in the immunocompromised host, with a mortality of over 50% despite the availability of effective antibiotics.

B. Acute interstitial pneumonitis: an acute illness characterized by infiltration of the alveolar septum by mononuclear cells

1. Etiology
   a) Viruses: influenza, para-influenza, respiratory syncytial virus, adenoviruses, cytomegalovirus, herpesviruses, measles, echo, and Coxsackie viruses
   b) Chlamydiae: Psittacosis
   c) Rickettsiae: *Coxiella burneti* (Q fever)
   d) *Mycoplasma pneumoniae*

2. Pathologic changes
   a) The alveolar septa are expanded by hyperemia and a cellular infiltrate composed of plasma cells and lymphocytes.
   b) The alveolar epithelium shows cytopathic changes.
      (1) Necrosis of pneumocytes: causes denudation, intra-alveolar hemorrhage, and the formation of hyaline membranes
      (2) Inclusion bodies: present in CMV, herpes simplex, varicella, adenovirus, measles, influenza, and psittacosis
      (3) Multinicleated giant cells: measles, respiratory syncytial virus infection

3. Clinical characteristics
   a) Usually mild; acute onset with fever, cough, and dyspnea
   b) Absence of alveolar exudate and consolidation
   c) Chest x-ray shows the pattern of interstitial inflammation in contrast to the well-defined opacity of lobar pneumonia

C. Acute necrotizing pneumonia

1. An extremely severe acute pneumonia characterized clinically by sudden onset of a severe illness and rapid progression with a high mortality, and pathologically, by extensive necrosis and intra-alveolar hemorrhage

2. Etiologic agents: very virulent organisms
    a) *Yersinia pestis* (pneumonic plague)
    b) *Bacillus anthracis* (anthrax)
    c) Legionnaire's disease
    d) Viral pneumonia (most commonly influenza and adenovirus)
D. Chronic lung infections
  1. Chronic lung abscess
    a) Commonly occurs in the following clinical settings:
        (1) Distal to an obstructed bronchus
        (2) After comatose states, where aspiration of pharyngeal secretions may occur: alcoholic coma, diabetic coma, epilepsy, after anesthesia
    b) Tendency of culture of pus from a chronic lung abscess to grow multiple bacteria (polybacterial), frequently anaerobes like Bacteroides
    c) Clinically, occurrence of persistent fever, weight loss, and chronic cough productive of much odorous sputum
  2. Pulmonary tuberculosis
    a) Primary (childhood) tuberculosis (fig. 10-4)
        (1) This occurs when a child who has not been previously exposed to tubercle bacilli inhales the organism.
        (2) It leads to the formation of the *primary complex*, composed of
            i) The ghon focus at the site of parenchymal infection. This is usually subpleural and may be located anywhere in the lung.
            ii) Enlarged regional (hilar) lymph nodes.
        (3) Before immunity is established, tubercle bacilli survive in macrophages and are transported via lymphatics and the blood stream throughout the body: preallergic lymphohematogenous dissemination.
        (4) Development of immunity against the tubercle bacillus causes
            i) macrophage activation (by lymphokines), leading to destruction of the tubercle bacilli and recovery from the primary infection.
            ii) inhibition of macrophage migration (lymphokine), which stops the free movement of infected macrophages.
            iii) delayed (type IV) hypersensitivity, which leads to caseation necrosis in the granulomas. It is also responsible for "tuberculin conversion," in which

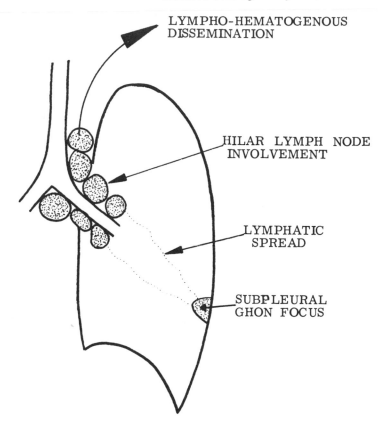

LYMPHO-HEMATOGENOUS
DISSEMINATION

HILAR LYMPH NODE
INVOLVEMENT

LYMPHATIC
SPREAD

SUBPLEURAL
GHON FOCUS

Fig. 10-4. Primary tuberculosis: the primary complex.

the individual demonstrates a positive skin test
with tuberculin (extract of tubercle bacilli).

(5) Clinically, this stage is usually asymptomatic or manifests as a mild flu-like illness.

(6) In 95% of cases, immunity stops disease progression,
leading to recovery. The lesions heal by fibrosis and
may calcify.

(7) Complications are rare, occurring in 5% of cases, and
include
  i) locally progressive pulmonary disease, causing

exensive caseous consolidation of the lung (caseous pneumonia).

ii) erosion of a caseous granuloma into a bronchus (tuberculous bronchopneumonia) or blood vessel (causing a severe bacteremia: miliary tuberculosis).

b) Recovery from primary tuberculosis: a recovered individual
   (1) is tuberculin positive
   (2) has partial immunity to tuberculosis
   (3) commonly harbors dormant tubercle bacilli in the lungs, brain, meninges, bone, kidneys, lymph nodes, intestines, etc., that are the result of preallergic lymphohematogenous dissemination of bacilli

c) Secondary (adult) tuberculosis (Fig. 10-5)
   (1) This may occur as a result of
      i) reinfection
      ii) reactivation of dormant foci of tubercle bacilli
   (2) Multiplication of tubercle bacilli evokes a brisk secondary immune response. This produces
      i) localized disease, due to inhibition of macrophage migration.
      ii) extensive caseation, due to delayed hypersensitivity.
   (3) Pathologic characteristics of secondary pulmonary tuberculosis include the following:
      i) The disease is commonly restricted to the apices of the lungs.
      ii) It is a solid, often large mass of caseous granulomatous inflammation with extensive fibrosis: "tuberculoma."
      iii) The granuloma liquefies and opens into a bronchus, leading to
         (A) the coughing up of large numbers of tubercle bacilli. The patient is now infective.
         (B) cavitation (cavitary fibrocaseous tuberculosis).
   (4) Clinical features include the following:
      i) Almost always symptomatic
      ii) Chronic cough, frequently with hemoptysis due to erosion of a blood vessel in the wall of the cavity; marked weight loss, low grade fever, and night sweats common

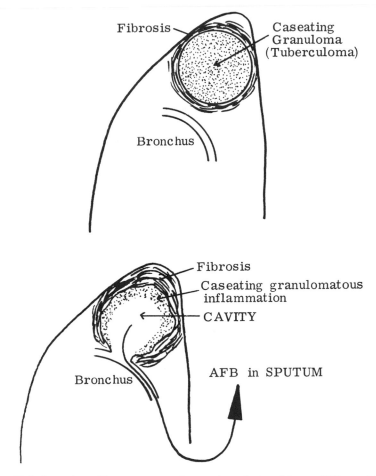

Fig. 10-5. Secondary fibrocaseous cavitary tuberculosis of lung. AFB = acid-fast bacilli = Mycobacteria.

    iii) Demonstration by physical examination and chest x-ray of the changes of apical fibrosis and cavitation

    iv) Finding of tubercle bacilli in sputum or tissue, on an acid-fast stained smear or in culture, which confirms diagnosis

3. Atypical mycobacterial infection
    a) Occurs in immunodeficient states, commonly in the acquired immunodeficiency syndrome.
    b) Pulmonary disease is very similar to pulmonary tuberculosis, and is distinguished only by culture.
4. Fungal granulomas of the lung
    a) Histoplasmosis is common in the Mississippi Valley, and Coccidioidomycosis in the Southwestern United States. Blastomycosis, Paracoccidioidomycosis and Sporotrichosis are very uncommon in the United States. Infection with Cryptococcus neoformans is common in the immunodeficient host.
    b) Pathologic lesions are chronic granulomas with extensive caseation and fibrosis, very similar to tuberculosis. Diagnosis depends on identifying the fungus in sputum or tissue (Fig. 10-6) or culture.
    c) Cryptococcal pneumonia is commonly characterized by numerous yeasts in alveoli without any inflammatory response.
    d) The types of disease are very similar to those seen in tuberculosis.
        (1) Primary infection, characterized by a parenchymal granulomatous focus and regional lymph node enlargement.
        (2) Progressive primary infection, characterized by widespread dissemination of fungus in the body.
        (3) Reactivation-type chronic cavitary lung disease, commonly seen in histoplasmosis and coccidioidomycosis.

DISEASES CAUSING AIRWAYS OBSTRUCTION

I. Bronchial asthma
    A. Definition
        1. Bronchial asthma is a clinical entity characterized by acute narrowing of bronchioles due to smooth muscle contraction and edema (bronchospasm). This produces expirational wheezing.
        2. Attacks are usually of short duration and reverse completely. Rarely they maybe severe and prolonged ("status asthmaticus"), and lead to acute ventilatory failure and even death.

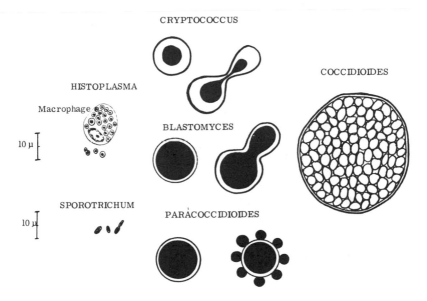

Fig. 10-6. Fungi in granulomas: differential features. Histoplasma and Sporothrix are 2–4 μ. Coccidioides appears as 20–100 μ spherules. Budding characterizes the intermediate-sized (10–25 μ) yeasts: Cryptococcus (single, narrow-based), Blastomyces (single, broad-based), Paracoccidioides (multiple).

B. Etiology
   1. Extrinsic allergic asthma
      a) Reagin-mediated, type I hypersensitivity (atopic) reaction
      b) Common in childhood; has a familial tendency
      c) Serum IgE increased and skin tests against the offending antigen positive
   2. Intrinsic asthma
      a) Nonreaginic; pathogenesis unknown, but it has been suggested that these patients have hyperreactive airways that constrict in response to a variety of nonspecific stimuli
      b) Occurs in older patients
      c) Common precipitants: aspirin, cold, exercise, and respiratory infections
      d) serum IgE normal; skin tests negative
C. Pathologic features of bronchial asthma not specific
   1. Mucus plugs in bronchioles that cause obstruction and increase susceptibility to secondary infection

2. Focal collapse of alveoli distal to obstructed bronchiole
3. Air-trapping and compensatory distension of alveoli
4. Inflammation in the bronchiolar wall, characterized by numerous eosinophils

II. Chronic obstructive pulmonary disease (COPD)
  A. Definition
    1. A clinically defined entity characterized by features of chronic obstruction to air flow in the lungs
    2. Diagnosed by abnormal tests of ventilatory function. FEV_1/FVC ratio the most widely used test (Fig. 10-7)
  B. Incidence: extremely common; incidence is increasing
  C. Clinical features
    1. Chronic cough, either dry or productive of mucoid sputum, progressive dyspnea, and wheezing
    2. Overinflated lung, increased anteroposterior diameter of the chest ("barrel chest"); flattened diaphragm
    3. Increased pulmonary arterial pressure, right ventricular hypertrophy and failure ("cor pulmonale") common
    4. Changes in blood gases variable
      a) They result from decreased alveolar ventilation and imbalanced ventilation and perfusion.
      b) One group of patients hyperventilate and maintain relatively normal arterial oxygen tension and normal or decreased CO_2 tension (type A COPD or "pink puffers").
      c) Other patients do not hyperventilate, are cyanotic, have increased arterial pCO_2 and right ventricular failure with peripheral edema (type B COPD or "blue bloaters").
      d) Most patients display a mixture of these findings.
      e) In patients with chronic hypercapnia, the respiratory center becomes insensitive to the pCO_2 stimulus and is driven by the hypoxemia. Administration of oxygen in these patients can remove the respiratory center drive and cause CO_2 retention and death ("carbon dioxide narcosis").
  D. Pathological features
    1. COPD is associated with chronic obstructive bronchitis, which is characterized by
      a) increased mucus secretion, leading to a chronic cough productive of mucoid sputum. Chronic bronchitis is defined by the presence of this clinical feature.

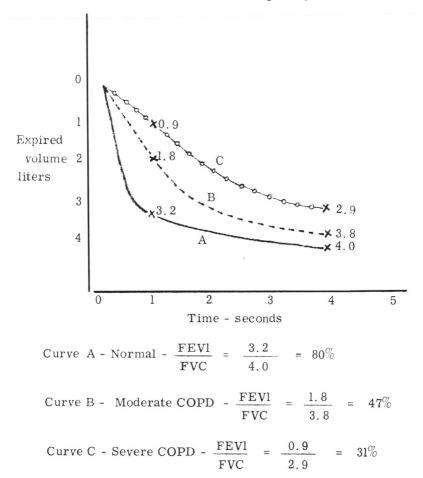

$$\text{Curve A - Normal -} \quad \frac{FEV1}{FVC} \quad = \quad \frac{3.2}{4.0} \quad = \quad 80\%$$

$$\text{Curve B - Moderate COPD -} \quad \frac{FEV1}{FVC} \quad = \quad \frac{1.8}{3.8} \quad = \quad 47\%$$

$$\text{Curve C - Severe COPD -} \quad \frac{FEV1}{FVC} \quad = \quad \frac{0.9}{2.9} \quad = \quad 31\%$$

Fig. 10-7. Chronic obstructive pulmonary disease. Forced expiration curves and FEV_1/FVC ratios in normal (A) and COPD (B,C). FEV_1 = forced expiratory volume in 1 second; FVC = vital capacity.

    b) hypertrophy of bronchial wall mucous glands. The Reid index (the ratio of mucous gland thickness to bronchial wall thickness) is increased above the normal value of 0.5.

    c) chronic inflammation and fibrous replacement of the

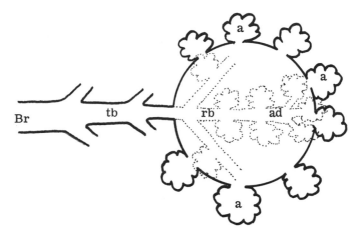

A. CENTRILOBULAR EMPHYSEMA

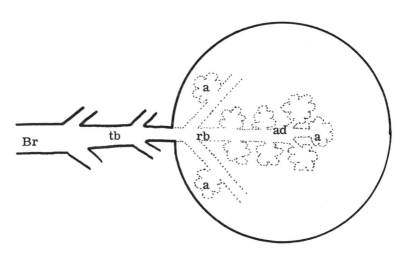

B. PANACINAR EMPHYSEMA

Fig. 10-8. Emphysema. Centrilobular emphysema involves the respiratory bronchioles (rb) and alveolar ducts (ad), but spares the alveoli (a). In panacinar emphysema, the whole acinus is destroyed. Br = bronchiole. tb = terminal bronchiole.

muscular wall of small bronchioles. The fibrosed bronchioles tend to collapse in expiration under the influence
of positive intrapleural pressure, resulting in ventilatory
obstruction.

2. It is also associated with emphysema (Figs. 10-8, 10-9).

   a) Emphysema is defined in anatomical terms as the per-

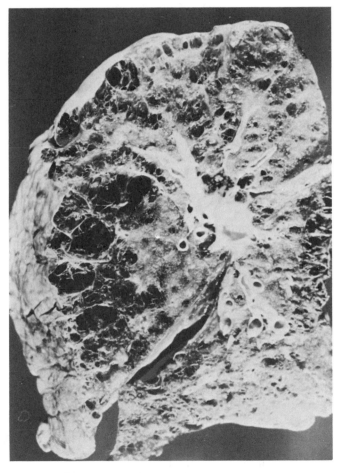

Fig. 10-9. Emphysema of the lung, severe.

manent dilatation of the air spaces distal to the terminal bronchiole with destruction of lung parenchyma. Involvement is diffuse in both lungs.

b) Two types of emphysema are recognized in COPD.

(1) Centrilobular emphysema: dilatation and destruction affects the central part of the acinus formed by the respiratory bronchioles. The periphery of the acinus is spared.

(2) Panacinar emphysema: the dilatation and destruction affects the entire acinus.

c) Gross and miscroscopic diagnosis of emphysema requires fixation of the lungs in a state of inflation before they are cut.

d) other types of emphysema (senile, bullous, etc.) are not associated with COPD.

E. Etiology of COPD
1. The etiology of COPD is unknown.
2. Destruction of lung parenchyma is believed to be the action of proteolytic enzymes. These are normally inactivated by plasma anti-trypsins.
3. Hypersecretion of mucus in chronic bronchitis favors inflammation and local leukocyte proteolytic enzyme release.
4. Cigarette smoking is the single most important etiologic factor.
5. Alpha-1-antitrypsin deficiency is associated with COPD.
   a) Plasma anti-proteolytic activity is dependent on the level of alpha-1-antitrypsin.
   b) The alpha-1-antitrypsin level is determined by inheritance at a single locus (Pi). A normal individual has two M genes (PiMM). The PiZZ homozygotes (rare) have a severe deficiency of alpha-1-antitrypsin and develop panacinar emphysema.
   c) The heterogygous PiMZ state occurs in 3–5% of the population and is associated with a moderate reduction in serum alpha-1-antitrypsin. There is no established association between emphysema and the PiMZ genotype.

III. Bronchiectasis
A. Definition: an abnormal and irreversible dilation of the bronchial tree proximal to the terminal bronchioles
B. Pathologic features
1. Bronchiectasis usually has a patchy distribution, commonly affecting one area.

2. The dilated bronchi and bronchioles maybe cylindrical, fusiform, or saccular. Intervening lung shows fibrosis.
3. The distended bronchi are inflamed and contain pus.
C. Etiology: the result of chronic infection with pulmonary parenchymal fibrosis. This is commonly seen in
   1. bronchial obstruction, e.g., by tumor or foreign body.
   2. mucoviscidosis (fibrocystic disease of the pancreas).
   3. bronchopneumonia, as that following measles and whooping cough.
   4. Kartagener's Syndrome, a congenital defect in ciliary motion that interferes with bronchial clearance of mucus and bacteria.
D. Clinically, chronic cough with profuse, purulent sputum is associated with fever, weight loss, and debility.

DIFFUSE INFILTRATIVE (RESTRICTIVE) LUNG DISEASES

I. This is a group of noninfectious lung diseases characterized by
   A. diffuse inflammation and fibrosis involving the interstitium of the alveolar septum.
   B. clinical presentation with chronic progressive dyspnea, tachypnea, and cyanosis.
   C. pulmonary function abnormalities of restrictive type. The vital capacity is reduced without airways obstruction. The FEV_1/FVC ratio is normal.
   D. thickening of the alveolar membrane affecting diffusion of oxygen leading to hypoxemia and normal or decreased $PaCO_2$ levels.
   E. a characteristic reticulonodular pattern of interstitial involvement on chest radiograph.
   F. association of the end stage with extensive parenchymal destruction, fibrosis, and the formation of abnormal cystic spaces ("honeycomb lung).
II. Etiology
   A. Physical and chemical agents
      1. Inhaled mineral dusts (pneumoconioses) and gases (oxygen)
      2. Ingested toxins and drugs: paraquat (a herbicide); cancer chemotherapeutic agents such as bleomycin, methotrexate, busulphan, and cyclophosphamide; nitrofurantoin (a urinary antiseptic).

      3. Radiation
   B. Immunologic injury
      1. Hypersensitivity pneumonitis
      2. Connective tissue diseases (systemic lupus erythematosus, progressive systemic sclerosis, rheumatoid arthritis)
      3. Goodpasture's syndrome and idiopathic pulmonary hemosiderosis
      4. Usual interstitial pneumonitis (UIP), desquamative interstitial pneumonitis (DIP), lymphocytic interstitial pneumonitis (LIP)
      5. Wegener's granulomatosis
   C. Neoplastic proliferations
      1. Malignant lymphoma
      2. Primary bronchioloalveolar carcinoma
   D. Diseases of unknown etiology
      1. Sarcoidosis
      2. Pulmonary alveolar proteinosis
III. Pneumoconioses (inorganic dust diseases)
   A. Noncollagenous pneumoconioses, which result from inhalation of dusts that do not stimulate fibrosis
      1. Coal-workers' pneumoconiosis (anthracosis)
         a) This is seen in its most extensive form in coal miners.
         b) The basic lesion is the "coal dust macule," a collection of carbon-laden macrophages around a respiratory bronchiole.
         c) Fibrosis is absent, and the patient has no symptoms or abnormality in lung function.
         d) Rarely, coal workers develop a complicated clinical disease known as progressive massive fibrosis (PMF), characterized by the formation of large black fibrous masses.
      2. Other noncollagenous pneumoconioses
         a) Stannosis (tin)
         b) Siderosis (iron)
         c) Graphite and clay pneumoconioses
   B. Collagenous pneumoconioses
      1. Silicosis
         a) Etiology
            (1) It is caused by inhalation of crystalline silicon dioxide (silica) dust particles in the 2–3 μ size range.
            (2) It exists in nature as quartz, chrystobalite, and tridymite.

(3) Occupations at increased risk are hard rock, gold, tin, and copper mining; sandblasting, and iron, steel, and granite work.

(4) Significant pulmonary disease usually occurs after 10–15 years exposure, but rarely after as little as 1 year.

b) Pathologic features

(1) The characteristic lesion is the silicotic nodule, which forms in the lung and hilar lymph nodes.

(2) Grossly, the silicotic nodule is black (due to associated carbon pigment), and hard (collagen and calcification).

(3) Microscopically, silica particles are recognized as birefringent needle-shaped crystals when examined by polarized light.

c) Clinicial features

(1) Silicosis may be asymptomatic.

(2) Rarely it produces acute lung disease (acute silicotic proteinosis) with massive exposure.

(3) It produces chronic pulmonary fibrosis with dyspnea and pulmonary hypertension (cor pulmonale).

(d) Complications

(1) Silicosis results in a greatly increased incidence of tuberculosis.

(2) There is slightly increased incidence of autoimmune disease, particularly progressive systemic sclerosis.

2. Asbestosis

a) Etiology

(1) Asbestos is found in nature as chrysotile, amosite, and crocidolite.

(2) It is present in such diverse materials of modern civilization as insulation and brake linings in vehicles, making low-grade exposure almost universal.

(3) Asbestos-related disease was first recognized in workers with high levels of exposure, e.g., workers in shipyards and construction.

(4) Lower levels of exposure are also associated with significant risk. Asbestos-related disease occurs in families of shipyard workers, and in communities with asbestos-based industries.

b) Pathologic characteristics

(1) It appears as diffuse interstitial fibrosis, maximal in the basal region.

(2) The parietal pleura becomes thickened by a plaque-like deposition of hyalinized collagen. This is maximal in the lateral chest and diaphragmatic pleura.

(3) Microscopically, ferruginous (asbestos) bodies are seen in the lung. They appear as long (50–100 μ) brown structures having a beaded appearance. While ferruginous bodies are most commonly seen in asbestosis, they can occur with any fibrous molecule of similar size and shape.

c) Clinical characteristics

(1) It appears as diffuse pulmonary fibrosis with progressive dyspnea.

(2) Incidental findings include fibrous, calcified plaques in the parietal pleura.

(3) Malignant neoplasms: asbestos exposure is associated with a greatly increased risk of

  i) bronchogenic (lung) carcinoma: this is the most common associated neoplasm. Cigarette smoking has a profound additive effect.

  ii) mesothelioma of pleura, peritoneum, and pericardium: though uncommon, this represents the most specific associated neoplasm.

IV. Immunologic diseases

  A. Hypersensitivity pneumonitis (extrinsic allergic alveolitis)

    1. Etiology

      a) This results from inhalation of small organic particles, most commonly spores of thermophilic fungi.

      b) These fungi grow best at 50–60°C in decaying vegetation such as hay and sugar cane and in heated water in air-conditioning and air heating systems.

      c) A variety of occupations are at risk, including farming (farmer's lung) and bird breeding (bird-breeder's lung).

      d) The pathologic reaction is caused by a combined type III and IV hypersensitivity to the inhaled spores.

    2. Pathologic characteristics

      a) This is an acute interstitial pneumonitis due to complement fixation. The alveolar septa are expanded by neutrophils, lymphocytes, and plasma cells.

      b) Ill-defined granulomas with giant cells in alveolar septa are present.

      c) If it is recognized early and the patient is removed from the source of spores, the disease is reversible.

    d) With continued exposure, diffuse interstitial fibrosis leads to end-stage honeycomb lung.

3. Clinical characteristics
    a) Acute dyspnea, fever, and cough occur 4–6 hours after exposure to the antigen. Initially, these symptoms subside spontaneously in 12–18 hours.
    b) As pulmonary fibrosis ensues, the disease goes into its chronic phase with all the features of diffuse interstitial fibrosis.

B. Idiopathic interstitial pneumonitis (fibrosing alveolitis; Hamman–Rich syndrome): a group of diseases characterized by diffuse interstitial pneumonitis and fibrosis without a recognizable cause. A good response to steroids is seen in the early stages, suggesting an immunologic basis. It is classified into three categories.

    1. Usual interstitial pneumonitis (UIP)
        a) In the acute phase, there is interstitial infiltration by lymphocytes, plasma cells, and macrophages, plus pulmonary edema and acute alveolar damage with hyaline membranes.
        b) The disease progresses at a variable rate with increasing interstitial fibrosis and hyperplasia of type II pneumocytes. The end result is a honeycomb lung.

    2. Desquamative interstitial pneumonitis (DIP)
        a) This is similar to UIP with aggregation of mononuclear cells in the alveoli. The desquamated cells are macrophages and type II pneumocytes.
        b) Controversy exists over whether DIP is a variant of UIP or a completely different disease.

    3. Lymphocytic interstitial pneumonitis (LIP; pseudolymphoma)
        a) This is characterized by extensive infiltration of the interstitium with lymphocytes.
        b) It may be diffuse or involve a single area of lung, producing a mass lesion ("pseudolymphoma").
        c) It has an increased incidence of malignant lymphoma.

C. Interstitial fibrosis in connective tissue diseases: indistinguishable from UIP; occurs in progressive systemic sclerosis and rheumatoid arthritis

D. Anti-basement membrane antibody diseases
    1. Goodpasture's syndrome
        a) Definition: a disease caused by antibodies against the

basement membrane of glomerular capillaries and pulmonary alveoli
b) Pathologic features
  (1) Anti-basement membrane antibody fixes on lung alveolar basement membrane, causing a complement mediated type II hypersensitivity reaction.
  (2) There is marked intra-alveolar hemorrhage, usually recurrent. With time, large numbers of hemosiderin-containing macrophages accumulate in the alveoli.
  (3) Immunofluorescence shows linear deposition of IgG and complement in the alveoli.
c) Clinical features
  (1) Goodpasture's syndrome has a striking male predominance. Its onset is most frequently in the second and third decades of life.
  (2) It includes recurrent hemoptysis, with chronic blood loss and anemia.
  (3) Progressive dyspnea, cough and cor pulmonale occur due to pulmonary fibrosis.
  (4) Chest radiograph shows pulmonary infiltrates due to the intra-alveolar hemorrhage in the acute phase. Changes of increasing pulmonary fibrosis dominate chronic disease.
  (5) Glomerulonephritis, often severe, occurs.
2. Idiopathic pulmonary hemosiderosis: morphologically identical to Goodpasture's syndrome; thought to be a variant of it without renal involvement
V. Sarcoidosis
  A. Definition: a systemic disorder of uncertain etiology that commonly manifests in the lungs
  B. Associated with many immunologic abnormalities
    1. Depressed cell-mediated immunity
      a) Decreased numbers of T cells in the peripheral blood
      b) Anergy (failure of delayed hypersensitivity to antigens injected in intradermal skin tests)
    2. Hyperactivity of humoral immunity
      a) Increased number of B lymphocytes in peripheral blood
      b) Hyperimmunoglobulinemia
  C. Pathologic characteristics
    1. Noncaseating epithelioid cell granulomas
    2. In the lung, granulomas found in the alveolar septa, associated with interstitial pneumonitis and fibrosis

3. Two types of inclusions seen in the epithelioid and giant cells; neither specific for sarcoidosis:
    a) Schaumann bodies: round, calcified, laminated bodies
    b) Asteroid bodies: small, with a central pink zone surrounded by a clear zone traversed by fine radial lines

D. Clinical characteristics
    1. Occurs typically in black females between 20 and 35 years
    2. Abnormality in the chest radiograph present in over 90% of patients with sarcoidosis
        a) Bilateral hilar lympadenopathy: common
        b) Pulmonary infiltrates due to interstitial pneumonitis and fibrosis
    3. Has a variable course: 65% of patients with hilar adenopathy alone undergo complete spontaneous remission; pulmonary parenchymal involvement usually signifies progressive disease

VASCULAR DISEASES OF THE LUNG

I. Pulmonary embolism
  A. Definition: an extremely common and serious disease that causes more than 50,000 deaths per year in the United States
  B. Etiology
    1. Pulmonary emboli originate in deep leg vein thrombi in over 90% of cases. Thrombi in pelvic veins are second in frequency.
    2. Deep-vein thrombosis and pulmonary embolism occur most commonly
        a) after surgery.
        b) after childbirth.
        c) in patients who are immobilized for any reason.
        d) in patients with cardiovascular disease, as after myocardial infarction, and in congestive heart failure.
        e) in users of oral contraceptives; users have a slightly increased risk.
    3. Slowing of the circulation and a hypercoagulable state in the blood (increased fibrinogen level, increased platelet count, etc.) are contributory mechanisms.
  C. Effects
    1. Sudden death is due to a large embolus that becomes impacted in the right ventricular outflow tract and main pulmonary artery.

2. Pulmonary infarction
   a) Pulmonary infarction occurs when a medium-sized embolus obstructs a peripheral pulmonary artery in a patient whose bronchial arterial circulation is impaired (patients with left heart failure and pulmonary hypertension).
   b) Pulmonary infarcts are wedge-shaped and hemorrhagic.
   c) Clinically, there is pleural-type chest pain, hemorrhagic pleural effusion, dyspnea, fever, and hemoptysis.
3. Multiple small emboli over a long period may cause pulmonary hypertension.

II. Pulmonary hypertension
   A. This is an elevation of pulmonary artery pressure.
   B. Secondary pulmonary hypertension is secondary to a known disease. This is common, and maybe caused by
      1. mitral valve disease: stenosis and incompetence.
      2. pulmonary diseases associated with emphysema and fibrosis ("cor pulmonale").
      3. multiple small pulmonary emboli.
   C. Primary pulmonary hypertension: a disease of unknown etiology occurring mainly in young females and frequently associated with collagen diseases

III. Adult respiratory distress syndrome (ARDS; "shock lung")
   A. A common complication in many seriously ill patients with
      1. hypovolemic shock (due to anoxia)
      2. sepsis (endotoxins)
      3. acute pancreatitis (circulating phospholipases)
      4. inhalation of toxic gases, e.g., oxygen (toxic free radicals)
   B. Pathologic characteristics
      1. Acute diffuse alveolar damage leads to pulmonary edema, hemorrhage, and formation of hyaline membranes.
      2. Grossly, the lungs are purple, heavy and solid. Hemorrhagic fluid exudes from the cut surface.
      3. In the recovery phase, there is hyperplasia of the type II pneumocytes and interstitial fibrosis.
   C. Clinical characteristics
      1. Rapidly increasing dyspnea
      2. Hypoxemia
      3. Cyanosis

IV. Vasculitis
   A. Systemic lupus erythematosus and other immune complex diseases may produce acute alveolar damage and small-vessel vasculitis.
   B. Wegener's granulomatosis

1. This is a necrotizing vasculitis of small arteries. The inflammatory reaction around the affected vessel is granulomatous with scattered neutrophils, eosinophils, and lymphocytes. Arterial necrosis and disruption is the rule.
2. The classical form of the disease has involvement of
   a) the nose, paranasal sinuses, and nasopharynx.
   b) the lungs.
   c) the kidneys: necrotizing glomerulitis.
3. Pulmonary involvement is characterized by a rapidly expanding infiltrate that tends to be bilateral, with multiple nodular mass lesions that tend to cavitate.
4. The etiology is unknown. A hypersensitivity immunologic reaction to an unknown antigen is postulated.

NEOPLASMS OF THE RESPIRATORY SYSTEM

I. Neoplasms of the upper respiratory tract
   A. Benign
      1. Squamous papilloma
         a) Papillary, wart-like excrescence in mouth, pharynx, and larynx
         b) Juvenile laryngeal papillomatosis caused by papilloma virus in children; characterized by multiple, recurrent lesions
         c) Inverted papilloma of the nasal cavity characterized by inward growth of the benign squamous epithelium; tends to recur
      2. Nasal angiofibroma presents as a polyp, mainly in young males
      3. Mixed tumors of salivary gland origin (pleomorphic adenoma)
         a) Benign; occur in both major and minor salivary glands
         b) Circumscribed but not encapsulated, firm mass
         c) Microscopically composed of small, polygonal epithelial cells and abundant myxoid stroma resembling cartilage
      4. Non-neoplastic "tumors"
         a) Allergic and inflammatory polyps in the nose: common
         b) Pyogenic granuloma: a polypoid mass of granulation tissue in the oral cavity; seen particularly in pregnancy
         c) Laryngeal ("singer's") nodule: trauma-induced lesion of the vocal cords characterized by vascular proliferation, stromal myxoid degeneration, and fibrosis

B. Malignant
  1. Squamous carcinoma
     a) Etiology unknown in most cases
        (1) Nasopharyngeal poorly differentiated squamous carcinoma is common in the Far East and has been etiologically related to the Epstein–Barr virus.
        (2) Oral carcinoma occurs frequently in India and Sri Lanka, where it is associated with the habit of chewing betel.
     b) Clinical features
        (1) chronic ulcer, with a hard everted edge
        (2) metastatic tumor in the cervical lymph nodes in a significant number of patients.
  2. Malignant salivary gland neoplasms
     a) May occur in the major and minor salivary glands
     b) A variety of different types recognized: mucoepidermoid carcinoma, adenoid cystic carcinoma, acinic cell carcinoma, carcinoma arising in mixed tumor, adenocarcinoma
     c) Present as infiltrative masses, usually slow growing
  3. Malignant lymphoma and plasmacytoma
II. Neoplasms of the bronchi and lung
  A. Carcinoma of the lung (bronchogenic carcinoma)
     1. Incidence
        a) It causes 85,000 deaths annually in the United States.
        b) Incidence is 100,000 cases per year; and is increasing.
        c) The male:female ratio was 7:1 in 1960 and is now 2.5:1 due to a dramatic increase in the incidence in females.
        d) It occurs in older individuals, and is rare in individuals under 40 years.
     2. Etiology
        a) Cigarette smoking: the strongest etiologic factor
        b) Industrial carcinogens: asbestos, heavy-metal mining
        c) Radiation exposure
        d) Urban pollution: an unknown risk factor
     3. Classification: four major and several minor types
        a) Squamous (epidermoid) carcinoma: 40–60%
        b) Adenocarcinoma: 10–25%
        c) Small-cell undifferentiated carcinoma ("oat-cell carcinoma") arises from bronchial neuroendocrine cells: 10–25%
        d) Large-cell undifferentiated carcinoma: 5–20%
        e) Other malignant neoplasms: bronchioloalveolar carci-

noma, bronchial carcinoid, mucoepidermoid carcinoma, adenoid cystic carcinoma

4. Pathologic characteristics
    a) Central (bronchogenic) carcinoma (Fig. 10-10)
        (1) 75% of lung carcinomas arise in the hilar bronchi and are accessible by bronchoscopy.

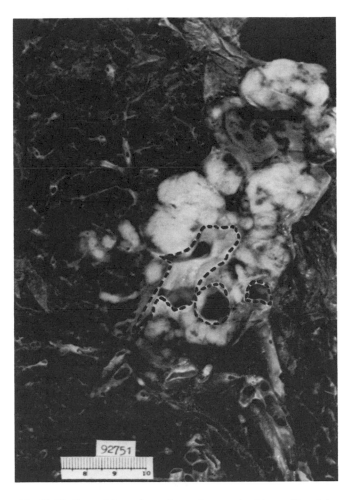

Fig. 10-10. Central bronchogenic carcinoma. A white multinodular mass surrounds the hilar bronchi (outlined).

(2) All histologic types occur.

(3) The tumor grows into the bronchial lumen as a nodular growth causing bronchial obstruction. In most cases, the neoplasm infiltrates the lung parenchyma to form a large hilar mass.

(4) Squamous carcinomas tend to keratinize and undergo central necrosis, leading to the formation of a cavity (Fig. 10-11).

b) Peripheral lung carcinoma

(1) This usually appears as a circumscribed mass in the periphery of the lung field, commonly in relation to a scar.

(2) It tends to be adenocarcinoma.

5. Clinical features

a) Many cases are detected at an asymptomatic stage by routine chest radiograph and, less commonly, by sputum examination.

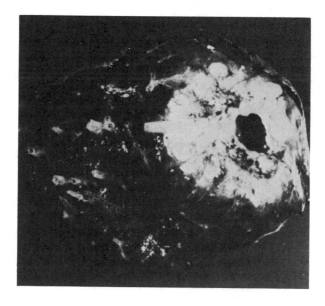

Fig. 10-11. Cavitary squamous carcinoma in a resected segment of lung.

b) Features include cough, hemoptysis, dyspnea, and chest pain.
c) Features of bronchial obstruction include unresolving pneumonia, lung abscess, and bronchiectasis.
d) Ectopic hormones are secreted.
   (1) ACTH, ADH and calcitonin: with oat cell carcinoma
   (2) Parathormone: with squamous carcinoma
e) Other nonmetastatic remote effects include
   (1) myopathy, peripheral neuropathy, and myasthenia-like syndrome.
   (2) finger clubbing and hypertrophic osteoarthropathy.
   (3) skin rashes of various types.
f) Effects of local invasion include
   (1) effusions in the pleura and pericardium.
   (2) superior vena caval obstruction.
   (3) chylothorax thoracic duct involvement
   (4) tracheoesophageal fistula
   (5) "Pancoast's syndrome": an apical lung carcinoma (usually squamous) that has invaded the T1 intercostal nerve and the cervical sympathetic trunk (causing Horner's syndrome).
g) Lymphatic metastasis to mediastinal nodes occurs early. Retrograde permeation of pleural lymphatics (pleural lymphatic carcinomatosis) occurs in advanced lesions.
h) Hematogenous metastasis occurs early, particularly in oat-cell carcinoma. Patients often present with a metastasis. Common sites of metastasis are adrenals, liver, brain and bone.

  6. Treatment and prognosis
    a) The overall 5-year survival is about 10%.
    b) Small-cell undifferentiated carcinoma is treated primarily by chemotherapy, which has improved median survival from less than 6 months to about 2 years.
    c) Non-small-cell carcinomas remain localized to the lung for longer periods and surgical resection is possible in about 30% of cases. Patients with resectable tumors less than 4 cm in size and without lymph node metastases have a 50% 5-year survival.

  B. Other primary tumors, many benign, e.g., sclerosing hemangioma and chondroid hamartoma, occur in the lung.
  C. Metastatic tumors of the lung are very common.
III. Neoplasms of the pleura: mesothelioma
  A. Benign fibrous mesothelioma

1. This is a rare benign neoplasm that presents as a localized growth of firm, dense, fibrous tissue on the visceral pleura, often attached to the lung surface by a pedicle. It may reach a large size.
2. Microscopically, it is composed of fibroblasts and collagen.

B. Malignant mesothelioma
   1. This is a rare neoplasm associated etiologically with asbestos exposure.
   2. It is common in the elderly, and presents with pleural effusion.
   3. Grossly, the tumor diffusely involves the pleura, encasing large areas of lung as a grayish, gelatinous mass.
   4. Microscopically, the tumor is biphasic with malignant spindle cells and epithelial cells that form tubules.
   5. Its prognosis is poor; 50% of patients are dead within one year.

11

The Gastrointestinal System

ESOPHAGUS

I. Functional abnormalities of deglutition (swallowing)
  A. Plummer–Vinson syndrome
    1. Severe iron deficiency, microcytic hypochromic anemia, koilonychia, atrophic glossitis, and dysphagia
    2. Marked female preponderance
    3. Web-like mucosal folds in upper esophagus
    4. Atrophy of the pharyngeal mucosa that interferes with the afferent arc of the deglutition reflex
    5. Precancerous lesion (esophageal carcinoma)
  B. Achalasia of the cardia
    1. Common; caused by an abnormal myenteric plexus in the esophagus
    2. Cause unknown; rarely caused by *Trypanosoma cruzi* (Chagas' disease)
    3. Failure of peristalisis and relaxation of cardia
    4. Dilation of the esophagus above the cardia; subsequent elongation and tortuosity ("sigmoid")
    5. Obstruction not complete; nutrition maintained
  C. Scleroderma (progressive systemic sclerosis) (see Chapter 18)
II. Inflammatory lesions of the esophagus
  A. Reflux esophagitis
    1. Common; caused by reflux of acid gastric juice through an incompetent cardiac sphincter
    2. Associated with hiatal hernia of sliding type
    3. Causes low retrosternal burning pain ("heartburn')
    4. Grossly: mucosa reddened with superficial erosions
    5. Histologically: hyperplasia of basal cells and neutrophil infiltration of the epithelium
    6. Possible consequences of prolonged reflux
      a) Barrett's esophagus: gastric metaplasia of epithelium
      b) Peptic ulceration of the esophagus
  B. Infections: uncommon

      1. *Candida albicans*: forms white plaques surrounded by erythema

      2. Herpes simplex: acute inflammation with ulceration

   C. Chronic fibrous strictures: May follow from the following:

      1. Reflux esophagitis and peptic ulceration

      2. Ingestion of lye (corrosive alkali) in attempted suicide

III. Traumatic lesions

   Esophageal laceration (Mallory-Weiss syndrome)

      1. Usually follows severe, prolonged vomiting

      2. Results from a longitudinal mucosal tear in the lower esophagus

      3. Causes acute, severe hemorrhage

IV. Neoplasms of the esophagus

   A. Benign neoplasms: uncommon

   B. Carcinoma of the esophagus

      1. Incidence

         a) 4% of cancer deaths in the United States

         b) Common after age 50 years

         c) Common in the Far East, Africa

      2. Etiology

         a) Chronic alcoholism and cigarette smoking

         b) Premalignant conditions: lye strictures and Plummer–Vinson syndrome

      3. Gross characteristics

         a) 50% occur in middle third; 30% in lower third

         b) May appear as a polypoid mass (rare), malignant ulcer (common), or stricture (common).

      4. Microscopic characteristics

         a) Over 90% are squamous carcinoma.

         b) Adenocarcinomas occur mainly at the lower end in metaplastic epithelium of Barrett's esophagus.

      5. Spread

         a) Local invasion of wall and adjacent mediastinum occurs first

         b) Lymphatic and blood stream spread occurs early.

      6. Five-year survival: less than 10%

   C. Other malignant neoplasms: rare

STOMACH

I. Congenital pyloric stenosis

   A. Hypertrophy of the pyloric muscle causes gastric outlet obstruction.

B. It is familial and common in males.

C. It manifests 1–2 weeks after birth with projectile vomiting.

II. Inflammatory lesions

  A. Acute gastritis

    1. This is very common; it causes mild epigastric pain, nausea, vomiting, and anorexia.

    2. It is caused by a variety of agents, including

      a) drugs: aspirin, steroids, and other anti-inflammatory agents.

      b) alcohol.

      c) stress: burn trauma, surgery, shock.

    3. The gastric mucosa shows edema, erythema, and erosions

    4. Rarely it produces severe bleeding and hematemesis.

    5. Microscopically, neutrophils and hyperemia can be seen in mucosa.

  B. Chronic nonspecific gastritis

    1. Characterized by an increase in lymphocytes and plasma cells in the mucosa.

    2. Of little clinical significance

  C. Chronic hypertrophic gastritis (Rugal hypertrophy, Menetrier's disease): rare

  D. Eosinophilic (allergic) gastroenteritis: rare

  E. Immunologically mediated chronic atrophic gastritis

    1. This is a progressive immunologic destruction of the gastric mucosa with loss of parietal cells.

    2. There is failure of secretion of acid (achlorhydria) and intrinsic factor.

    3. Vitamin B_{12} is not absorbed, causing megaloblastic anemia (pernicious anemia).

    4. The disease is common in older age groups.

    5. Autoantibodies are present against

      a) gastric parietal cells (in 90%): not specific.

      b) intrinsic factor (IF) blocking and binding antibodies (in 70%): specific.

    6. Histologic examination shows lymphocytic infiltration of the mucosa with progressive loss of parietal cells and mucosal atrophy.

    7. Chronic atrophic gastritis predisposes to development of carcinoma.

III. Peptic ulcer disease

  A. Incidence: common. 98% of peptic ulcers occur in the duodenum and stomach.

  B. Pathogenesis

1. Hypersecretion of acid
   a) Increased acid secretion occurs in duodenal ulcer, but not in gastric ulcer.
   b) Characteristics of Zollinger–Ellison syndrome include the following.
      (1) Pancreatic islet cell tumor secreting gastrin; often malignant
      (2) Marked gastric hypersecretion of acid
      (3) Multiple, recurrent peptic ulcers in stomach, duodenum, and jejunum
2. Decreased mucosal resistance: the primary factor in the genesis of gastric ulcer.

C. Site of chronic peptic ulcers
   1. Duodenal: first part
   2. Stomach: pyloric antrum and lesser curvature

D. Gross characteristics
   1. Chronic peptic ulcer is usually solitary, often large, round to oval, with a punched-out appearance (Fig. 11-1).
   2. The margins are flush with the mucosa; the floor is smooth.
   3. The base is fibrous and frequently extends into the muscle wall.

E. Histological characteristics
   1. The ulcer base shows granulation tissue and fibrosis
   2. The epithelium at the ulcer edge may show considerable cytologic atypia.

F. Symptoms: burning epigastric pain related to meals

G. Complications
   1. Bleeding: due to erosion of blood vessels

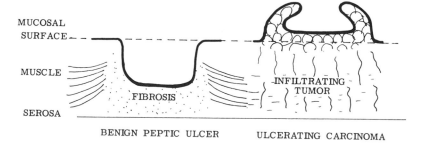

Fig. 11-1. Benign vs malignant ulcers of the stomach. The benign ulcer is punched out, below the level of the mucosa, and has a firm fibrotic base. The malignant ulcer has a raised, everted margin and a hard base of infiltrating tumor.

     a) Slow: causing iron deficiency anemia
     b) Rapid: causing hematemesis and melena
  2. Perforation into the peritoneal cavity
  3. Obstruction, usually pyloric, occurring with ulcers in the duodenum and pyloric antrum
  4. Penetration of the ulcer through gastric wall into adjacent organs
  5. Malignant transformation
     a) Does not occur in duodenal ulcers
     b) Occurs in gastric ulcers, probably rarely (1–5%)
IV. Neoplasms of the stomach
  A. Benign
    1. Mucosal polyps: adenomatous, hyperplastic
    2. Intramural solid masses: leiomyoma
  B. Malignant
    1. Carcinoma of the stomach
      a) Incidence
        (1) Common; accounts for over 90% of gastric malignancies
        (2) Has declined in the United States since 1940
        (3) High incidence in Japan, Chile, and Iceland
      b) Gross characteristics
        (1) Site: pyloric antrum most common site; can arise anywhere
        (2) "Early" gastric cancer: thickening or nodule or superficial ulcer in the mucosa
        (3) "Late" gastric cancer: May present as
           i) a fungating mass
           ii) a malignant ulcer with elevated, everted margins and irregular edges and floor (Fig. 11-1)
           iii) an excavated ulcer closely resembling a peptic ulcer
           iv) a diffusely infiltrating cancer that causes thickening and contraction of the stomach with minimal mucosal change ("linitis plastica")
      c) Microscopic characteristics: adenocarcinomas of varying degrees of differentiation; a fibrotic response commonly occurs around the cancer cells
      d) Spread of gastric carcinoma
        (1) Invasion of gastric wall
           i) Carcinoma restricted to the mucosa and submucosa ("early" gastric carcinoma) has a 5-year survival of around 90%.

     ii) Carcinoma which invades the muscle wall has a 5-year survival of around 20%.

    (2) Early lymphatic spread to regional lymph nodes

    (3) Transcelomic spread with implantation of tumor in the peritoneum or ovaries ("Krukenberg tumors")

    (4) Early blood stream metastasis

  e) Clinical features

    (1) Early gastric carcinoma is asymptomatic or has symptoms that mimic peptic ulcer disease.

    (2) Late cancer presents with anorexia, weight loss, and anemia.

    (3) Bleeding and pyloric obstruction occur late.

2. Lymphoma of the stomach: rare

  a) Both Hodgkin's and non-Hodgkin's—commonly B-cell—lymphomas occur.

  b) Forms nodular masses with thickening of mucosal folds.

  c) With treatment, 5-year survival is 70%.

3. Leiomyosarcoma of the stomach: rare; present as bulky masses with mucosal ulceration

INTESTINES

I. Malabsorption syndrome

  A. Definition: a clinical syndrome characterized by increased fecal excretion of fat (steatorrhea) and the effects of malabsorption of vitamins, minerals, protein, and carbohydrates

  B. Clinical features

    1. Steatorrhea: passage of soft, yellowish, greasy stools containing increased fat (more than 6 g per 24 hrs)

    2. Deficiencies of fat-soluble vitamins

    3. Protein malnutrition leading to weight loss

    4. Anemia common; due to combined deficiency of iron, vitamin B_{12}, and folic acid

  C. Causes of malabsorption syndrome

    1. Deficiency of bile resulting from

      a) obstruction of bile duct

      b) bile acid deconjugation due to bacterial overgrowth in the lumen of the small intestine caused by

        (1) intestinal stasis: diverticula, blind loops, scleroderma

        (2) fistulae, particularly enterocolic

    2. Intestinal mucosal abnormalities

    3. Intestinal enzyme deficiency

D. Intestinal mucosal abnormalities
1. Gluten-induced enteropathy
   a) May manifest in childhood (celiac disease) or adulthood (idiopathic steatorrhea)
   b) Due to the effect of the wheat protein gluten on the mucosa
   c) Jejunal histology shows villous atrophy; shortened and blunted villi with increased lymphocytes in the epithelium
   d) Dramatic improvement in both clinical symptoms and histologic abnormalities after withdrawal of gluten from the diet
2. Tropical sprue
   a) Common in the Caribbean, Far East, and India
   b) Characterized by villous atrophy
   c) Is thought to result from chronic bacterial contamination of the small intestine; treatment with broad-spectrum antibiotics often successful
   d) Marked folic acid deficiency present
3. Whipple's disease ("intestinal lipodystrophy")
   a) Characterized by macrophages with abundant pale, foamy cytoplasm in the lamina propria of the small intestine
   b) On electron-microscopy large numbers of bacilli seen in the macrophages
   c) Relief of symptoms as well as disappearance of the bacillary bodies on treatment with antibiotics
   d) Occurrence of similar macrophages in lymph nodes, spleen, and rarely, other sites
II. Infections of the intestine
   A. Enterotoxin-mediated disease (see Chapter 5)
   1. *Vibrio cholerae*, toxigenic *Escherichia coli*, and *Staphylococcus aureus* produce enterotoxins that cause increased mucosal secretion leading to diarrhea.
   2. The lesion is biochemical; no gross or microscopic changes occur in the intestinal mucosa.
   3. The organism does not invade the mucosa or the blood.
   B. Invasive intestinal infections
   1. Viral gastroenteritis
      a) Common; caused by rotaviruses and parvoviruses
      b) Causes acute diarrhea, vomiting, and fever; self-limited
   2. Salmonella gastroenteritis
      a) Salmonellae other than *S. typhi* are a common cause of "bacterial food poisoning.

b) Acute inflammation of the small intestinal mucosa occurs, with superficial ulceration and neutrophil infiltration.

c) It is characterized by fever, abdominal pain, and diarrhea; it is usually mild and self-limited.

3. Typhoid fever
   a) This is caused by *S. typhi*, ingested with food or water contaminated with the feces of a case or carrier of typhoid.
   b) *S. typhi* multiplies in the intestinal lymphoid tissue in the 1–3 week incubation period.
   c) After incubation, the bacilli enter the blood stream (bacteremic phase), causing fever.
   d) Symptoms include splenomegaly, a skin rash, bradycardia, and peripheral blood neutropenia.
   e) The diagnosis is made in the first week by blood culture, which is positive in 95% of cases.
   f) In the second week *S. typhi* re-enters the intestine (intestinal phase), causing diarrhea.
   g) Ulceration of the lymphoid (Peyer's patches) causes longitudinal ulcers in the terminal ileum.
   h) Histologic examination shows necrosis and a chronic inflammatory cell infiltrate.
   i) Stool and urine culture are positive in the second week.
   j) Complications of typhoid enteritis include
      (1) hemorrhage from the ulcers, which can be severe.
      (2) perforation of the intestine.

4. Shigella colitis (bacillary dysentery)
   a) This is caused by Shigella, which infects the colon, producing an acute inflammation.
   b) Bacteremia is rare.
   c) The colonic mucosa is hyperemic with multiple superficial ulcers. Neutrophils are the dominant cells.
   d) Clinically, Shigella colitis is an acute illness with high fever and diarrhea with blood and mucus ("dysentery").
   e) *Shigella dysenteriae* type I produces an exotoxin that causes systemic neurotoxic and vasculotoxic effects.

5. *Entamoeba histolytica* (amebic colitis)
   a) *E. histolytica* is a common cause of colitis in endemic areas.
   b) Trophozoites invade the colonic mucosa; the rectum and cecum are most frequently involved.
   c) The amebae multiply in the submucosa, producing enzy-

matic necrosis and acute inflammation, leading to abscesses.

d) Ulceration of the overlying mucosa leads to flask-shaped ulcers with extensive undermining of the residual mucosa.

e) Clinical characteristics include a low-grade fever and diarrhea with blood and mucus.

f) The diagnosis is made by finding amebae in the stools or in a biopsy specimen.

g) In severe cases, extensive ulceration may be associated with severe hemorrhage and perforation.

6. Acute appendicitis
   a) This is a common condition that occurs most frequently in young adults.
   b) Its causes include infection by *Escherichia coli, Streptococcus faecalis*, and anaerobes.
   c) Mucosal ulceration with neutrophilic infiltration spreads rapidly to involve the muscularis and serosa.
   d) Clinically, there is fever, pain in the right lower quadrant of the abdomen, vomiting, and peripheral blood leukocytosis.
   e) Grossly, at surgery, the inflamed appendix appears swollen, red, dull, and often has a fibrinous exudate.
   f) Complications include the following:
      (1) The inflamed tissue may form a localized inflammatory mass in the right lower quadrant ("phlegmon").
      (2) Suppuration and perforation may produce an abscess or generalized peritonitis.
      (3) Infection of the portal venous radicles may lead to abscesses in the liver (pylephlebitis suppurativa).

7. Intestinal tuberculosis
   a) Primary: very rare after pasteurization of milk
   b) Secondary
      (1) This still occurs fairly commonly.
      (2) It is caused by swallowing infected sputum (in patients with pulmonary disease) or reactivation of dormant intestinal lesions.
      (3) The terminal ileum and cecum are maximally involved.
      (4) Grossly, the mucosa shows transverse ulcers and thickening of wall by fibrosis.

(5) Microscopically, the mucosa shows caseating granulomatous inflammation.

(6) In the acute phase, the patients develop diarrhea that is occasionally bloody and low-grade fever.

(7) Complications include
    i) extension to involve large areas of ileocccal mucosa forming an inflammatory mass.
    ii) intestinal strictures causing obstruction.
    iii) intestinal fistulae.
    iv) tuberculous peritonitis.

8. Acute membranous enterocolitis (pseudomembranous colitis)
    a) This is a severe, necrotizing acute inflammation that occurs mainly in patients who are on antibiotic therapy (clindamycin).
    b) Antibiotics alter the luminal microbial flora and permit proliferation of *Clostridium difficile.*
    c) *Clostridium difficile* produces an exotoxin that causes superficial mucosal necrosis and acute inflammation.
    d) Grossly and microscopically, the necrotic mucosa and inflammatory exudate form adherent membranous plaques on the surface.
    e) Clinically, the disease is an acute severe diarrhea with bleeding and mucus.
    f) Untreated, mortality is high; vancomycin is effective.

9. Enteroinvasive *Escherichia coli*
    a) Causes neonatal necrotizing enterocolitis
    b) Causes adult infective diarrhea

10. *Campylobacter fetus*
    a) Common, particularly in children; usually mild
    b) Causes acute inflammation of small and large intestine

C. Parasitic infestations of the intestine
1. Very common, affecting 25% of the world population
2. Giardiasis (*Giardia lamblia*)
    a) Common protozoan flagellate parasite
    b) Attaches by a ventral sucker to small intestinal mucosal epithelium; the duodenum is maximally affected
    c) Occurrence of severe diarrhea and abdominal cramps with heavy infestations
    d) Common occurrence of partial villous atrophy
3. Nematodes (*roundworms*)
    a) Ascariasis (*Ascaris lumbricoides*)
        (1) Ascariasis is usually asymptomatic.

       (2) Symptoms may result from

          i) intestinal obstruction by a coiled mass of worms.

          ii) migration of worms up the pancreatic duct (pancreatitis) and biliary tract (gall stones, cholangitis).

   b) Enterobiasis (pinworm, *Enterobius vermicularis*)

       (1) Adult worms in the region of the appendix do not cause symptoms.

       (2) The eggs laid in the perianal region cause intense pruritus.

   c) Whipworms: (*Trichuris trichiura*) a common, harmless infestation of the colon

   d) Hookworms infestation (*Ancylostoma duodenale; Necator americanus*)

       (1) The worms attach themselves to the mucosa and actively suck blood.

       (2) Iron deficiency anemia, often profound, develops secondary to the blood loss.

   e) Strongyloidiasis (*Strongyloides stercoralis*)

       (1) Its symptoms are related to lung migration (mild cough with blood-tinged sputum) and intestinal infection (abdominal pain, diarrhea with blood).

       (2) In immunosuppressed patients, hyperinfection occurs with numerous migrating worms in the blood.

   f) Trichinosis (*Trichinella spiralis*)

       (1) This is an unnatural parasite of man, contracted by ingestion of undercooked, infected meat.

       (2) The intestinal phase of parasite multiplication causes mild abdominal pain and diarrhea.

       (3) The phase of larval dissemination in the blood is characterized by an acute, severe illness with high fever and peripheral blood eosinophilia.

       (4) The larvae settle in

          i) skeletal muscle, resulting in acute inflammation with eosinophils that causes severe muscle pain, swelling, and tenderness.

          ii) cardiac muscle, resulting in myocarditis.

          iii) brain, resulting in encephalitis.

4. Cestodes (tapeworms)

   a) Four adult tapeworms infest the intestine of man, causing no symptoms.

       (1) *Taenia solium* (pork tapeworm)

(2) *Taenia saginata* (beef tapeworm)
(3) *Hymenolepis nana* (dwarf tapeworm)
(4) *Diphyllobothrium latum* (fish tapeworm)
  b) *D. latum* causes vitamin B_{12} deficiency.
  c) *Taenia solium* larvae may enter the blood and cause cysticercosis (brain, muscle, skin, etc.).
5. Trematodes (flukes)
  a) Schistosomiasis
    (1) Two species, *S. Mansoni* (colon) and *S. japonicum* (small intestine), cause intestinal disease.
    (2) Adult worms in peri-intestinal venous plexuses do not cause symptoms.
    (3) Pathologic changes are due to migration of ova
      i) across the wall of the intestine, resulting in intestinal inflammation and ulceration, which causes bleeding.
      ii) to the liver, producing fibrosis around the portal tracts and portal hypertension.
  b) Intestinal fluke infestation (*Fasciolopsis buski*): rare
III. Idiopathic inflammatory bowel disease (Table 11-1)
  A. Crohn's disease ("regional enteritis"; "granulomatous colitis") (Fig. 11-2)

Table 11-1. Differences between Ulcerative Colitis and Crohn's Disease

	Ulcerative Colitis	Crohn's Disease
Colon involvement	++++	++
Ileal involvement	10% (only terminal)	+++
Rectal involvement	+++	±
Skip lesions	−	+++
Perianal lesions	+	+++
Acute mucosal inflammation	++	++
Crypt abscesses	++	+
Transmural inflammation	−	+++
Fissures	−	+++
Fistulae	±	+++
Fibrosis and stenosis	±	+++
Granulomas in intestine and nodes	−	++ (60%)
Risk of cancer	+++	+

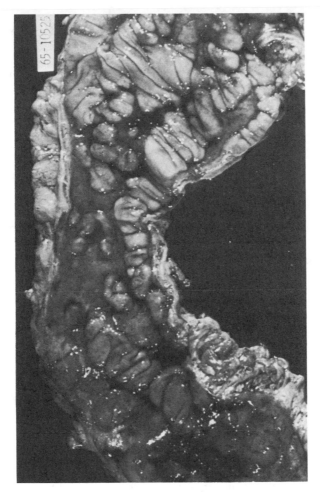

Fig. 11-2. Crohn's disease showing irregular ulceration ("cobblestone" effect).

1. Incidence
   a) Occurs predominantly in the United States and Western Europe
   b) Most commonly in young adults; slight familial tendency; commonest in whites, particularly Jewish, both sexes
2. Etiology

      a) Unknown; no infectious agent has been found

      b) Strong but not conclusive evidence that the injury is immunological

3. Sites of involvement

      a) Combined ileal and colonic (50%); ileum alone (30%); colon alone (20%).

      b) Perianal disease common

      c) Involvement of oral cavity, larynx, esophagus, stomach, perineum, and vulva rare

4. Gross characteristics

      a) Involvement is typically segmental with skip areas; involved segments are sharply demarcated from normal areas.

      b) In the acute phase the bowel is swollen and hyperemic in all its layers. The mucosa shows reddening and ulceration.

      c) In the chronic phase

         (1) the affected segment of bowel is markedly thickened and rigid ("lead-pipe") with luminal narrowing.

         (2) the mucosa shows longitudinal, serpiginous ulcers separated by edematous mucosa ("cobblestone" appearance) (Fig. 11-2).

         (3) fissures and fistulae may be present.

5. Histologic characteristics

      a) Noncaseating epithelioid cell granulomas are present in 60% of cases.

      b) Transmural chronic inflammation with fibrosis is present.

      c) The regional lymph nodes may show enlargement and noncaseating epithelioid cell granulomas.

6. Clinical features

      a) It is extremely variable.

      b) In the acute phase there is fever, diarrhea, and right lower quadrant pain.

      c) Chronic disease is manifested by variable diarrhea and intermittent abdominal pain.

7. Complications

      a) Intestinal obstruction

      b) Fistula formation between intestinal loops, bladder, vagina

      c) Extraintestinal manifestations: arthritis, uveitis

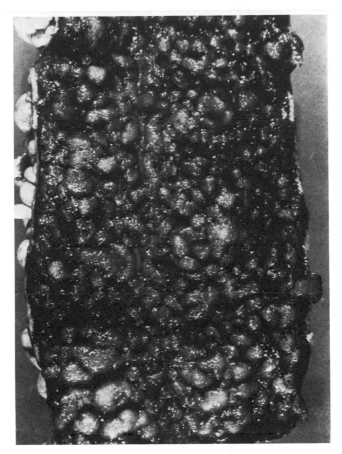

Fig. 11-3. Acute ulcerative colitis. The mucosa is hyperemic and ulcerated. The intervening mucosa is edematous, giving the appearance of pseudopolyps.

B. Ulcerative colitis (Fig. 11-3)
 1. Incidence
    a) 25,000 new cases per year in the United States
    b) Common in 20-25 year age group, whites, particularly Jewish, both sexes
 2. Etiology
    a) Unknown; no infectious agent identified
    b) Probably an immunologically mediated disease

    c) Symptoms frequently precipitated by psychologic stress
3. Sites of involvement
    a) Tends to spread proximally from the rectum without skip areas.
    b) Total colonic involvement not uncommon
    c) 10% of cases show mild inflammation of the terminal ileum ("backwash ileitis")
4. Pathologic characteristics (Fig. 11-3)
    a) In the acute phase, the mucosa is diffusely hyperemic with superficial ulcers. Neutrophils are present in the lamina propria and dilated glands ("crypt abscesses").
    b) With chronic disease, the mucosal crypts show atrophy and distorted architecture.
    c) The muscle wall and serosa are usually normal.
5. Clinical characteristics
    a) In the acute phase, there is fever, leukocytosis, lower abdominal pain, and diarrhea with blood and mucus.
    b) It usually follows a chronic course with exacerbations and remissions.
    c) Extraintestinal manifestations include arthritis, uveitis, skin lesions, and sclerosing pericholangitis.
6. Complications
    a) Severe bleeding and toxic megacolon in the acute phase
    b) Carcinoma
        (1) High (10%) risk of carcinoma
        (2) Risk greatest with
            i) long-standing (10 yrs) disease
            ii) early age of onset of disease
            iii) chronic continuous disease
            iv) total colonic involvement
        (3) Epithelial dysplasia precedes carcinoma
IV. Vascular lesions of the intestine
  A. Acute intestinal infarction
    1. Usually caused by sudden occlusion of the superior mesenteric artery
    2. May occur in severe hypotension and shock (Nonocclusive intestinal infarction)
    3. Rarely caused by mesenteric venous thrombosis
    4. Intestinal infarcts hemorrhagic; followed by infection (gangrene)
    5. Clinically: intestinal obstruction, bleeding and peritonitis due to perforation or leakage from gangrenous bowel

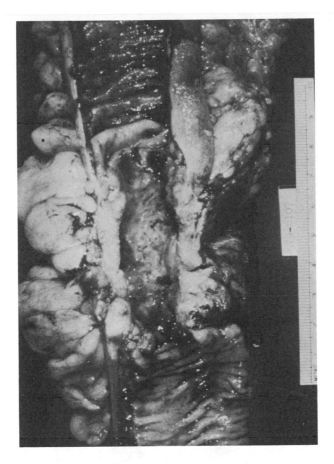

Fig. 11-4. Annular, circumferential, constrictive carcinoma of the left side of the colon. White tumor tissue has infiltrated the wall.

B. Ischemic colitis
   1. Caused by extensive atherosclerotic narrowing of intestinal arteries
   2. Usual sites: splenic flexure and rectosigmoid
   3. An acute illness with fever, left-sided abdominal pain, and bloody diarrhea

V. Neoplasms of the intestines
A. Carcinoma of the colon and rectum (Figs. 11-4, 11-5)
1. Incidence
a) Accounts for over 90% of malignant intestinal tumors
b) Incidence in the United States: 110,000 cases per year
c) The second most common cause of cancer mortality in the United States
d) 90% of cases occur after age 50 years
2. Etiology

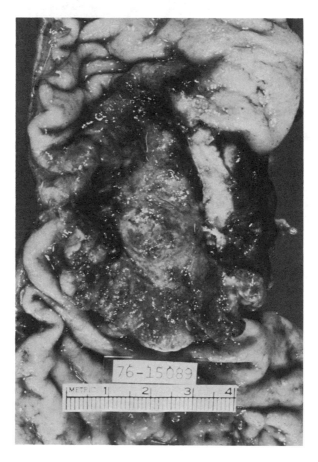

Fig. 11-5. Ulcerative carcinoma of the rectum.

a) Unknown
b) Dietary factors: low fiber content and high content of animal fats
3. Gross characteristics
   a) The rectosigmoid region is the site of 60% of colon cancers.
   b) 5% of cases have multiple carcinomas
   c) Right-sided colonic cancers tend to be fungating, polypoid masses that project into the lumen.
   d) Left-sided colonic cancers tend to be annular, constricting (napkin ring) lesions (Fig. 11-4).
   e) Rectal carcinomas tend to present as malignant ulcers with hard, everted edges (Fig. 11-5).
4. Microscopic evaluation reveals most colon cancers are adenocarcinomas
5. Clinical characteristics
   a) Change in bowel habit and bleeding per rectum
   b) Intestinal obstruction: common in left-sided carcinomas
   c) Symptoms of right-sided carcinoma: abdominal mass, pain, blood loss anemia, weight loss
6. Clinicopathologic stages of disease (Duke's stage) (5-year survival rates in parentheses)
   a) Stage A: cancer limited to mucosa (100%)
   b) Stage B_1: infiltrating muscle partially; no lymph node involvement (67%)
   c) Stage B_2: Infiltrating full thickness of colon wall; no lymph node involvement (55%)
   d) Stage C_1: infiltrating muscle partially; lymph node involved (40%)
   e) Stage C_2: infiltrating full thickness; lymph node involved (20%)
   f) Stage D: distant metastases (10%)
7. Premalignant lesions
   a) Chronic ulcerative colitis: Responsible for 1% of colon cancers
   b) Heredofamilial polyposis syndromes: Account for about 1% of colon cancer
      (1) Familial polyposis coli
          i) Autosomal dominant inheritance
          ii) Presence of innumerable adenomatous polyps in the colon
          iii) Polyps are not present at birth, but appear at about 15–20 years of age

             iv) Carcinoma supervenes in 100% of cases if colectomy is not performed

             v) Carcinoma usually occurs between 30–40 years

     (2) Gardner's syndrome: similar to polyposis but has extracolonic soft tissue lesions: epidermal cysts (skin), osteomas (bone), fibromatosis (soft tissue)

     (3) Turcot's syndrome

             i) Extremely rare; autosomal recessive

             ii) Colonic polyposis associated with central nervous system glial neoplasms

     (4) Peutz–Jegher's syndrome

             i) Fairly common; autosomal

             ii) Hamartomatous polyps occur mainly in small intestine

             iii) Associated with circumoral and buccal melanin pigmentation

             iv) Risk of malignant disease low

  c) Benign epithelial neoplasms (adenomas) (Fig. 11-6)

     (1) Common; the precursor lesion in many, if not most, colon carcinomas

     (2) Villous adenoma

             i) Usually single, large, sessile polyps in the rectosigmoid or cecum

             ii) Soft velvety, papillary growths that project into the lumen

             iii) High risk of carcinoma (30–70%)

     (3) Polypoid adenoma (adenomatous polyp; tubular adenoma)

             i) Accounts for over 90% of colonic polyps; commonly multiple

             ii) Are usually pedunculated with a well-defined stalk.

             iii) Histologically: composed of benign neoplastic glands; epithelial dysplasia common

             iv) Malignancy in a polyp manifested by invasion of the stalk by tumor cells

             v) Malignant transformation uncommon (2–5%)

B. Adenocarcinoma of the small intestine: rare

C. Malignant lymphoma

  1. The intestine is a common site of primary extranodal lymphoma.

  2. Most of these are B-cell lymphomas.

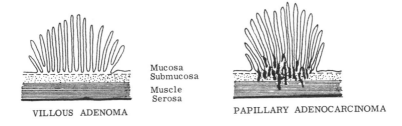

VILLOUS ADENOMA   Mucosa / Submucosa / Muscle / Serosa   PAPILLARY ADENOCARCINOMA

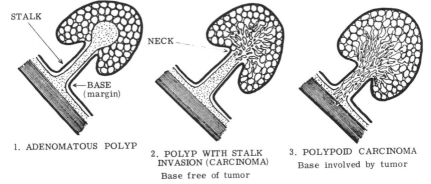

STALK   NECK   BASE (margin)

1. ADENOMATOUS POLYP
2. POLYP WITH STALK INVASION (CARCINOMA)
Base free of tumor
3. POLYPOID CARCINOMA
Base involved by tumor

Fig. 11-6. Colonic neoplasms. A villous adenoma differs from a papillary adenocarcinoma by its lack of infiltration at the base. A benign adenomatous polyp (1) has no stalk invasion. A polyp with stalk invasion and a free base (2) is usually cured by polypectomy. Involvement of the base by carcinoma (3) is equivalent to a polypoid adenocarcinoma.

   3. The ileocecal region is a favored site for Burkitt's lymphoma.
  D. Smooth muscle tumors: rare
  E. Carcinoid tumors
   1. Arise in neuroendocrine cells in the mucosa
   2. Sites
    a) Appendix: most common site; benign in over 95% of cases
    b) Ileum: tend to be malignant in 60% of cases

    c) Rectum: intermediate in frequency and malignant potential (15%)

  3. Gross characteristics: firm, yellowish intramural masses; may be multiple

  4. Microscopic characteristics

    a) Composed of nests, cords and sheets of small, round cells separated by vascular channels

    b) Early occurrence of muscular and vascular involvement; not evidence that the tumor is malignant

    c) Dense-core neurosecretory granules on electron microscopy

  5. Clinical characteristics

    a) Local fibrosis causing intestinal obstruction

    b) Carcinoid syndrome

      (1) Secretion of serotonin (5HT) causing abdominal cramps, diarrhea, bronchospasm, cardiac valve fibrosis

      (2) Occurs only with malignant intestinal carcinoids that have metastasized to the liver, usually extensively

      (3) Increase in urinary 5-hydroxy-indole acetic acid (5HIAA)

F. Nonneoplastic mucosal polyps of the intestine

  1. Not all mucosal polyps are adenomas.

  2. Other kinds of polyps include hyperplastic, hamartomatous, retention, inflammatory, and lymphoid polyps.

  3. These have no increased incidence of malignancy.

VI. Intestinal obstruction

  A. Congenital

    1. Intestinal atresia: failure to develop a lumen

    2. Imperforate anus: common

    3. Hirschsprung's disease (congenital megacolon)

      a) Failure of development of the myenteric plexus

      b) Dilation of the colon proximal to the aganglionic segment, which remains narrow

  B. Acquired

    1. Neoplasms: notably carcinoma

    2. Nonneoplastic lesions

      a) Adhesive bands: from previous abdominal surgery, trauma, or peritonitis

      b) Hernias

        (1) A hernia is the protrusion of a sac of peritoneum through a defect in the abdominal wall.

    (2) Protrusion of a loop of intestine into the hernia sac may be followed by obstruction.

  c) Intussusception

    (1) This is a telescoping of one segment of intestine (usually ileum) into another.

    (2) The blood supply of the intussuscepted bowel becomes obstructed at the neck, leading to hemorrhagic infarction and gangrene.

    (3) Patients present with intestinal obstruction and bleeding per rectum.

  d) Volvulus

    (1) This is a twisting of the intestine about the axis of its mesentery.

    (2) It commonly occurs in the sigmoid colon in elderly individuals.

VII. Intestinal diverticula

  A. (Congenital) Meckel's diverticulum

    1. This is a vestigial remnant of the omphalomesenteric duct.

    2. It occurs in 2% of the population, within 2 feet of the ileocecal valve, and is about 2 inches long.

    3. The mucosa is small intestinal but frequently shows heteropic gastric mucosa and pancreatic tissue.

    4. It may produce chronic peptic ulceration and bleeding.

  B. (Acquired) jejunal diverticulosis: rare cause of malabsorption

  C. (Acquired) colonic diverticulosis

    1. This is seen predominantly in the sigmoid colon in elderly patients.

    2. It is very common in Western countries.

    3. The diverticula are false diverticula: mucosal herniations through points of weakness in the muscle wall.

    4. Diverticulosis is asymptomatic.

    5. Inflammation in relation to the diverticula (diverticulitis) causes fever and left-sided abdominal pain.

    6. Pericolic abscesses, fistulae, and gastrointestinal hemorrhage may occur.

    7. In the chronic phase there is marked mural fibrosis, leading to strictures and intestinal obstruction.

12

The Liver, Extrahepatic Biliary System, and Pancreas

LIVER

I. Manifestations of liver disease
  A. Jaundice (see Chapter 3); causes include the following:
    1. Defective hepatocellular uptake due to abnormalities in intracellular transport proteins, resulting in unconjugated hyperbilirubinemia (Gilbert's syndrome)
    2. Defective conjugation of bilirubin
      a) Neonatal jaundice: immaturity of hepatic enzyme systems
      b) Crigler–Najjar syndrome: congenital (autosomal recessive) absence of UDP glucuronyl transferase
      c) Hepatocellular jaundice in liver cell failure
    3. Decreased excretion of bilirubin
      a) A congenital defect in transferring bilirubin from the cell into the biliary canaliculus (Dubin–Johnson and Rotor syndromes)
      b) Intrahepatic cholestasis: due to viral hepatitis or drugs
      c) Bile duct obstruction (obstructive jaundice)
  B. Hepatocellular failure
    1. Acute hepatic failure
      a) Etiology
        (1) Massive liver cell necrosis
        (2) Acute fatty liver: occurs in Reye's syndrome, acute fatty liver of pregnancy, and tetracycline toxicity
      b) Effects
        (1) Jaundice
        (2) Hypoglycemia
        (3) Bleeding tendency
        (4) Hepatic encephalopathy
    2. Chronic hepatic failure

a) Cirrhosis accounts for most cases
b) Effects
    (1) Portal hypertension
    (2) Hepatic encephalopathy
    (3) Hepatorenal syndrome
    (4) Endocrine changes: testicular atrophy and gynecomastia
    (5) Decreased serum albumin: edema and ascites
    (6) Hypoprothrombinemia and a tendency to bleed
C. Portal hypertension
    1. Causes
        a) Sinusoidal: cirrhosis of the liver accounts for 90% of cases
        b) Presinusoidal: rare
            (1) Extrahepatic: obstruction of the main portal vein
            (2) Intrahepatic: obstruction of portal venous radicals in the liver due to schistosomiasis, congenital hepatic fibrosis
            (3) Idiopathic portal hypertension (mechanism unknown)
        c) Postsinusoidal: rare; obstruction of hepatic venous outflow (Budd–Chiari syndrome)
    2. Effects
        a) Splenomegaly: due to passive congestion
        b) Varices: development of collateral venous channels between portal and systemic veins in the
            (1) lower esophagus and stomach
            (2) rectum, producing hemorrhoids
            (3) umbilicus ("caput medusae")
        c) Ascites
D. Hepatic encephalopathy
    1. Occurs in both acute and chronic hepatic failure; characterized by confusion, drowsiness, convulsions, coma, and death
    2. Unknown toxic agent acting on the brain; produced from nitrogenous substances in the intestine by bacteria and absorbed in the portal vein
E. Hepatorenal syndrome
    1. The occurrence of renal failure in a patient with liver disease
    2. No pathologic changes identified in the kidney; renal failure is of "pre-renal" type
    3. Cause unknown

II. Hepatocellular necrosis: classification (Fig. 12-1)
  A. Focal necrosis: Necrosis of single liver cells, or small groups of cells, occurring randomly in the liver
  B. Zonal necrosis
    1. Necrosis of liver cells in the identical region of each liver lobule
    2. Centrizonal (centrilobular) necrosis
      a) Severe congestion secondary to cardiac failure
      b) Viral hepatitis
      c) Carbon tetrachloride and chloroform poisoning
    3. Midzonal: seen in yellow fever
    4. Peripheral zonal (periportal)
      a) Phosphorous poisoning
      b) Eclampsia

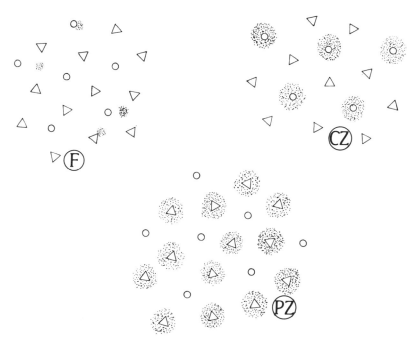

Fig. 12-1. Types of hepatocellular necrosis (stippled areas indicate necrosis). Triangles = portal areas; circles = central veins. PZ = peripheral zonal; CZ = centrizonal. F = Focal.

C. Massive necrosis
   1. This is necrosis involving large areas of the liver.
   2. It is caused by hepatitis viruses, drugs (halothane, acetaminophen, isoniazid), and toxins (mushrooms, insecticides).
   3. Degrees of liver cell necrosis less than massive necrosis are compatible with survival (submassive necrosis).
   4. Massive necrosis is characterized by decrease in size of the liver, which appears yellow, soft and flabby. The capsule is wrinkled (acute yellow atrophy).
   5. In submassive necrosis, the yellow necrotic areas contrast with surviving red-brown liver parenchyma.
   6. Survival is associated with regeneration of the liver.
III. Infections of the liver
   A. Viral hepatitis
      1. Causes
         a) Hepatitis A virus (infectious hepatitis).
            (1) Etiology: a 27nm-sized virus particle identified in stools of patients
            (2) Transmission
                i) Usually by the fecal–oral route
                ii) Parenteral transmission is rare
                iii) Incubation period: 2–6 weeks (short)
                iv) Characteristics: mild, rarely fatal, and does not produce chronic hepatitis
         b) Hepatitis B virus (serum hepatitis).
            (1) Etiology
                i) The virus particle (Dane particle) is a 42-nm particle with a central core and surface capsid.
                ii) Three distinct antigens: HBcAg (core antigen); HBsAg (surface antigen), and HBeAg.
                iii) Hepatitis B virus imparts a "ground glass" appearance to liver cells. It can be demonstrated by orcein stains (Shikata) and immunohistologic methods.
            (2) Transmission
                i) Transmitted mainly by the parenteral route: increased incidence among IV drug abusers and patients on renal dialysis
                ii) Transmitted nonparenterally by
                    (A) sexual intercourse: prostitutes, homosexual males
                    (B) transplacental infection of the fetus

(C) insect vectors (?)
    iii) Incubation period: 2–6 months (long)
  c) Hepatitis non-A, non-B.
    (1) Virus not identified; no screening test
    (2) Responsible for over 90% of post-transfusion hepatitis in the United States.
    (3) Incubation period: 7–8 weeks (intermediate)
  d) Other viruses, including
    (1) cytomegalovirus.
    (2) Epstein–Barr virus (infectious mononucleosis).
    (3) yellow fever virus.
    (4) herpes simplex and herpes varicella-zoster virus.
2. Clinical syndromes associated with viral hepatitis
  a) Acute viral hepatitis
    (1) Acute onset with fever, severe loss of appetite, and vomiting (preicteric phase)
    (2) Soon followed by jaundice, bilirubinuria, and tender enlargement of the liver (icteric phase).
    (3) Elevation of liver enzymes (transaminases (GOT, GPT): occurs in the preicteric phase
    (4) Anicteric hepatitis common
    (5) Microscopic characteristics
        i) Diffuse swelling ("ballooning") of liver cells
        ii) Focal necrosis, which tends to occur around the central veins
        iii) Lymphocytic infiltrate in the portal tracts
    (6) Recovery within weeks in most cases
  b) Cholestatic hepatitis
    (1) A variant of acute hepatitis in which marked intrahepatic cholestasis occurs
    (2) Benign course; recovery is the rule
  c) Subacute hepatic necrosis (impaired regeneration syndrome)
    (1) Rare; a severe protracted illness lasting several months; has a high mortality
    (2) Occurs in hepatitis B and non-A, non-B
    (3) Histologic characteristics
        i) Bridging necrosis: bands of necrosis linking central veins and portal areas
        ii) Regenerative activity absent
  d) Fulminant hepatitis
    (1) Rare; massive or submassive necrosis with acute liver failure

(2) Most common in hepatitis B and non-A, non-B
   e) Chronic persistent viral hepatitis
      (1) Common; caused by Hepatitis B (40%-60%) and non-A, non-B
      (2) Patient may be asymptomatic (slight abnormalities in liver function tests) or have mild symptoms over a period exceeding 6 months
      (4) Benign and self-limiting; does not progress to cirrhosis
      (5) Histologically, increased numbers of lymphocytes and plasma cells in the portal tracts
      (6) In cases due to hepatitis B, the virus (HBsAg) is present in liver cells and blood; represents the carrier state
   f) Chronic active viral hepatitis
      (1) Occurs with hepatitis B and non-A, non-B
      (2) Histologic characteristics
         i) Focal necrosis of liver cells
         ii) Widening of the portal tracts by mononuclear cell infiltration and fibrosis
         iii) Extension of the inflammation into the liver lobule
         iv) Piecemeal necrosis: active destruction of liver cells at the periphery of the lobule by the inflammatory process.
      (3) Clinical characteristics
         i) Acute hepatitis
         ii) Portal hypertension and chronic liver failure
         iii) Very high serum transaminases
      (4) Progresses to cirrhosis at a variable rate
   g) Viral-induced cirrhosis of the liver (see VI, below).
   h) Viral-induced hepatocellular carcinoma (see VIII, below).
B. Bacterial infections of the liver; may occur as a result of
   1. systemic bacteremia
   2. ascending cholangitis (inflammation of biliary tree), usually secondary to extrahepatic biliary obstruction
   3. pylephlebitis suppurativa
      a) A suppurative thrombophlebitis of the portal vein
      b) Caused by spread of infection from a focus in the intestine
C. Parasitic infections of the liver
   1. Amebic "hepatitis" and amebic liver abscess

a) Entry of amebae (*Entamoeba histolytica*) into the portal venous branches in the colonic submucosa
b) Enzymatic necrosis of liver cells is produced.
  (1) Multiple micro-"abscesses" ("amebic hepatitis") develop.
  (2) Large "abscess" cavities develop.
c) Amebic "pus" has a typical reddish-brown (anchovy sauce) appearance and is composed of enzymatically liquefied necrotic liver cells and amebae.
d) Clinically, patients develop fever, right hypochondrial pain, liver enlargement and marked tenderness.
e) Serum levels of amebic antibodies are elevated.
f) Complications include
  (1) rupture through the diaphragm to pleural cavity or lung. A bronchohepatic fistula may result in coughing out the pus.
  (2) rupture into the pericardial sac.
  (3) intraperitoneal rupture.
  (4) systemic spread of organisms.
2. Schistosomiasis
  a) Intestinal schistosomes (*S. mansoni* and *S. japonicum*) liberate their eggs into the portal venous system.
  b) The eggs produce portal fibrosis causing portal hypertension.
3. Hydatid cysts (*Echinococcus granulosus*)
  a) The liver is the most common site for hydatid cysts.
  b) Large, cystic masses develop.
  c) Histologic examination shows the parasite and the typical laminated wall.
4. Oriental cholangiohepatitis (usually *Clonorchis sinensis*): rare
IV. Toxic and metabolic injuries
  A. Alcoholic liver disease
    1. Acute alcoholic liver disease (acute sclerosing hyaline necrosis)
      a) This is characterized by sudden onset of fever, jaundice, tender hepatomegaly, and ascites, usually occurring after a recent bout of heavy drinking.
      b) Histologic changes vary from case to case, and include
        (1) fatty change, cholestasis.
        (2) neutrophil infiltration of sinusoids.
        (3) focal lytic necrosis of liver cells.

    (4) sclerosis around the central veins, creeping along sinusoids.

    (5) hyaline necrosis; alcoholic hyaline is a bright pink irregular mass of material in the cytoplasm (Mallory body).

  2. Chronic alcoholic liver disease

    a) Precirrhotic disease is characterized by

      (1) increased collagen in both portal tracts and central areas.

      (2) lack of true regenerative nodules; in this way it differs from cirrhosis.

      (3) clinical appearance of chronic liver disease.

      (4) a halt in progression if alcohol is discontinued.

    b) Alcoholic cirrhosis (see VI, below)

B. Drug and toxin-induced liver disease

  1. Predictable hepatocellular toxicity (dose-related)

    a) Agents that produce liver cell necrosis in all individuals at a predictable dose level

    b) Agents: poisonous mushroom (*Amanita phalloides*), chloroform, carbon tetrachloride, accetaminophen

  2. Unpredictable liver injury due to chemicals

    a) A hypersensitivity response to a drug; dosage not a factor

    b) Cholestatic jaundice (common): phenothiazines, steroid hormones

    c) Acute hepatitis: similar clinicopathologically to viral hepatitis

    d) Granulomatous hepatitis: occurs with many drugs; small epithelioid cell granulomas in liver lobule

    e) Hepatocellular necrosis, often massive

      (1) Halothane: usually after multiple exposures to the anesthetic

      (2) Isoniazid (INH): rare; risk increases with age over 35 years

    f) Chronic active hepatitis: methyldopa, oxyphenisatin

    g) Focal nodular hyperplasia, liver cell adenoma: oral contraceptives

C. Nutritional liver disease

  1. Malnutrition (Kwashiorkor) (see Chapter 5) may cause fatty liver and cirrhosis

  2. Treatment of obesity with ileoileal bypass causes fatty liver and sclerosing hyaline necrosis that is similar to acute alcoholic liver disease.

V. Immunologic (?) diseases of the liver
  A. Chronic active hepatitis
    1. Nonviral chronic active hepatitis (hepatitis B negative, no history of transfusion of blood products) presents a clinical and pathologic picture identical to viral chronic active hepatitis.
    2. Autoantibodies are present: anti smooth muscle antibody and antinuclear antibodies.
    3. It affects females predominantly; it may respond to steroid therapy.
  B. Primary biliary cirrhosis (PBC)
    1. This is a disease predominantly seen (90%) in middle-aged females.
    2. The etiology is probably immunological; antimitochondrial antibody is present in serum, often in high titer.
    3. Clinically, patients present with progressive biliary obstruction.
      a) The onset is insidious, with hepatomegaly, elevation of alkaline phosphatase, and pruritus.
      b) Hyperlipidemia (cholesterol) with skin xanthomata develops.
      c) Jaundice appears 6–18 months after the onset.
    4. The progress is slow with portal hypertension and liver failure 5–15 years after onset.
    5. Histologically,
      a) the small bile ducts are surrounded by a dense infiltrate of lymphocytes and plasma cells. Epithelioid cell granulomas occur in 30%.
      b) the bile ductules, after an initial phase of proliferation, show progressive destruction and are absent in the final stage.
      c) portal fibrosis, usually mild, is present.
VI. Cirrhosis of the liver (Fig. 12-2)
  A. Definition: a chronic liver disease caused by a large number of etiologic agents in which the liver shows
    1. progressive necrosis of liver cells.
    2. fibrosis, which causes distortion of lobular architecture.
    3. regenerative nodules, that are the result of hyperplasia of the surviving liver cells. Depending on whether the nodules are less or more than 3 mm, cirrhosis is classified as micronodular, macronodular, or mixed.
  B. Grossly, the liver may be enlarged or contracted; it is firm and nodular.

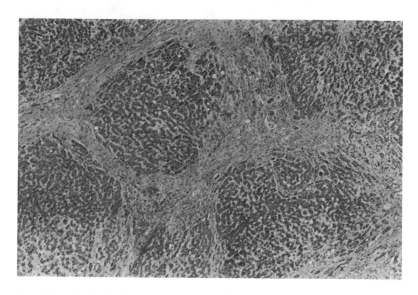

Fig. 12-2. Cirrhosis, low-power microscopic appearance, showing regenerative nodules separated by broad bands of fibrosis.

   C. Clinically, it is manifested by chronic liver failure and portal hypertension.

   D. Types of cirrhosis include the following.

     1. Alcoholic cirrhosis (30–60% of cases of cirrhosis)

       a) This is commonly associated with fatty change, sinusoidal collagen, neutrophils, and hyaline.

       b) Cirrhosis is typically micronodular (fatty micronodular cirrhosis), but may be macronodular or mixed.

       c) Fibrosis is initially fine but later becomes broad.

       d) It tends to have a slow rate of progression.

     2. Viral-induced cirrhosis (10–30%)

       a) This is caused by hepatitis B and non-A, non-B viruses.

       b) Typically, this is macronodular cirrhosis with broad bands of collagen separating the nodules.

       c) Features of chronic active hepatitis and ground glass hepatocytes may be present. Orcein or immunoperoxidase stain identifies hepatitis B virus.

       d) Progress to chronic liver failure is rapid.

     3. Cryptogenic cirrhosis (15–20%): no etiology found after

complete evaluation; may include cirrhosis following auto-immune chronic active hepatitis or non-A, non-B virus
4. Hemochromatosis (2–5%) (see Chapter 3): the liver has a brown color due to hemosiderin in liver cells and Kupffer cells
5. Wilson's disease: rare, occurs in young adults
6. Cirrhosis in alpha-1-antitrypsin deficiency: rare; onset in early childhood in PiZZ individuals (see Chapter 10); liver cells contain eosinophilic globules of alpha-1-antitrypsin.
7. Cirrhosis in galactosemia: rare; occurs in the neonatal period
8. Biliary cirrhosis
   a) Primary (See V.B, above)
   b) Secondary biliary cirrhosis
      (1) End stage of large bile duct obstruction
      (2) Cirrhosis superimposed on changes of biliary obstruction
         i) Marked cholestasis with bile plugs and bile lakes
         ii) Bile ductule dilatation and proliferation
         iii) Cholangitis, with neutrophils around bile ductules
         iv) Portal fibrosis: micronodular cirrhosis
VII. Vascular lesions of the liver
   A. Chronic venous congestion—in right heart failure—causes tender enlargement due to centrizonal congestion; fibrosis may occur in chronic cases ("cardiac cirrhosis").
   B. Budd–Chiari syndrome: rare; it is the result of obliteration of hepatic venous radicles by fibrosis, thrombosis, or rarely, neoplasm.
   C. Infarction of the liver: this is rare, because of the dual blood supply by hepatic artery and portal vein.
VIII. Neoplasms of the liver
   A. Benign neoplasms: rare
      1. Bile duct adenoma: small subcapsular nodule found incidentally at surgery
      2. Cavernous hemangioma: small, red nodule found incidentally at surgery
      3. Biliary cystadenoma: mainly in adult females; forms a large cystic mass filled with mucin
      4. Focal nodular hyperplasia
         a) This occurs predominantly in women using oral contraceptives.

b) It presents as a firm, circumscribed, often large mass in the liver; it is commonly subcapsular.

c) On cut section there is a central scar with nodules of hyperplastic liver cells and proliferating bile ductules.

d) The lesion is benign.

5. Liver cell adenoma

a) This is very rare; it occurs in women using oral contraceptives.

b) It is a solid, circumscribed brownish mass with areas of hemorrhage and necrosis.

c) Microscopically, it is composed of cytologically benign hepatocytes arranged in thickened cords.

d) It is benign; surgery is curative.

B. Malignant neoplasms

1. Primary hepatocellular carcinoma (hepatoma)

a) Incidence

(1) Rare in the United States and Europe

(2) Common in the Far East and parts of Africa

b) Etiologic factors

(1) Aflatoxins

(2) Cirrhosis predisposes to hepatocellular carcinoma

(3) Hepatitis B virus infection

c) Gross characteristics (Fig. 12-3)

(1) May present as a large solitary tumor, multiple nodules, or an infiltrative mass

(2) Cirrhosis present in 80% of cases

d) Histological characteristics

(1) Composed of malignant cells that resemble liver cells arranged in cords

(2) Immunohistologic determination for alpha-fetoprotein positive

e) Early occurrence of lung metastases

f) Clinical characteristics

(1) Should be suspected when a patient with cirrhosis shows new symptoms such as pain, loss of weight, fever, increasing ascites, or change in liver size.

(2) Hemorrhagic infarction of the tumor followed by severe intraperitoneal hemorrhage

(3) Elevated serum levels of alpha-fetoprotein (AFP) in 70% of patients

(4) Prognosis bad; average survival after diagnosis: 2 months

2. Cholangiocarcinoma

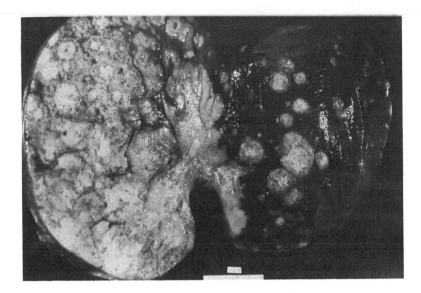

Fig. 12-3. Hepatocellular carcinoma with a dominant mass in right lobe and multiple smaller masses in the left lobe.

a) Rare in the United States and Europe
b) Grossly, presents features similar to hepatocellular carcinoma
c) Histologically, presents as a well-differentiated adenocarcinoma
3. Metastatic tumors (Fig. 12-4)
a) The most common neoplasm in the liver
b) Produces multiple nodules with massive liver enlargement
c) Grossly, may be differentiated from hepatocellular carcinoma by the presence of central necrosis (umbilication)

EXTRAHEPATIC BILIARY SYSTEM

I. Congenital malformations
A. Biliary atresia
1. Most common cause of neonatal obstructive jaundice

   2. Commonly affects only extrahepatic bile ducts; rare involvement of intrahepatic ducts
  B. Choledochal cyst
   1. Most common cause of obstructive jaundice in children beyond infancy
   2. Characterized by focal dilatation, often to massive size, of the common bile duct, with obstruction of the biliary system.
II. Cholelithiasis (Fig. 12-5)
  A. Formation of gall stones in the gall bladder; rarely, stone formation in the common bile duct
  B. Types of stones
   1. Mixed stones (80%)
      a) Composed of cholesterol, calcium bilirubinate, and calcium carbonate
      b) Usually multiple, variable in size and shape, commonly faceted
      c) Laminated on cut section
   2. Combined stones (10%)
      a) Have a pure center and mixed shell, or the reverse
      b) Characteristically large, oval, and single
   3. Pure cholesterol stones
      a) Single, large, round, or oval stones
      b) Cut section has a radiating crystalline structure
   4. Pure calcium bilirubinate (pigment) stones, multiple, very small, faceted, black stones.
   5. Pure calcium carbonate stones: very rare
  C. Fewer than 20% of gall stones have sufficient amounts of calcium to make them visible on plain radiographs.
  D. Etiology
   1. Cholesterol-based stones, both pure and mixed, are formed when bile has
      a) increased amounts of cholesterol and/or
      b) decreased levels of bile salts.
   2. Cholesterol stones are found with increased frequency in
      a) women: associated with obesity, multiparity ("fat fertile females of forty or fifty"), and the use of oral contraceptives.
      b) American Indians.
   3. Pigment stones form in patients who have
      a) chronic hemolytic processes.
      b) parasitic infestation of the bile ducts: *Clonorchis sinensis, Ascaris lumbricoides.*
  E. Clinicopathologic effects of cholelithiasis

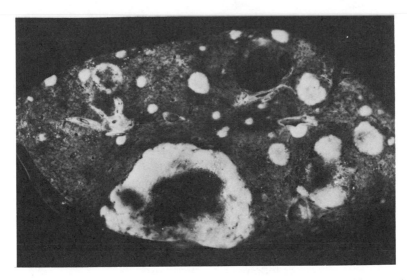

Fig. 12-4. Metastatic carcinoma in liver showing multiple nodules with central necrosis.

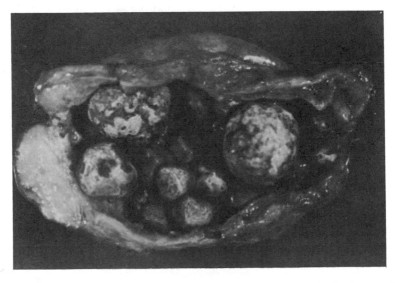

Fig. 12-5. Gall bladder filled with multiple mixed gallstones. A focal area of thickening in the fundus represents a carcinoma.

1. Asymptomatic gall bladder stones (estimated 30%)
2. Chronic cholecystitis (40%)
   a) Almost never occurs without gall stones
   b) Symptoms: biliary colic and vague abdominal symptoms
   c) Pathologic characteristics: thickening of the wall by fibrosis and the presence of chronic inflammatory cells; calcification may occur
3. Acute cholecystitis (30%)
   a) Usually (80%) a stone is found obstructing the cystic duct.
   b) Acute inflammation is bacterial (due to bile stasis) and chemical (due to concentration of bile).
   c) Clinical characteristics include an acute onset with fever and right hypochondrial pain.
   d) Pathologically, the gall bladder is congested and swollen with large numbers of neutrophils.
   e) Necrosis of the gall bladder wall (gangrenous cholecystitis) may be followed by perforation.
4. Movement of the gall stones
   a) Causes cystic duct obstruction, which may lead to
      (1) acute cholecystitis
      (2) dilatation of the gall bladder, which becomes filled with mucus (mucocele of the gall bladder)
   b) Causes common bile duct obstruction, which leads to biliary colic, intermittent obstructive jaundice, and fever due to cholangitis (Charcot's triad)
   c) Causes cholecystoenteric fistula, in which the gall stone passes into the small intestine through a fistula between it and the gallbladder; in the small intestine, gall stone may produce intestinal obstruction (gallstone ileus).
III. Benign strictures of the bile ducts
   A. A cause of obstructive jaundice
   B. Etiology
      1. Postsurgical trauma: most common
      2. External trauma: rare
      3. Postinflammatory: usually secondary to choledocholithiasis (stone in bile duct)
      4. Sclerosing cholangitis: a rare disease of unknown etiology with irregular fibrosis of bile ducts; associated with ulcerative colitis
IV. Neoplasms of the biliary system
   A. Benign: rare
   B. Malignant

1. Carcinoma of the gall bladder (Fig. 12-5)
   a) 80% of cases associated with gall stones
   b) Preceded by epithelial dysplasia
   c) Common in American Indians, Mexicans; mainly in older females.
   d) Gross characteristics
      (1) Fungating, papillary lesions that grow into the lumen
      (2) Scirrhous (hard fibrotic), infiltrative lesions that produce thickening of the wall
   e) Histological characteristics: adenocarcinomas with sclerosis
   f) Main prognostic indicator: stage of the disease; extension through the wall of the gall bladder, metastatic disease associated with an almost zero 5-year survival.
2. Carcinoma of bile ducts
   a) Uncommon; causes obstructive jaundice
   b) May involve the common bile duct or main hepatic ducts at the porta hepatis ("Klatskin tumor")
   c) Gross characteristics: tend to be small, firm, with circumferential thickening and narrowing of the bile duct
   d) Histological characteristics: adenocarcinomas with dense reactive fibrosis
   e) Tend to grow very slowly; ultimate prognosis poor

PANCREAS

I. Congenital diseases of the pancreas
   A. Fibrocystic disease ("mucoviscidosis")
      1. Common in Caucasians; autosomal recessive inheritance
      2. Characterized by abnormally viscous exocrine secretions
      3. Fundamental defect in mucus unknown; increased sodium, chloride and calcium content, abnormal glycoproteins
      4. Pathologic changes dependent on obstruction of ducts by the viscid mucus.
         a) Pancreatic changes are present in 80%. The ducts are dilated with atrophy of exocrine glands and fibrosis (chronic pancreatitis in childhood).
         b) Pulmonary changes, bronchial obstruction causing bronchiectasis and lung abscess, are the most serious.
         c) Intestinal obstruction, secondary to viscid mucus in the lumen, may occur in the neonatal period (meconium-ileus).

5. Clinical characteristics
   a) Most patients present in the first year of life wtih steator-
      rhea and/or recurrent pulmonary infections.
   b) The outlook for survival has improved.
   c) In adults, infertility (due to vas deferens obstruction) is a
      problem.
6. Diagnosis by examination of sweat electrolyte levels

B. Ectopic pancreatic tissue
1. Found in about 2% of all patients
2. Sites of ectopic pancreas (in descending frequency) stomach,
   duodenum, jejunum, Meckel's diverticulum

II. Acute pancreatitis
A. Definition: an acute inflammation of the pancreas characterized
   by necrosis and hemorrhage caused by the escape of digestive
   pancreatic juice

B. Etiology
1. Unknown
2. Factors commonly involved
   a) Gall stones (50%)
   b) Alcoholism (20%)
3. Infectious agents usually not involved; occurrence in mumps
   and cytomegalovirus of a mild, nonnecrotizing, acute pancreatitis

C. Pathologic changes
1. Necrosis of pancreatic parenchyma: patchy or diffuse
2. Hemorrhage, frequently extensive
3. Inflammation with neutrophils dominating
4. Characteristic fat necrosis due to enzyme release
   a) Appears as chalky white foci that may become calcified
   b) Presents in and around the pancreas, omentum, me-
      sentery, and rarely in fat outside the abdominal cavity
5. Peritoneal cavity often contains a brownish serous fluid
   composed of altered blood, fat globules, and very high levels
   of amylase
6. In severe cases: occurrence of extensive liquefaction of the
   gland (pancreatic abscess).

D. Clinical characteristics
1. An acute illness; a common medical emergency
2. Severe epigastric pain and vomiting
3. Shock due to peripheral circulatory collapse
4. Laboratory test results
   a) Transient glucosuria and hypocalcemia
   b) Increased serum amylase (immediate) and lipase (after 72
      hours)

E. Complications
   1. Pancreatic abscess
   2. Pseudocyst of the pancreas: common late complication
      a) Collection of hemorrhagic fluid in the pancreas, often large
      b) Cyst lined by granulation tissue; no epithelium
      c) May rupture into stomach, colon
III. Chronic pancreatitis (Fig. 12-6)
   A. Etiology
      1. Unknown
      2. Etiologic associations
         a) Alcoholism (40%)
         b) Biliary tract disease (20%)
      3. No etiologic factors are identified in 30–40% of cases
   B. Pathologic characteristics
      1. Atrophy of acinar structures
      2. Intralobular and interlobular fibrosis
      3. Irregular narrowing and dilatation of ducts that are filled with protein plugs or calculi.
      4. Variable chronic inflammatory cell infiltrate
      5. Gross characteristics: the gland is hard with foci of cal-

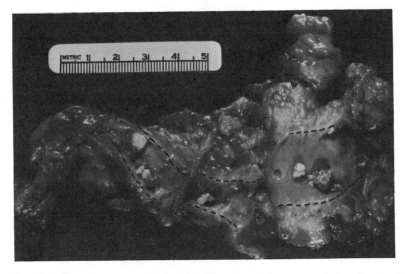

Fig. 12-6. Chronic pancreatitis showing dilatation of the pancreatic duct (outlined) in which are numerous calculi. The parenchyma is atrophic and fibrotic.

cification; cut section reveals dilated ducts containing calculi

6. Involvement frequently diffuse; may be localized

C. Clinical characteristics

1. Pain: often severe: may be constant or intermittent

2. Pancreatic insufficiency

    a) Deficiency of pancreatic juice leading to steatorrhea, fat-soluble vitamin deficiency, and weight loss

    b) Diabetes mellitus (islet deficiency): occurs in about 30% of patients

IV. Neoplasms of the pancreas

A. Mucinous cystadenoma and cystadenocarcinoma

1. Arises from the ducts

2. Usually solitary and multilocular; often very large

3. Mucinous cystadenomas: lined by a cytologically benign mucin-secreting columnar epithelium

4. Cystadenocarcinomas (malignant): lined by an epithelium that is stratified, disorganized, and infiltrating the capsule.

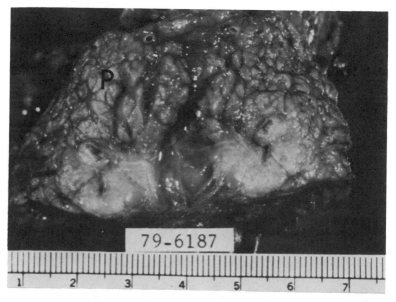

Fig. 12-7. Carcinoma of the pancreas. Cut surface of gland showing an ill-defined white tumor replacing the lobular appearance of normal pancreas (P).

5. Cystadenocarcinomas: 60% 5-year survival after surgical treatment.
B. Carcinoma of the pancreas (Fig. 12-7)
   1. Definition: malignant neoplasm of the exocrine pancreas (95% in ducts; 5% in acini)
   2. Epidemiology
      a) 20,000 patients die from pancreatic cancer in the United States annually (6% of all cancer deaths)
      b) Incidence increasing
      c) 90% occur over age 50 years; more common in males
      d) 70% occur in the head of pancreas
   3. Pathologic characteristics
      a) Gross characteristics
         (1) Solid, hard, infiltrative masses that expand the gland; frequently invade surrounding structures
         (2) Carcinomas of the head: tend to be detected when they are small because of bile duct obstruction; body and tail tumors: large
      b) Histologic characteristics
         (1) 90% adenocarcinomas, frequently well-differentiated with marked sclerosis
         (2) 10% mixed adenosquamous carcinomas or anaplastic carcinomas with giant cells, and spindle cells
         (3) Acinar cell carcinoma resembles the cells of the acini (rare)
         (4) Perineural invasion very common
      c) Spread
         (1) Direct invasion into duodenum, stomach, transverse colon
         (2) Lymphatic spread to regional nodes: occurs early
         (3) Blood stream metastasis to liver: occurs early
   4. Clinical characteristics
      a) Manifests as
         (1) painless obstructive jaundice
         (2) Weight loss, abdominal mass, anemia
         (3) lipase production by an acinar cell carcinoma, which causes fat necrosis in skin and joints (rare)
         (4) frequently elevated serum levels of carcinoembryonic antigen (not specific)
      b) Prognosis dismal: mean survival 6 months after diagnosis
C. Islet cell neoplasms (see Chapter 13).

13

The Endocrine System

PITUITARY (HYPOPHYSIS)

I. Diseases of the anterior pituitary
  A. Hypersecretion of hormones
    1. Etiology
      a) Most cases of anterior pituitary hypersecretion are due to benign neoplasms of a single cell type: Pituitary adenoma.
      b) The adenoma may be large or very small (microadenoma). Nonfunctioning adenomas tend to be large.
      c) Adenomas are composed of uniform round cells arranged in nests or trabeculae separated by highly vascular stroma.
      d) Cells may be chromophobic (nonfunctioning), acidophilic (growth hormone, prolactin), or basophilic (ACTH). The correlation between the hormone secreted and histologic appearance is not exact.
      e) Identification of cell type is by immunoperoxidase and electron microscopy.
    2. Clinicopathologic effects of pituitary adenomas
      a) Local effects due to growth of tumor
        (1) Pituitary adenomas are usually well-circumscribed. They rarely invade surrounding structures (invasive adenoma).
        (2) The sella turcica becomes enlarged and erosion of bone occurs.
        (3) Visual defects due to compression of the optic nerves, chiasma or tracts (bitemporal hemianopia is typical) occur.
        (4) Third ventricle is compressed and hydrocephalus may be present.
        (5) Other pituitary cells atrophy.
      b) Systemic effects due to hormone secretion by tumor

    (1) Growth hormone excess (acromegaly and gigantism)
        i) Bone growth: in children this causes gigantism; in adults it causes enlargement of bones (acromegaly).
        ii) Cartilage growth leads to increase in size of nose and ears and joint abnormalities.
        iii) All the viscera are increased in size.
        iv) Glucose tolerance is impaired.
        v) Infertility, amenorrhea, and impotence occur due to compression atrophy of gonadotrophin-producing cells.
    (2) Prolactin excess
        i) Amenorrhea and infertility occur in females; impotence and infertility occur in males.
        ii) Galactorrhea (milk secretion) occurs.
    (3) ACTH excess
        i) Cortisol secretion by the adrenal is increased (Cushing's syndrome).
        ii) Pigmentation of the skin is increased due to melanocyte-stimulating activity associated with ACTH excess.
    (4) TSH and gonadotrophin excess: rare

  B. Hyposecretion of anterior pituitary hormones (hypopituitarism)
    1. Etiology
      a) Ischemic necrosis of the pituitary in pregnancy (Sheehan's syndrome)
        (1) Ischemic necrosis of a gland that has undergone physiologic hyperplasia in pregnancy; over 90% of the pituitary becomes infarcted
        (2) Associated with postpartum hemorrhage and shock
      b) Chromophobe (nonsecreting) pituitary adenoma: the most common cause in the adult
      c) Craniopharyngioma
        (1) An epithelial tumor derived from Rathke's pouch
        (2) Common in childhood
        (3) Benign neoplasm, but has a tendency to recur after (incomplete) surgical removal; located in suprasellar region; may be solid or cystic; calcification present in most cases; may reach a large size
        (4) Cyst contains an oily fluid with cholesterol crystals
        (5) Microscopically, major component is benign squamous epithelium

    d) Other types of destructive lesions: rare

2. Clinical effects depend on whether the patient is a child or an adult.

    a) Dwarfism: failure of growth hormone action in childhood

    b) Simmond's disease: in adults, is characterized by

      (1) gonadotrophin deficiency, leading to amenorrhea, infertility, and impotence.

      (2) TSH deficiency, leading to hypothyroidism with thyroid atrophy.

      (3) ACTH deficiency, leading to decreased cortisol secretion.

      (4) weight loss (pituitary "cachexia").

    c) Isolated growth hormone deficiency produces little effect in adults.

II. Diseases of the posterior pituitary

    A. Failure of ADH secretion: diabetes insipidus

      1. ADH deficiency leads to failure of renal water reabsorption. Urine volume is increased (polyuria), with increased serum osmolarity, which induces thirst and polydipsia (excessive intake of water). Deprivation of water fails to induce a concentrated urine.

      2. Diabetes insipidus commonly results from lesions of the base of the brain that involve the hypothalamopituitary axis such as

      a) neoplasms (e.g., metastatic cancer)

      b) tuberculous meningitis, sarcoidosis

      c) Hand–Schuller–Christian disease (histiocytosis X)

    B. Excessive ADH secretion

      1. By the pituitary in cases of inappropriate ADH secretion (SIADH; Schwartz–Bartter syndrome)

      a) Common

      b) Caused by a large variety of underlying diseases

        (1) Pulmonary disorders: tuberculosis, pneumonia

        (2) Cerebral neoplasms and trauma

        (3) Drugs such as chlorpropamide, vincristine

        (4) Numerous other conditions such as cirrhosis of the liver, adrenal insufficiency, porphyria

      c) Characterized by increased serum levels of ADH, water retention in the kidneys, dilutional hyponatremia, and decreased serum osmolarity

      2. Ectopic ADH secretion by neoplasm: commonly oat cell carcinoma of lung

THYROID

I. Synthesis of thyroid hormone (Fig. 13-1)
II. Excessive secretion of thyroid hormone (hyperthyroidism; thyrotoxicosis)
  A. Graves' disease (diffuse toxic goiter): common
  1. Etiology
    a) Graves' disease is an autoimmune disease characterized by the presence of thyroid-stimulating immunoglobulins (TSI), usually IgG.
      (1) LATS (long-acting thyroid stimulator)
      (2) HTS (human thyroid stimulator)
      (3) LATS-P (LATS-protector)
    b) The combination of TSI with the thyroid cell membrane causes increased hormone secretion.
  2. Pathological characteristics
    a) The thyroid gland is diffusely and symmetrically enlarged.
    b) The gland is extremely vascular, with a typical deep red, "beefy" appearance on cut section.
    c) Thyroid cells are increased in number (hyperplasia) as well as in size (hypertrophy).
    d) The follicles are small and closely packed; colloid is scant and shows peripheral vacuolation.
    e) Lymphocytic infiltration is common.
  3. Associated lesions
    a) Exophthalmos (forward protrusion of the eyeball)
      (1) Occurs in 70% of cases; unrelated to severity of thyrotoxicosis
      (2) Due to edema and accumulation of mucopolysaccharides in the connective tissue of the orbit
    b) Pretibial myxedema (in 5% of patients): accumulation of mucopolysaccharide material in the pretibial skin
    c) Thymic hyperplasia
  4. Clinical characteristics
    a) Females 15–30 years old are most commonly affected.
    b) All of the following clinical characteristics are caused by thyroid hormone excess.
      (1) Nervousness, anxiety, insomnia, fine tremors
      (2) Weight loss despite a good appetite
      (3) Heat intolerance and increased sweating
      (4) Visual changes: staring eyes protruding out of their sockets, impaired eye muscle function

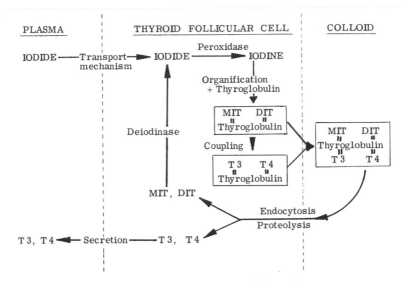

MIT, DIT = mono- and di-iodotyrosine; T 3 = tri-iodothyronine
T 4 = thyroxine

Fig. 13.1 Synthesis of thyroid hormones

      (5) Palpitations, tachycardia, cardiac arrhythmias, and heart failure
      (6) Amenorrhea and infertility
      (7) Muscle weakness (proximal myopathy), osteoporosis with bone pain
   c) The thyroid gland is enlarged diffusely.
   d) Laboratory confirmation of diagnosis includes
      (1) Elevated total T4 and T3
      (2) Elevated free thyroxine index
      (3) Increased uptake of radioiodine
   c) T3 toxicosis is thyrotoxicosis with normal serum T4 levels and elevated T3 levels.
 B. Other causes of hyperthyroidism: rare
   1. Toxicity in multinodular goiter and follicular adenoma
   2. TSH secreting pituitary adenoma
   3. Trophoblastic neoplasms—hydatidiform mole and choriocarcinoma—due to secretion of TSH-like hormones
   4. Thyroiditis

III. Decreased secretion of thyroid hormones (hypothyroidism)
    A. Results in
        1. cretinism if deficiency is present from birth
        2. myxedema if it occurs in adults
    B. Confirmed in the laboratory by
        1. decreased total T4 and T3 in serum
        2. decreased free thyroxine index
        3. serum TSH levels are invariably elevated in primary hypothyroidism
    C. Cretinism
        1. Etiology
            a) Abnormal development: thyroid agenesis
            b) Failure of hormone synthesis due to "inborn errors of metabolism" (enzyme deficiency)
            c) Failure of hormone action (abnormal receptors in the target organs): very rare
            d) Dietary iodine deficiency
            e) Presence of goitrogens in the diet (substances that block thyroid hormone synthesis)
        2. Clinical characteristics
            a) Thyroid gland enlargement (goitrous cretinism) except in congenital agenesis or hypoplasia of the thyroid (nongoitrous cretinism)
            b) Lethargy, somnolence, feeding problems, hypothermia
            c) Persistent neonatal jaundice
            d) Hoarse cry, hypotonic muscles, large tongue, umbilical hernia
            e) Growth retardation ("failure to thrive")
            f) Mental retardation: replacement of thyroid hormone from an early age will prevent mental retardation
    D. Myxedema
        1. Clinical characteristics
            a) Lethargy, cold intolerance, constipation, menorrhagia
            b) Deposition of mucopolysaccharides in connective tissue of
                (1) skin: producing myxedema
                (2) larynx: causing hoarseness
                (3) heart: causing cardiac enlargement
             c) Pleural and pericardial effusions
            d) Increased serum cholesterol and an increased incidence of atherosclerotic vascular disease
            e) Normochromic, normocytic anemia
            f) Psychomotor retardation and overt psychosis (myxedema madness)

2. Causes
  a) Iatrogenic hypothyroidism
    (1) Due to ablation of the thyroid by surgery or radiation
    (2) Due to antithyroid drugs
  b) Secondary hypothyroidism
    (1) Due to pituitary failure of TSH secretion
    (2) Distinguished from other causes of myxedema by the low serum TSH level
  c) Primary hypothyroidism: Hashimoto's autoimmune thyroiditis
    (1) Responsible for the majority of cases of adult hypothyroidism
    (2) A disease of middle-aged females.
    (3) Etiology of Hashimoto's thyroiditis
      i) An autoimmune disease, with IgG antibodies against
        (A) thyroglobulin
        (B) a colloid component other than thyroglobulin
        (C) microsomal antigen
      ii) T-cell-mediated hypersensitivity
    (4) Pathologic characteristics
      i) The thyroid is enlarged symmetrically; the pyramidal lobe is frequently prominent.
      ii) The gland is firm and rubbery, and has a coarse nodular ("bossellated") appearance.
      iii) In the final stages, the gland becomes atrophic and replaced by collagen.
      iv) Microscopic examination reveals extensive lymphoid infiltration with fibrosis and atrophy of thyroid follicles.
      v) Surviving follicle cells show Hurthle cell (large cells with abundant pink cytoplasm) metaplasia.
    (5) Clinical characteristics
      i) Gradual enlargement of the thyroid in middle-aged females.
      ii) Thyroid function is variable; it is commonly euthyroid or mildly hypothyroid at presentation; hypothyroidism progressively worsens.
      iii) Thyroid autoantibodies are present in high titer.
IV. Thyroid diseases with normal hormone production
  A. Abnormalities of thyroglossal duct descent

1. Thyroglossal duct cysts
   a) Common; epithelial-lined cyst
   b) Develop in the midline of the neck in the line of descent of the thyroglossal duct
2. Ectopic thyroid tissue
   a) May occur in the midline at any point from the tongue to the thyroid
   b) May be present with or without a normal thyroid gland
3. Mediastinal thyroid: excessive descent of thyroid

B. Diffuse nontoxic or multinodular goiter
   1. Definition
      a) This is compensatory hyperplasia of the thyroid that results from increased TSH stimulation.
      b) This follows deficiency of thyroid hormone production.
      c) The patient is euthyroid, because the compensatory hyperplasia represents a mechanism to increase hormone output.
      d) There is a fine balance between thyroid enlargement, TSH level, and hormone output to maintain euthyroidism.
   2. Etiology
      a) Endemic goiter
         (1) Occurs mainly in inland mountainous regions of the world: Alps, Andes, Himalayas
         (2) Due to chronic iodine deficiency and/or dietary goitrogens
      b) Sporadic goiter
         (1) Increased physiologic demand for thyroxine (physiologic goiter) at puberty or pregnancy
         (2) Mild deficiency in enzymes of thyroid hormone synthesis
   3. Pathologic characteristics
      a) Diffuse colloid goiter
         (1) Initial phase of TSH induced hyperplasia, where the gland is diffusely enlarged.
         (2) Followed by the involution phase, where follicles progressively enlarge and become filled with large amounts of colloid, and the epithelium becomes flattened.
      b) Multinodular goiter (Fig. 13-2)
         (1) This is a continuation of the process that causes diffuse colloid goiter (above), representing
            i) irregular hyperplasia and involution.
            ii) hemorrhage, necrosis, cyst formation, and fibrosis leading to multiple nodules.

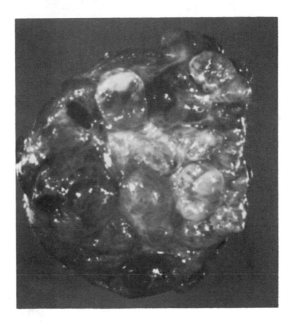

Fig. 13.2 Multinodular goiter. Cut surface of enlarged thyroid lobe showing multiple nodules, some showing hemorrhage.

> (2) The thyroid is enlarged, and often massive.
> 4. Clinical characteristics
>   a) Caused by enlargement of the thyroid
>   (1) Cosmetic effect: the most common reason for surgery
>   (2) Pressure effects: may be severe in a retrosternal (mediastinal) thyroid
>   b) Patients clinically and biochemically euthyroid
>   c) Risk of developing cancer very small
> C. Subacute thyroiditis (Synonyms: DeQuervains thyroiditis; giant cell thyroiditis; granulomatous thyroiditis)
>   1. Definition: a self-limited inflammatory disease of the thyroid characterized by a granulomatous inflammation with giant cells
>   2. Etiology
>   a) Viral etiology very likely; the disease frequently follows an upper respiratory infection

        b) Autoimmunity suggested but unlikely

3. Pathologic characteristics
   a) The gland is enlarged diffusely and very firm.
   b) Microscopic examination reveals
      (1) extensive follicle destruction.
      (2) aggregates of macrophages and giant cells around fragments of colloid.
      (3) fibrosis, which may be extensive.

4. Clinical characteristics
   a) It has an acute onset with painful thyroid enlargement and fever.
   b) Transient hyperthyroidism is common (acute release of hormone from the damaged gland).
   c) It is self-limited; recovery is the rule in weeks to months.

D. Riedel's thyroiditis: a rare disorder of unknown etiology in which there is extensive fibrosis of the thyroid gland

E. Neoplasms of the thyroid

1. Follicular adenoma
   a) Common; presents clinically as a solitary thyroid nodule that does not take up iodine ("cold" nodule on a thyroid scan)
   b) Occurs at any age; most common in young females
   c) Pathologic characteristics
      (1) Gross examination reveals a solitary, encapsulated, firm nodule.
      (2) Microscopic examination reveals it to be composed of follicular cells arranged in different patterns and surrounded by a complete fibrous capsule.
      (3) If capsular invasion or vascular invasion is identified, the lesion is malignant (follicular carcinoma).

2. Carcinoma of the thyroid
   a) Incidence: uncommon; responsible for about 1000 deaths annually in the United States
   b) Papillary carcinoma
      (1) Most common type of thyroid carcinoma (60–70%)
      (2) Male:female ratio of 1:3; tends to affect younger individuals
      (3) Gross pathologic characteristics
         i) Range in size from microscopic to massive lesions over 10 cm in diameter; infiltrative nodules
         ii) Frequently multifocal
         iii) May invade surrounding structures

        iv) Metastasis to cervical lymph nodes occurs commonly

(4) Microscopic pathologic characteristics
    i) Papillary structure
    ii) The nuclei have a clear appearance
    iii) Psammoma bodies, laminated calcific bodies, present in 50% of cases: diagnostic of papillary carcinoma
    iv) Biologic behavior of mixed papillary and follicular carcinoma similar to that of papillary carcinoma.

(5) Clinical progression
    i) Papillary carcinoma grows very slowly.
    ii) Spread occurs via lymphatics to cervical lymph nodes.
    iii) Blood stream spread occurs rarely.
    iv) Even with widespread metastatic papillary carcinoma, patients remain well clinically for several years.

(6) Treatment and prognosis
    i) Disease restricted to the thyroid and cervical lymph nodes is curable by surgery.
    ii) Papillary carcinomas are TSH-dependent; suppression of TSH controls tumor.
    iii) Radioiodine therapy is used.
    iv) The overall prognosis is 90% survival at 5 years and 80–85% at 20 years.

c) Follicular carcinoma
  (1) 25% of thyroid carcinomas
  (2) Females affected more than males
  (3) Gross pathologic characteristics
    i) A circumscribed lesion, grossly indistinguishable from an adenoma, but showing capsular or vascular invasion microscopically
    ii) A firm, pale, invasive mass that irregularly enlarges a lobe
    iii) Possible extension through the thyroid capsule
    iv) Multifocal lesions rare
  (4) Microscopic characteristics
    i) Composed of variably sized thyroid follicles; well-differentiated tumors closely resemble normal thyroid

   ii) Invasion of thyroid parenchyma and vascular invasion

  (5) Clinical progression

   i) Slow-growing, but more rapid than papillary carcinoma

   ii) Lymphatic spread to cervical lymph nodes uncommon

   iii) Blood stream spread to bone and lungs common and occurs early

  (6) Treatment and prognosis

   i) Total thyroidectomy

   ii) Radioiodine therapy

   iii) 5-year survival: 65%; 20-year survival: 30%

 d) Medullary carcinoma

  (1) Rare, accounting for 10% of thyroid carcinoma

  (2) Derived from the "parafollicular" C cells of the thyroid

  (3) 90% solitary sporadic thyroid lesions

  (4) 10% familial (autosomal dominant); associated with

   i) pheochromocytoma and adrenal medullary hyperplasia

   ii) Parathyroid adenoma or hyperplasia (Sipple syndrome, multiple endocrine adenomatosis type II, MEA-II)

  (5) Secrete calcitonin

  (6) Gross characteristics: a hard, grayish-white mass that is poorly circumscribed and may involve a large portion of the gland

  (7) Microscopic characteristics

   i) Small cells arranged in nests and sheets

   ii) Stroma stains for amyloid

  (8) Electron microscopy shows neurosecretory dense-core granules

  (9) Clinical progression

   i) Slow but progressive

   ii) Local invasion of neck structures common

   iii) Both lymphatic and blood stream spread common

  (10) Treatment: surgery the only available treatment

  (11) Prognosis: 5 year survival: 40–50%

 e) Undifferentiated carcinoma

  (1) Rare, represents 10% of thyroid carcinoma

  (2) Commonly seen in patients over 50 years

(3) Gross characteristics
- i) Very large with extensive involvement of the thyroid and extension beyond the capsule into surrounding neck structures
- ii) Hard and gritty, grayish-white with frequent necrosis and hemorrhage

(4) Microscopic characteristics: composed of large cells with extreme pleomorphism and numerous bizarre giant cells and high mitotic activity (giant cell carcinoma)

(5) Highly malignant, with a rapid rate of progression

(6) Death due to local invasion of neck structures before widespread metastases occur

(7) The prognosis is terrible; 5-year survival: close to zero.

PARATHYROID

I. Excess PTH secretion (hyperparathyroidism)
  A. Classification and etiology
  1. Primary hyperparathyroidism: an autonomous inappropriate secretion of PTH by the parathyroid gland. This may be due to
     a) single adenoma (80–90%).
     b) multiple adenomas (1–4%).
     c) hyperplasia involving all glands (3–15%).
     d) carcinoma (1–4%).
  2. Secondary hyperparathyroidism: diffuse hyperplasia of the parathyroids with increased PTH secretion as a compensation for lowered ionized calcium. This occurs in
     a) chronic renal failure.
     b) malabsorption syndromes.
     c) vitamin D deficiency.
  3. Ectopic PTH production by tumors: squamous cell carcinoma of the lung and adenocarcinoma of the kidney are the most common causes of ectopic PTH production.
     duction.
  B. Clinical effects
  1. Changes in blood chemistry
     a) Increased serum calcium, decreased serum phosphate
     b) Increased urinary calcium and phosphate
     c) Increased alkaline phosphatase

2. Renal disease
   a) Renal calculi
   b) Nephrocalcinosis: deposition of calcium in the renal interstitium, leading to renal failure
3. Bone disease
   a) Osteoporosis, due to resorption of bone
   b) Fibrosis and cyst formation
   c) "Brown tumors": solid masses composed of osteoclastic giant cells, fibroblasts, and collagen
4. Metastatic calcification
5. Neurologic dysfunction with very high serum calcium levels
C. Parathyroid adenoma
   1. Usually single and small
   2. Well-circumscribed, with a rim of compressed parathyroid tissue
   3. Composed of a mixed cell population as a rule, with chief cells, oxyphil cells, and water clear cells
   4. Cells arranged in sheets and cords
D. Parathyroid carcinoma: rare
E. Primary parathyroid hyperplasia: rare
   1. This is hyperplasia of all parathyroid glands without a known provocative factor.
   2. All glands may be enlarged uniformly or one gland may be disproportionately large.
   3. Distinction between adenoma and nodular hyperplasia is difficult without examining at least two parathyroid glands.
   4. Chief cell hyperplasia may be familial and associated with multiple endocrine adenomatosis (MEA syndromes).
F. Secondary parathyroid hyperplasia: common; grossly and microscopically indistinguishable from primary hyperplasia
II. Decreased PTH secretion (hypoparathyroidism)
   A. Etiology
      1. Accidental surgical removal of parathyroids in the course of thyroidectomy: most common cause
      2. Infarction of parathyroids
      3. Idiopathic hypoparathyroidism
         a) Rare; more common in females
         b) Believed to have an autoimmune basis; organ-specific parathyroid antibodies demonstrable in about 40% of patients
      4. Congenital absence of parathyroids: associated with thymic agenesis (Nezelof's syndrome): rare
      5. Pseudohypoparathyroidism: rare

a) Features of hypoparathyroidism with normal serum PTH levels
b) Believed to be due to end-organ unresponsiveness to PTH
c) Skeletal abnormalities commonly associated: short stature, short neck, and abnormal hand bones

B. Clinical effects
1. Decreased serum calcium
2. Increased serum phosphate
3. Tetany due to hypocalcemia: carpopedal spasms, increased irritability of nerves and muscles, convulsions, laryngospasm
4. Metastatic calcification due to hyperphosphatemia: increased bone density, cataracts, calcification in the basal ganglia

ADRENAL CORTEX

I. Excess secretion of adrenocortical hormones
A. Excess cortisol secretion (Cushing's syndrome; hypercortisolism)
1. Etiology
a) With high ACTH levels in the serum
(1) Excessive pituitary ACTH secretion by a basophil adenoma (60%)
(2) Ectopic ACTH secretion by nonpituitary neoplasms, most commonly oat-cell carcinoma of the lung (15%)
b) With low ACTH levels in the serum
(1) Functioning adrenal adenoma or carcinoma (25%)
(2) Iatrogenic: large doses of glucocorticoids in the treatment of nonendocrine diseases
2. Clinical effects
a) Obesity with central redistribution of fat: "moon" facies and truncal obesity with thin extremities
b) Increased gluconeogenesis leading to protein (muscle) wasting; growth retardation in children
c) Thinning of the skin (with striae), easy bruising, and slow wound healing: consequences of protein catabolism
d) Increased susceptibility to infections
e) Hypertension, sodium retention, and potassium loss (hypokalemia) due to the minerallocorticoid effect of cortisol
f) Diabetes mellitus due to the effect of cortisol on glucose metabolism

g) Osteoporosis

h) Mental disturbances: steroid encephalopathy

i) Associated androgen excess leading to hirsuitism, acne, and menstrual disturbances in females

3. Diagnosis

   a) Diagnosis of the presence of Cushing's syndrome is by

     (1) elevated plasma cortisol.

     (2) loss of diurnal rhythm of cortisol secretion.

     (3) failure to suppress cortisol secretion with the low-dose (0.5 mg every 6 hrs for 2 days) dexamethazone test.

   b) Diagnosis of the cause of Cushing's syndrome is by

     (1) plasma ACTH level

     (2) the high-dose (2 mg every 6 hrs) dexamethazone suppression test: suppression of cortisol secretion indicates pituitary ACTH excess; no suppression occurs with adrenal neoplasms and in the ectopic ACTH syndrome.

4. Adrenocortical neoplasms (adenoma and carcinoma)

   a) These are single masses having a distinctive yellow-orange color (Fig. 13-3)

   b) Adenomas are usually well circumscribed. Carcinomas tend to infiltrate surrounding tissues extensively.

   c) Adenomas are small (usually under 50 g). Carcinomas are larger (over 100 g).

   d) Microscopically,

     (1) adenomas are composed of regular large cells filled with lipid and small, central nuclei.

     (2) carcinomas frequently display

       i) capsule invasion and invasion of adjacent structures.

       ii) vascular invasion.

       iii) anaplasia and high mitotic rate.

       iv) metastasis.

5. Adrenocortical hyperplasia (bilateral)

   a) These are associated with excess ACTH stimulation, either pituitary or ectopic.

   b) They are characterized by enlargement of both glands, either diffuse or nodular, with an aggregate weight of over 8 g.

   c) Microscopically, the hyperplasia involves the zona fasciculata and reticularis.

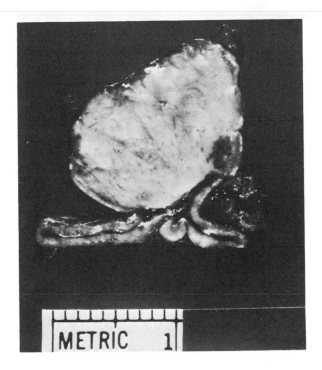

Fig. 13.3 Adrenocortical adenoma

B. Excess aldosterone secretion (hyperaldosteronism)
   1. Primary hyperaldosteronism (low-renin aldosteronism; Conn's syndrome)
      a) Etiology
         (1) Adrenocortical adenoma: large majority
         (2) Primary hyperplasia of the zona glomerulosa and adrenal carcinoma: very rare
      b) Clinical characteristics
         (1) Hypertension
         (2) Sodium retention in kidney in exchange for potassium and hydrogen
         (3) Hypokalemia and alkalosis
         (4) Elevated plasma aldosterone levels; low plasma renin
      c) Morphologic characteristics
         (1) Adrenal adenomas associated with hyperaldosteron-

ism are similar to those in Cushing's syndrome
(2) Hyperplasia microscopically involves the zona glomerulosa.
2. Secondary hyperaldosteronism
   a) This is caused by high renin output by the juxtaglomerular apparatus of the kidney in
      (1) renal ischemia: renal artery stenosis, malignant hypertension.
      (2) states of reduced effective plasma volume: cardiac failure, nephrotic syndrome.
      (3) Bartter's syndrome: juxtaglomerular hyperplasia with increased renin production.
      (4) renin-secreting renal tumors: very rare.
   b) Hyperplasia of the zona glomerulosa leads to excessive aldosterone secretion.
C. Excess androgen secretion: may result from the following:
   1. Androgen secreting adrenal neoplasms: most commonly adrenal carcinomas
   2. Congenital adrenal hyperplasia (CAH)
      a) This is the consequence of enzyme deficiency in adrenal steroid synthesis.
      b) Decreased cortisol production stimulates pituitary ACTH secretion and bilateral adrenal cortical hyperplasia.
      c) Grossly and microscopically, the hyperplasia is indistinguishable from that seen in Cushing's syndrome.
      d) Clinical effects depend on the enzyme that is deficient (Fig. 13-4).
         (1) Complete 21-hydroxylase deficiency (30%)
            i) Failure of cortisol synthesis (Addison's disease)
            ii) Failure of aldosterone synthesis (marked sodium loss in the urine)
            iii) Increased androgen synthesis
         (2) Partial 21-hydroxylase deficiency (60%)
            i) Cortisol and aldosterone levels normal
            ii) Conversion of 17-hydroxy-progesterone to androgenic hormones (virilization)
         (3) 11-hydroxylase deficiency (5%): elevated levels of 11-deoxycortisol and deoxycorticosterone leading to sodium retention and hypertension
         (4) others: rare
D. Excess feminizing hormone secretion
   1. Very rare
   2. Almost invariably associated with adrenal carcinoma

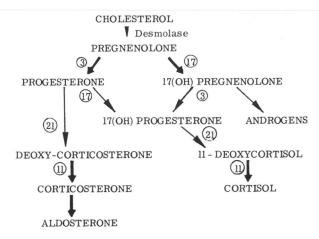

Fig. 13.4 Synthesis of adrenocortical hormones

3 = 3 beta hydroxysteroid dehydrogenase
11 = 11 - hydroxylase
17 = 17 - hydroxylase
21 = 21 - hydroxylase

II. Decreased secretion of cortisol
   A. Acute destruction of the adrenals
     1. Neonatal hemorrhagic necrosis: rare
     2. Bacteremia (Waterhouse–Friderichsen syndrome)
       a) Most commonly seen in meningococcal infections
       b) Both adrenals destroyed by necrosis and hemorrhage
       c) Fulminant illness with shock, coma, a hemorrhagic skin rash, and high mortality
   B. Chronic destruction of the adrenals (Addison's disease)
     1. Etiology
       a) "Idiopathic" atrophy (autoimmune Addison's disease)
         (1) Antiadrenal antibody is present in the serum.
         (2) The glands are small and contracted by fibrosis, with an aggregate weight less than 4 g.
         (3) Histologically there is loss of cortical cells and a heavy lymphocytic infiltrate in both adrenals.
       b) Tuberculous and fungal granuloma: rare today
       c) Metastatic cancer, particularly lung carcinoma: rare

    d) Amyloidosis, hemochromatosis: rare

    e) Congenital adrenal hyperplasia (see above)

  2. Clinical characteristics

    a) Minerallocorticoid deficiency leading to increased sodium excretion in the distal renal tubules with

      (1) decreased serum sodium and chloride, causing hypotension

      (2) hyperkalemia and acidosis

    b) Decreased cortisol levels in plasma

    c) Pigmentation of the skin due to increased pituitary ACTH

    d) Absent corticosteroid response to stress (Addisonian crisis)

C. Adrenal atrophy secondary to deficiency of pituitary ACTH

ADRENAL MEDULLA

  I. Hyperplasia of the medulla (Fig. 13-5): very rare

 II. Neoplasms of the medulla

  A. Pheochromocytoma (Fig. 13-5)

    1. Definition and general features

      a) Pheochromocytoma is defined as a catecholamine-producing neoplasm of the adrenal medulla and extra-adrenal sympathetic ganglia.

      b) 10% of pheochromocytomas are extra-adrenal, arising in

        (1) paravertebral sympathetic ganglia.

        (2) ganglia at the bifurcation of the aorta ("organ of Zuckerkandl").

        (3) sympathetic ganglia in the wall of the urinary bladder.

      c) 10% of patients have multiple pheochromocytomas.

      d) 10% of pheochromocytomas are malignant.

      e) Familial occurrence of pheochromocytomas in:

        (1) Multiple endocrine adenomatosis (MEA) IIa: medullary carcinoma of the thyroid and parathyroid adenoma or hyperplasia

        (2) MEA IIb: mucocutaneous neuromas, medullary carcinoma of the thyroid and parathyroid lesions

        (3) Generalized neurofibromatosis (von Recklinghausen's disease)

    2. Clinical characteristics

      a) Hypertension

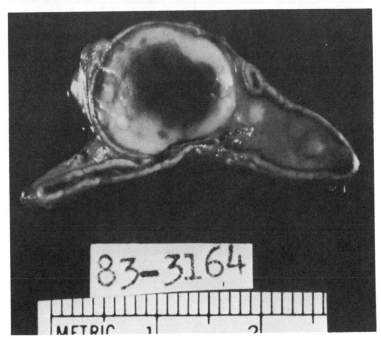

Fig. 13.5 Section of adrenal showing a pheochromocytoma and hyperplasia of the medulla in the region not involved by tumor. From a patient with multiple endocrine adenomatosis (type IIa).

  b) Palpitations, tachycardia, excessive sweating, and a feeling of apprehension
  c) Impaired glucose tolerance (diabetes mellitus)
3. Laboratory diagnosis
  a) Increased urinary metanephrine and vanillyl-mandelic acid (VMA)
  b) Increased plasma and urinary catecholamines
  c) Localization of the tumor before surgery by
    (1) computerized axial tomography (CT scan) of the abdomen
    (2) nuclear medicine scan using radioisotopes taken up specifically by the cells of the adrenal medulla
    (3) selective adrenal vein sampling and catecholamine assay

4. Treatment: surgical removal of the tumor
5. Pathologic characteristics
   a) Gross characteristics: vary in size from microscopic to large masses; round, well circumscribed, and solid
   b) Microscopic characteristics
      (1) Composed of large cells (pheochromocytes) arranged in nests and cords separated by a vascular connective tissue
      (2) Contains abundant cytoplasm that is granular and stains positively with chromium salts (chromaffin cells)
      (3) Cellular and nuclear pleomorphism with frequent bizarre giant cells common even in benign tumors
   c) Diagnosis of malignant pheochromocytoma
      (1) Cannot be made on the basis of gross or microscopic examination of the adrenal tumor
      (2) Made only when distant metastases are demonstrated

B. Neuroblastoma
   1. General characteristics
      a) Neuroblastoma is a malignant neoplasm derived from primitive neural crest cells, most commonly in adrenal medulla.
      b) Neuroblastoma is the third most common malignant neoplasm in childhood, after leukemia–lymphoma and nephroblastoma.
   2. Clinical characteristics
      a) 80% of cases occur under the age of 5 years. It is rare after 15 years.
      b) Most cases present as an abdominal mass.
      c) 75% of patients have increased secretion of catecholamines.
      d) Good prognostic factors include
         (1) young age.
         (2) early clinical stage of the disease.
         (3) histologic evidence of ganglion cell differentiation.
      e) Hematogenous metastasis occurs early to bone (Hutchinson-type) and liver (Pepper-type); extensive bone marrow involvement is common.
   3. Pathologic characteristics
      a) Gross characteristics: large, soft, hemorrhagic masses
      b) Microscopic characteristics
         (1) Small, round cells having dark nuclei and scant cytoplasm; arranged in sheets and "rosettes"

(2) Ganglionic differentiation characterized by large, multinucleated cells scattered in the tumor

c) Electron microscopy: shows dense-core neurosecretory granules

ENDOCRINE PANCREAS
(ISLETS OF LANGERHANS)

I. Hyperfunction of pancreatic islets
  A. Pathologic characteristics
    1. Diffuse hyperplasia of the islets: very rare
    2. Islet cell adenoma: common
      a) Commonly solitary, 10–15% of cases have multiple adenomas.
      b) Grossly, they are firm, encapsulated nodules that vary in size from microscopic (microadenomas) to huge masses.
      c) Microscopically, they are composed of uniform, small cells arranged in nests and trabeculae.
      d) The diagnosis of the cell type is made by
        (1) evaluation of serum for hormone excess.
        (2) immunologic demostration of hormone in the tumor cells.
        (3) electron microscopy to demonstrate the characteristic granules of the cell types.
    3. Islet cell carcinoma
      a) Islet cell carcinoma commonly resembles adenomas.
      b) The diagnosis of carcinoma can be made when the tumor infiltrates beyond the confines of the pancreas or when distant metastases are present.
  B. Clinical characteristics
    1. Hyperinsulinism (B cell lesions): common
      a) 70% solitary adenomas (insulinoma); 10% multiple adenomas; 10% carcinomas; 10% diffuse islet cell hyperplasia
      b) Increased insulin secretion causes Whipple's triad:
        (1) Hypoglycemic attacks, precipitated by fasting
        (2) Plasma glucose level of less than 40 mg/dl during an attack
        (3) Prompt relief of symptoms by glucose administration
      c) Symptoms of hypoglycemia: dizziness, confusion, excess sweating, leading to convulsions, coma and death

    d) Diagnosis established by an inappropriately high level of serum insulin during a hypoglycemic episode

  2. Glucagon excess (A cell lesions)

    a) 70% malignant islet cell neoplasms (glucagonoma)

    b) Clinical characteristics

      (1) Mild diabetes mellitus

      (2) A necrotizing migratory erythematous skin rash

      (3) Evidence of metastatic tumor in two-thirds of cases

    c) Diagnosis: high level of glucagon in the serum

  3. Somatostatinoma (D cell tumor): very rare; the majority (80%) are malignant

  4. Gastrinoma (G cell tumor): common

    a) Secretion of gastrin leads to the Zollinger–Ellison syndrome:

      (1) Hypersecretion of gastric acid

      (2) Unrelenting, recurrent peptic ulceration which occurs in the stomach, duodenum, esophagus, and jejunum

      (3) Severe diarrhea and hypokalemia

    b) 70% are malignant with lymph node and hepatic metastases.

    c) Diagnosis is by high serum gastrin levels that respond paradoxically to intravenous secretin and calcium injection.

  5. Diarrheogenic tumors (VIPomas) (Verner–Morrison syndrome): rare

    a) Caused by excessive secretion of vasoactive intestinal polypeptide (VIP)

    b) Clinical characteristics: produces watery diarrhea, hypokalemia, and achlorhydria (WDHA syndrome)

  6. Pancreatic polypeptide (PP) producing tumors: rare

II. Hypofunction of pancreatic islets: diabetes mellitus is the only clinical disease associated with hypofunction of the endocrine pancreas.

  A. Definition: a chronic disorder characterized by relative or actual deficiency of insulin, causing glucose intolerance.

  B. Etiology of diabetes mellitus

    1. Primary diabetes

      a) Insulin-dependent diabetes mellitus (IDDM) (type I)

        (1) Occurs mainly in juveniles (under 30 years, peak 12 years) (juvenile-onset diabetes)

        (2) No association with obesity

        (3) Associated with HLA-B8 and HLA-DW3

        (4) Prone to ketosis

        (5) Reduction in number of islets, and specifically B cells

        (6) Insulin markedly reduced or absent; exogenous insulin administration necessary to prevent ketosis

        (7) Presents with classical symptoms of polyuria, polydipsia, weight loss, thirst

        (8) Etiology unknown; some evidence for autoimmunity and viral infection

    b) Non-insulin-dependent diabetes mellitus (NIDDM) (type II)

        (1) Onset usually in adults over 40 years (maturity-onset diabetes); less commonly, the identical illness occurs in younger (20–25 years) individuals

        (2) Comprises 85% of patients with diabetes

        (3) Obesity frequently present

        (4) No association with HLA system

        (5) Glucose intolerance usually mild; ketosis rare

        (6) Islet mass and B cell mass usually normal

        (7) Insulin present in serum, in either reduced, normal, or even increased amounts

        (8) Control of diabetes may be achieved without insulin by diet or oral agents

        (9) Etiology unknown; probably peripheral resistance to action of insulin

  2. Secondary diabetes

    a) Pancreatic destruction

        (1) Chronic pancreatitis

        (2) Hemochromatosis

        (3) Acute pancreatitis, rarely

        (4) Total pancreatectomy

    b) Excess production of other diabetogenic hormones

        (1) Growth hormone (acromegaly)

        (2) Cortisol (Cushing's syndrome)

        (3) Thyroid hormone (thyrotoxicosis)

        (4) Catecholamines (pheochromocytoma)

        (5) Glucagon (glucagonoma)

C. Metabolic effects of insulin deficiency

  1. Abnormal glucose metabolism

    a) Hyperglycemia, especially after a glucose load

    b) Glucosuria: causes loss of water in kidneys (osmotic diuresis) leading to polyuria, increased serum osmolarity, and thirst

    c) Glucose tolerance test always abnormal

2. Abnormal protein metabolism
   a) Muscle breakdown occurs to provide amino acids for stimulated gluconeogenesis.
   b) Severe muscle wasting and loss of weight is usual in IDDM.
3. Abnormal lipid metabolism
   a) Fat oxidation is stimulated.
   b) The entry of acetyl CoA into the citric acid cycle is impaired
   c) Accumulating acetyl CoA is converted into ketone bodies (acetoacetate, beta-hydroxybutyrate), which are increased in plasma and urine, causing acidosis (ketoacidosis)
   d) Increased ketogenesis occurs in IDDM. In NIDDM the insulin levels are usually sufficient to prevent ketosis.
D. Pancreatic islet changes in diabetes mellitus
   1. Variable from case to case and not diagnostic of diabetes
   2. Islet and beta cell number reduced in IDDM
   3. "Insulitis": a lymphocytic infiltration of islets seen in some cases of early IDDM
   4. Deposition of collagen ("hyaline change") in the islets: occurs in both IDDM and NIDDM
   5. Amyloid change of the islets: commonly seen in long-standing NIDDM
E. Complications of diabetes mellitus
   1. Ketoacidotic coma: in IDDM
   2. Hyperosmolar nonketotic coma
      a) The result of extreme hyperglycemia, renal water loss and increased plasma osmolarity
      b) Usually occurs in elderly patients
   3. Microangiopathy and basement membrane thickening (BMT)
      a) Occurs in all forms of diabetes mellitus
      b) Diffuse basement membrane thickening results from increased deposition of glycoprotein; appears microscopically as a thick homogeneous hyaline widening of the membrane
      c) Thickening of the basement membrane of small blood vessels (microangiopathy) affects kidneys, retina, nerves, skin, etc.
   4. Hyperlipidemia and atherosclerosis
      a) Hypertriglyceridemia with and without hypercholesterolemia

b) Diabetes mellitus is one of the major risk factors for atherosclerotic vascular disease

5. Renal complications
   a) Glomerular lesions
      (1) Diffuse glomerular basement membrane thickening associated with proteinuria
      (2) Nodular glomerulosclerosis (Kimmelsteil–Wilson disease)
      (3) Progressive nephron loss, contraction of the kidney, and chronic renal failure
   b) Renal infections: often severe; may be associated with renal papillary necrosis and gas formation in the kidney (emphysematous pyelonephritis)
   c) Glycogen nephrosis (the Armanni–Ebstein lesion): glycogen accumulation in the cytoplasm of proximal tubular cells; of no significance

6. Eye changes
   a) Retinopathy
      (1) The fourth leading cause of blindness in the United States
      (2) Occurs in long-standing diabetes, both IDDM and NIDDM; a manifestation of microangiopathy
      (3) Nonproliferative retinopathy: characterized by capillary microaneurysms, retinal edema, exudates, and hemorrhages
      (4) Proliferative retinopathy
         i) Is the type of disease most frequently associated with visual impairment
         ii) Characterized by proliferation of small vessels, hemorrhage, fibrosis, and retinal detachment
   b) Other eye changes: cataracts, refractive errors, glaucoma

7. Nervous system changes
   a) Cerebrovascular accidents, usually infarcts, are common in diabetes due to accelerated atherosclerotic disease.
   b) Peripheral neuropathy due to myelin degeneration and, at a later stage, axon degeneration.

8. Skin changes
   a) Increased susceptibility to infections; frequent occurrence of carbuncles
   b) Necrobiosis lipoidica diabeticorum (NLD): a degeneration of dermal collagen that produces nodular lesions, usually in the pretibial region

Table 13-1. "Apudomas" (Tumors of Neuroendocrine Cells)

Site	Tumor	Secretory Products
Anterior pituitary	Pituitary adenoma	GH, ACTH, prolactin, FSH, LH, TSH
Bronchus	Carcinoid, oat-cell carcinoma	5HT, ACTH, ADH, Parathormone
GI tract	Carcinoid	5HT, VIP, gastrin
Pancreas	Islet cell adenoma, carcinoma	Insulin, glucagon, VIP, PP, somatostatin, 5HT, ACTH, bombesin
Thyroid	Medullary carcinoma	Calcitonin
Parathyroid	Adenoma, carcinoma	Parathormone
Adrenal medulla and autonomic ganglia	Pheochromocytoma, Neuroblastoma	Catecholamines
Paraganglia, glomus jugulare, carotid body	Paraganglioma, glomus tumor, chemodectoma	Catecholamines
Skin	Merkel cell tumor	Calcitonin, parathormone

F. Clinical course of diabetes melltius
  1. Average life expectancy is reduced, particularly with onset at a young age.
  2. Causes of death in diabetics, in order of frequency, are myocardial infarction, renal failure, cerebrovascular accidents, infections, ketoacidosis, and hyperosmolar coma.

DIFFUSE NEUROENDOCRINE SYSTEM (THE "APUD" CONCEPT)

I. Diffuse neuroendocrine "APUD" cells
  A. derive from the neural crest (neuroendocrine cells)
  B. have the ability to take up and decarboxylate certain amino acids that are the precursors of fluorogenic amines; hence APUD (amine precursor uptake and decarboxylation) cells
  C. are capable of secreting amines or peptide hormones
  D. contain dense-core neurosecretory granules visible upon electron microscopy

II. The concept of an APUD system is not entirely satisfactory and is beginning to fall into disfavor.

III. "APUDomas" or neuroendocrine tumors arise from cells of the APUD system (Table 13-1). These have certain common features:

A. Excessive amine and/or peptide hormone production, frequently leading to clinical effects

B. Common histologic appearance, characterized by nests and trabeculae of uniform round cells separated by a highly vascular stroma

C. Dense-core neurosecretory granules visible on electron microscopy

D. Positive staining for neuron-specific enolase by immunoperoxidase technique

E. Classified by the cell of origin or the principal substance it produces

14

The Breast

STRUCTURE AND FUNCTION

I. The adult female breast is composed predominantly of fibroadipose stroma, the glands comprising about 10% of the bulk.
II. During pregnancy, there is marked glandular hyperplasia.
III. The lactating breast is composed of closely packed, secreting glands with very little intervening stroma.
IV. After menopause, glands and ducts atrophy, and fibrosis occurs.

CONGENITAL ANOMALIES

I. Supernumerary breast and nipple (polymazia; polythelia) is common, and occurs along the milk line, which extends from the axilla to the pubis.
II. Amastia, absence of the breast, is very rare.

INFLAMMATORY LESIONS

I. Acute mastitis and breast abscess
  A. These commonly occur in the postpartum period at the onset of lactation.
  B. Cracks in nipples provide the portal of entry to bacteria.
  C. *Staphylococcus aureus* is the common agent.
II. Mammary duct ectasia (plasma cell mastitis)
  A. This is uncommon, and tends to occur in perimenopausal women.
  B. Obstruction of lactiferous ducts by inspissated luminal secretions causes dilatation (ectasia) and periductal inflammation.
  C. The segment of breast undergoes chronic inflammation, with plasma cells (plasma cell mastitis) or histiocytes (granulomatous mastitis).
  D. Grossly, the area is indurated and nipple retraction may occur, giving it a resemblance to breast cancer.

III. Fat necrosis
  A. This is uncommon and has an unknown etiology.
  B. The necrotic fat is surrounded by foamy histiocytes, lymphocytes, granulation tissue, and fibrosis.
  C. The localized area of scarring produces a firm, irregular mass, sometimes with skin retraction, that clinically mimics cancer.

FIBROCYSTIC DISEASE

Fibroadenosis, cystic hyperplasia, mammary dysplasia, chronic cystic mastitis, and cystic mastopathy are synonymous with fibrocystic disease.
  I. Incidence
  A. Fibrocystic disease is the most common breast lesion, affecting about 10% of females as a clinically apparent disease. Occurrence of subclinical disease is more frequent.
  B. It occurs after puberty, reaches its maximum severity during reproductive life, and persists into the postmenopausal period.
  II. Etiology
  A. The cause is unknown; it is thought to be an abnormal breast reaction to sex hormones, although no constant endocrine abnormality has been identified.
  B. Oral contraceptives do not increase the risk of fibrocystic disease.
  III. Pathologic changes (Fig. 14-1)
  A. Fibrosis
  B. Cystic change
    1. Cyst formation is considered abnormal when macrocysts (over 3 mm in diameter) are present. These frequently attain a large size, becoming palpable lesions.
    2. Unopened, the cysts appear blue due to the presence in them of a translucent turbid fluid (blue-domed cysts of Duguid).
    3. Cysts are lined by cuboidal, frequently apocrine, epithelium.
  C. Apocrine metaplasia: a change of ductal epithelium into apocrine cells. Apocrine cells have deep eosinophilic cytoplasm and show decapitation secretion.
  D. Adenosis
    1. This is a nonneoplastic proliferation of ductules and glands in the breast lobule.
    2. Sclerosing adenosis has marked fibrosis associated with the epithelial proliferation, resulting in distortion of the glands and an appearance that mimics carcinoma microscopically.

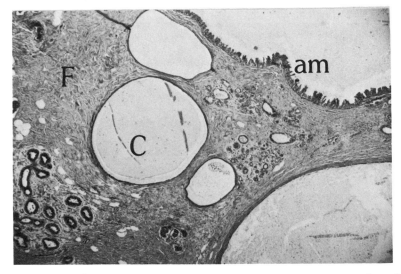

Fig. 14.1 Fibrocystic disease, showing cysts (C) and extensive fibrosis (F). One of the cysts is lined by epithelium that has undergone apocrine metaplasia (am).

    E. Papillomatosis ("epitheliosis")
       1. This is an epithelial proliferation in the ducts that may fill the duct and expand it.
       2. Cellular atypia may be present.
       3. Differentiation from intraductal carcinoma may be difficult.
  IV. Clinical significance of fibrocystic disease
    A. It may produce pain, nipple discharge, and breast masses that must be differentiated from carcinoma.
    B. It represents an increased risk of carcinoma.
       1. The risk is small, estimated at 2–3 times normal.
       2. Increased risk is present where there are
         a) gross (over 3mm) cysts.
         b) papillomatosis.

NEOPLASMS OF THE BREAST

  I. Fibroadenoma
    A. This is a very common benign neoplasm, most commonly occurring in young females.

B. It presents as a discrete, firm, freely movable nodule in the breast.

C. Grossly, it appears as an encapsulated, firm nodule that may be large (giant fibroadenoma).

D. Microscopically, it is composed of a dual population of neoplastic cells: a glandular component and a stromal component. (Fig. 14-2).

E. A lactating adenoma shows hyperplasia of the glands in a fibroadenoma with active secretion.

II. Cystosarcoma phyllodes (phyllodes tumor)

A. This is characterized, like fibroadenoma, by a dual population of cells: epithelial and stromal.

B. The stroma is highly cellular, and may show cytologic atypia and increased mitotic activity.

C. Most phyllodes tumors are benign; 10–20% of phyllodes tumors are malignant with development of metastases.

D. Grossly, they tend to be large, bulky masses with areas of cystic degeneration.

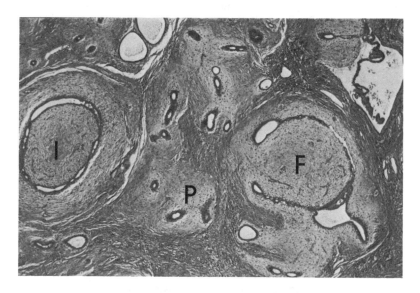

Fig. 14.2. Fibroadenoma. The fibrous component is initially around the epithelial component (pericanalicular (P)), but gradually encroaches on it (F) and finally becomes surrounded by it (intracanalicular (I)).

III. Duct papilloma
    A. This is a benign neoplasm arising commonly in the main lactiferous ducts.
    B. It is usually small (less than 1 cm), forming a delicate papillary growth of benign ductal cells projecting into the duct lumen.
    C. Clinically, the patient with duct papilloma presents with
        1. nipple discharge: serous or bloody.
        2. a subareolar mass, usually small.

IV. Nipple adenoma: rare

V. Carcinoma of the breast
    A. Incidence
        1. Until 1983, carcinoma of the breast was the leading cause of cancer deaths among females. In 1983, it was overtaken by lung cancer.
        2. 100,000 new cases are diagnosed per year in the United States; 35,000 deaths occur every year.
        3. One of seven women in the United States will develop breast carcinoma.
        4. There is a marked geographic variation in incidence; it is most common in the United States and Western Europe, but rare in Japan.
        5. Occurrence of breast cancer is rare before 25 years, uncommon before 30 years, but increases sharply in frequency after age 30.
    B. High-risk factors
        1. Nulliparity, late menopause, first pregnancy after age 30, and early onset of menarche
        2. Fibrocystic disease: slight risk
        3. Family history of breast cancer
        4. Cancer of one breast: increases the risk of a subsequent cancer of the other breast
        5. High-dose estrogen contraceptive pills: slight risk
    C. Etiology of breast cancer
        1. Unknown
        2. Genetic factors: uncertain
        3. Hormonal factors
            a) Estrogens are of questionable importance.
            b) Many breast cancers have estrogen, progesterone and other steroid receptors on their surface, and are "hormone-dependent."
        4. Viral agents
            a) The Bittner milk virus in mice.

b) Antigens similar to mouse mammary tumor virus are present on human breast cancer cells.
D. Clinical characteristics
1. Painless mass
2. Nipple discharge, often bloody
3. Skin retraction, dimpling and ulceration, and nipple retraction: late features
4. Nipple eczema or Paget's disease (see below)
E. Early detection
1. Early detection is important because the early stages of carcinoma have a greater chance of cure than advanced stages.
2. Methods used
a) Self-examination of the breast
b) Mammography: currently recommended for high-risk groups
(1) Patients with a prior breast carcinoma
(2) Patients with a history of breast cancer in the immediate family
(3) All females over 40 years of age
F. Diagnosis
1. Pathologic examination of a biopsy of the mass is the definitive diagnostic technique.
2. Cytologic examination of a sample obtained by fine needle aspiration is increasing in popularity.
G. Treatment
1. Surgery
a) Radical mastectomy
b) Modified radical mastectomy: spares the pectoral muscles; the current standard method
c) Simple mastectomy or "lumpectomy": adequate in selected cases
2. Radiotherapy: breast carcinoma is a moderately radiosensitive tumor.
3. Chemotherapy: routinely used after radical surgery because it has been realized that breast carcinoma is a systemic disease at a very early stage.
4. Hormonal therapy: most useful for estrogen and progesterone receptor-positive breast carcinomas. These represent 60–70% of breast cancers in premenopausal women.
H. Factors affecting prognosis in breast carcinoma
1. Pathologic type of tumor
a) In-situ (noninfiltrating) carcinomas

(1) Lobular carcinoma in situ (LCIS)
  - i) LCIS is neoplastic proliferation of lobular epithelial cells that fill and distend the lobule but are confined within the basement membrane.
  - ii) It tends to be multifocal and bilateral.
  - iii) LCIS increases the risk of developing invasive breast carcinoma; both breasts are at risk.

(2) Ductal carcinoma in situ (DCIS: intraductal carcinoma)
  - i) DCIS is a neoplastic proliferation of ductal epithelial cells, confined within the basement membrane of the duct.
  - ii) Invasion occurs early in most cases. The presence of even minimal invasion (Fig. 14-3) may be associated with metastasis.
  - iii) It is frequently multifocal and bilateral.

b) Invasive breast carcinomas
  (1) Infiltrating ductal carcinoma (IDC)

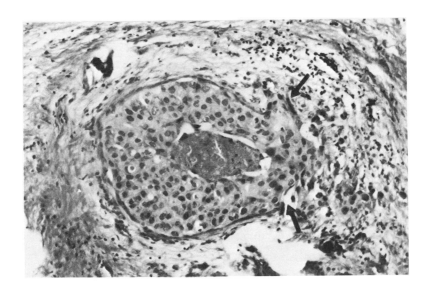

Fig. 14.3. Ductal carcinoma. Malignant cells have distended the duct. There is central necrosis ("comedocarcinoma"). Though predominantly contained by the basement membrane, there is focal invasion through it on one side (arrows).

       i) IDC is most common type of breast cancer (75–80%).

      ii) Grossly, they are hard, gritty, unencapsulated masses.

     iii) Microscopically, large malignant duct cells infiltrate into the fibrous stroma.

     iv) An in-situ component may be associated. This may be DCIS or LCIS.

(2) Infiltrating lobular carcinoma (ILC)

       i) ILC comprises 5–10% of all invasive carcinomas.

      ii) Grossly, they are indistinguishable from infiltrating ductal carcinoma.

     iii) Microscopically, they are distinguished by

        (*A*) smaller, more uniform cells.

        (*B*) the arrangement of tumor cells in single file, separated by fibrosis ("Indian file" arrangement).

        (*C*) the arrangement of tumor cells in concentric rings around normal ducts ("targetoid arrangement").

     iv) The prognosis of ILC is similar to that of infiltrating ductal carcinoma.

c) Breast carcinomas with a better prognosis than IDC

  (1) Medullary carcinoma

       i) Well-circumscribed, soft masses with necrosis and hemorrhage

      ii) Marked lymphocytic reaction around the tumor

     iii) Undifferentiated malignant cells in syncytial sheets

     iv) 5-year survival of over 90%

  (2) Mucinous carcinoma

       i) Secretion of mucin by the cancer cells; the mucin forms large pools in which are groups of small, well-differentiated epithelial cells.

      ii) Slow growing; high 5-year survival

  (3) Tubular carcinoma

       i) Histologically well-differentiated small tubular structures formed by the neoplastic ductal cells

      ii) High 5-year survival rate

  (4) Paget's disease of the nipple

       i) Presents as an eczematoid change in the nipple and skin around it

        ii) Characterized by the presence of carcinoma cells in the epidermis, due to intraepithelial spread of carcinoma

       iii) Invariably associated with carcinoma in the large ducts of the breast.

  d) Breast carcinoma with prognosis worse than IDC

    (1) Inflammatory carcinoma

      i) Characterized by the presence of extensive permeation of dermal lymphatics by carcinoma (dermal lymphatic carcinomatosis)

      ii) Has a very bad prognosis with few patients surviving one year.

    (2) Signet ring cell carcinoma: rare

2. Clinicopathologic stage of the disease

  a) Stage I: tumor less than 5 cm in size without axillary node involvement

  b) Stage II: tumor less than 5 cm in size with axillary node involvement, but without fixation of the nodes (i.e., no invasion through capsule of nodes)

  c) Stage III: tumor involves skin or chest wall; tumor exceeds 5 cm in size; fixation of involved axillary lymph nodes

  d) Stage IV: disseminated metastases irrespective of any other factor

I. Prognosis

1. The overall 5-year survival rate for breast carcinoma is about 60–70%.

2. The prognosis must be individualized according to tumor type and stage of disease. It then varies between 0% 5-year survival for inflammatory carcinoma and 95% for stage I medullary carcinoma.

VI. Other malignant tumors of the breast: extremely rare

  A. Sarcoma: among various kinds of sarcoma occurring in the breast, angiosarcoma is the most common.

  B. Lymphoma

DISEASES OF THE MALE BREAST

I. Gynecomastia

  A. Enlargement of the male breast, unilateral or bilateral

  B. Causes

    1. "Idiopathic": for no apparent reason

    2. Klinefelter's syndrome

3. Increased estrogen levels
   a) Cirrhosis of the liver
   b) Testicular tumors: stromal tumors secreting estrogenic substances
   c) Testicular destruction as occurs in lepromatous leprosy
4. Increased gonadotrophin levels: choriocarcinoma of the testis
5. Increased prolactin levels associated with diseases of the pituitary-hypothalamic axis
6. Drugs such as digitalis

C. Histologically, characterized by dense hyaline collagen and hyperplasia of the ducts.
D. Is a benign condition with no increased risk of carcinoma

II. Carcinoma of the male breast
A. Very rare
B. Behaves in a manner that is identical to infiltrating ductal carcinomas in the female
C. Diagnosis usually made later than in females; 50% of cases have axillary lymph node metastases at time of diagnosis
D. Overall prognosis for carcinoma of the male breast worse than for carcinoma of the female breast

The Urinary System

KIDNEY

I. Clinical manifestations of renal disease
   A. Hematuria: may be painful or painless
   B. Proteinuria: very common finding in many renal diseases.
   C. Acute nephritic syndrome (nephritis): oliguria, hematuria, mild proteinuria, azotemia, hypertension, and mild edema
   D. Nephrotic syndrome: massive proteinuria (over 5 g/24 hours), hypoproteinemia, and edema
   E. Acute renal failure: a marked diminution of urine output (less than 400 ml/day) and azotemia
   F. Chronic renal failure (chronic uremia): characterized by
      1. elevated serum creatinine and urea (azotemia)
      2. inability to concentrate urine, leading to polyuria
      3. metabolic acidosis
      4. failure of renal activation of vitamin D, causing bone changes (renal osteodystrophy)
      5. anemia: normochromic, normocytic, due to failure of erythropoietin production
      6. hypertension
      7. abnormal platelet function
II. Congenital malformations
   A. Renal agenesis: bilateral (fatal) or unilateral (asymptomatic)
   B. Renal hypoplasia: rare; usually unilateral; kidney has five or fewer calyces and is small (below 50 g in an adult), but otherwise normal in structure
   C. Ectopic kidney: common; usually just above the pelvic brim or in the pelvis
   D. Fusion of the kidneys
      1. This occurs in about 0.4% of individuals.
      2. Most commonly the lower poles of the kidneys are fused across the midline by a broad band of renal tissue (horseshoe kidney).
   E. Renal dysplasia
      1. Total renal dysplasia: rare; fatal

      2. Segmental dysplasia: rare; involved area shows cysts and abnormal tubules

F. Cystic disease of the kidney

    1. Adult polycystic disease

      a) Relatively common autosomal dominant disorder

      b) Bilaterally enlarged kidneys whose parencyma is replaced by a mass of cysts of varying size.

      c) Microscopically: cysts are lined by renal tubular epithelium

      d) Clinically: patients present in adult life (40 years) with hypertension and progressive chronic renal failure

    2. Infantile polycystic disease

      a) Rare, autosomal recessive disorder; death from renal failure very early in life

      b) Kidneys bilaterally enlarged; show innumerable, radially oriented, fusiform cysts

    3. Medullary cystic disease: rare

    4. Simple renal cysts: common, insignificant

III. Glomerular diseases

A. Definition

    1. A group of renal diseases characterized by primary abnormality of the glomerulus

    2. Abnormality structural (inflammation, cellular proliferation, basement membrane thickening, fibrosis, epithelial cell changes) and functional (increased permeability causing proteinuria or hemorrhage of glomerular origin)

    3. May be acute or chronic

B. Classification of glomerular diseases

    1. Congenital glomerulonephritis: very rare

      a) Hereditary nephritis, including Alport's syndrome

      b) Congenital nephrotic syndrome

    2. Primary acquired glomerulonephritis: common

      a) Diffuse glomerulonephritis

        (1) Minimal change glomerulonephritis

        (2) Proliferative glomerulonephritis

          i) Poststreptococcal glomerulonephritis

          ii) Mesangial proliferative glomerulonephritis

          iii) Anti-glomerular basement membrane disease (Goodpasture's syndrome)

          iv) Crescentic glomerulonephritis

        (3) Membranous glomerulonephritis

        (4) Mesangiocapillary glomerulonephritis

        (5) Chronic glomerulonephritis

      b) Focal glomerulonephritis

      c) Focal glomerulosclerosis

   3. Secondary acquired glomerulonephritis: common

      a) Systemic lupus erythematosus

      b) Progressive systemic sclerosis

   4. Other glomerular diseases: common

      a) Diabetic glomerulopathy

      b) Amyloidosis

C. Terminology

   1. Focal vs. diffuse: focal glomerular disease shows abnormality in some glomeruli; diffuse affects all

   2. Segmental vs. global: segmental glomerular disease involves only a portion of the glomerulus; global involves the entire glomerulus

   3. Primary vs. secondary: primary glomerular lesion is the main manifestation of disease; secondary lesion is part of a systemic disease

D. Minimal change glomerulonephritis (epithelial cell disease) (Fig. 15-1)

   1. This occurs predominantly in children.

   2. They present with nephrotic syndrome.

   3. The proteinuria is almost always highly selective, with loss of only small molecular weight proteins.

   4. Light microscopy shows no abnormality (hence "minimal change").

   5. Immunofluorescence shows no immunoglobulin or complement deposition.

   6. Electron microscopy shows fusion of the foot processes of the epithelial cells (nonspecific change).

   7. Its pathogenesis is unknown.

   8. Its prognosis is excellent; most patients show complete remission within 8 weeks after starting corticosteroid therapy.

E. Postinfectious glomerulonephritis (Fig. 15-2): synonyms: acute diffuse proliferative glomerulonephritis; post streptococcal glomerulonephritis

   1. One of the most common renal diseases in childhood

   2. Pathogenesis

      a) An infection (commonly Group A, beta-hemolytic streptoccal) precedes the nephritis by 1-3 weeks.

      b) Organisms other than streptococci may be involved.

      c) Immune complexes formed between antigens in the organism and host antibody are deposited in the glo-

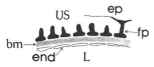

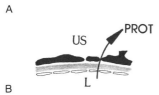

A

B

Fig. 15-1. (A) Normal glomerular filtration membrane. L = capillary lumen, US = urinary space, end = endothelial cell, bm = basement membrane, ep = epithelial cell, fp = foot processes. (B) Minimal change glomerulonephritis; there is fusion of epithelial cell foot processes associated with protein (Prot) leakage.

merular basement membrane, fix complement, and lead to inflammation.

3. Light microscopy
   a) A diffuse glomerulonephritis with edema
   b) The glomeruli show increased cellularity due to proliferation of endothelial and mesangial cells, and infiltration with neutrophils.
   c) Epithelial crescents may be present in a few glomeruli.
   d) Characteristic "humps" appear.
4. Electron microscopy shows large, dome-shaped, electron dense, subepithelial immune complex deposits ("humps").
5. Immunofluorescence shows a granular ("lumpy-bumpy") deposition of IgG and C3 along the glomerular basement membrane.
6. Clinical characteristics
   a) Onset of nephritic syndrome is abrupt. Periorbital edema is typical.
   b) A few patients present with nephrotic syndrome.
   c) Anti-streptolysin O and anti-hyaluronidase are elevated.
   d) Serum C3 is decreased in the acute phase.
7. Prognosis

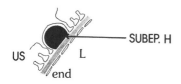

Fig. 15-2. Poststreptococcal glomerulonephritis, showing the subepithelial hump (Subep. h). This is composed of immune complex and fixed complement.

    a) The short-term prognosis is excellent, most patients returning to normal renal function and blood pressure within a year.

    b) The long-term prognosis is excellent (controversial).

F. Mesangial proliferative glomerulonephritis

  1. With mesangial IgG

    a) Common; characterized by increased number of mesangial cells

    b) May occur as an isolated finding or may represent the healing phase of postinfectious glomerulonephritis

  2. With mesangial IgA

    a) IgA Nephropathy (Berger's disease)

      (1) Common; occurs mainly in males between 10 and 30 years

      (2) Presents with hematuria, often recurrent; proteinuria (mild)

      (3) Light microscopy: mesangial hypercellularity and increased matrix; sclerosis common with progressive disease

      (4) Immunofluorescence: IgA in the mesangium as confluent masses or discrete granules

      (5) Electron microscopy: mesangial hypercellularity, sclerosis, and deposits

      (6) Progression very slow; chronic renal failure after a mean period of 6 years

    b) Henoch–Schönlein purpura (HSP)

      (1) Rare: mainly affects children

      (2) Characterized by a systemic vasculitis (skin, joints, intestine, kidneys)

      (3) Pathologic changes similar to Berger's disease

G. Goodpasture's syndrome: synonyms: anti-glomerular basement membrane disease; proliferative glomerulonephritis with pulmonary hemorrhage

  1. Rare; affects young adults, males more than females

  2. Clinical characteristics

    a) Proteinuria and hematuria followed by progressive renal failure

    b) Recurrent hemoptysis with dyspnea, cough, and bilateral pulmonary infiltrates on radiograph

  3. Serum contains anti-glomerular basement membrane antibodies of IgG type that cause type II hypersensitivity disease

  4. Light microscopy

a) Focal and diffuse proliferative glomerulonephritis
b) Necrosis and epithelial crescent formation and fibrosis
5. Immunofluorescence: IgG and C3 deposited in a diffuse linear pattern along the basement membrane
6. Prognosis poor
H. Proliferative glomerulonephritis with extensive crescent formation: synonyms: rapidly progressive glomerulonephritis; subacute glomerulonephritis
1. Characterized by the presence of epithelial crescents in more than 80% of the glomeruli
2. An epithelial crescent
a) is a proliferation of epithelial cells in Bowman's space.
b) is evidence of severe irreversible glomerular damage.
c) is caused by the release of fibrin into Bowman's space.
3. Etiology: usually unknown
a) Occasionally secondary to other diseases such as post-infectious glomerulonephritis
b) Anti-glomerular basement membrane antibodies present in the serum of some cases
4. Present with acute or rapidly progressive renal failure
5. Prognosis very poor
I. Membranous glomerulonephritis: synonyms: membranous nephropathy; epimembranous glomerulonephritis (Fig. 15-3)
1. Commonly occurs in adults (mean 35 years)
2. Clinically, nephrotic syndrome progressing to chronic renal failure
3. Etiology usually unknown
4. Light and electron microscopy: three stages:
a) Stage I: deposition of dome-shaped subepithelial electron-dense deposits (only seen on electron microscopy)
b) Stage II: spikes of basement membrane material protrude toward the epithelial side between the deposits
c) Stage III: the spikes enlarge and fuse on the epithelial side of the deposits, appearing as a thickened basement membrane
d) No hypercellularity
e) With progression, increasing thickness of the basement membrane converts glomerulus into hyaline mass
5. Immunofluorescence: granular deposits of IgG and C3
6. Prognosis: slow progression to chronic renal failure
J. Mesangiocapillary glomerulonephritis (MCGN): synonyms: membranoproliferative glomerulonephritis

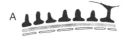

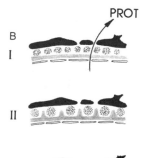

Fig. 15-3. (A) Normal glomerulus. (B) Membranous glomerulonephritis. In stage I there is fusion of foot processes and immune complex deposition on the epithelial side of the basement membrane. In stage II, spikes of basement membrane material protrude outward between deposits and in stage III, the spikes fuse on the epithelial side of the deposits. Prot = protein leakage.

1. Characterized by thickening of the glomerular capillary wall plus proliferation of mesangial cells
2. Two distinct patterns recognized
   a) MCGN Type I (65%).
      (1) A disease of children and young adults, who present with nephrotic syndrome or a mixed nephrotic–nephritic pattern
      (2) Light microscopy: shows proliferation of mesangial cells; basement membrane appears to be thickened and split
      (3) Electron microscopy: shows subendothelial deposits (IgG and C3)
      (4) Serum C3 levels frequently low
      (5) Prognosis poor
   b) Type II MCGN ("Dense deposit disease") (35%)
      (1) Occurs in children and young adults
      (2) Characterized by an intramembranous, dense ribbon-like deposit, leading to basement membrane thickening
      (3) Serum C3 levels low, often markedly
      (4) Prognosis poor

K. Focal glomerulosclerosis: synonyms: focal sclerosing glomerulonephritis; segmental hyalinosis
   1. Characterized by the presence of a focal, segmental sclerotic area in the peripheral part of the glomerulus, frequently near the hilum
   2. Causes nephrotic syndrome in children and young adults
   3. Electron microscopy: in the areas of sclerosis, an increase in the amount of mesangial matrix and collapse of the glomerular capillaries
   4. Prognosis poor
   5. Etiology unknown; a few cases have occurred in heroin addicts and patients with the acquired immunodeficiency syndrome
L. Secondary acquired glomerulonephritis
   1. Systemic lupus erythematosus (SLE) (see Chapter 18)
      a) Causes a variety of clinical effects; renal failure is common
      b) Light microscopic characteristics
         (1) Proliferative glomerulonephritis: focal, diffuse, mesangial, crescentic
         (2) Basement membrane thickening; may be diffuse (resembling membranous glomerulonephritis) or focal
      c) Electron microscopic characteristics: deposition of mesangial, subendothelial, and intramembranous immune complexes
      d) Immunofluorescence: granular IgG and C3 in glomerular capillaries and mesangium
   2. Progressive systemic sclerosis (scleroderma) (see Chapter 18)
      a) Light microscopic characteristics
         (1) Afferent arterioles show fibrinoid necrosis
         (2) Intralobular arteries show "onion skin"-type intimal fibrosis
         (3) Glomeruli show fibrinoid necrosis and segmental basement membrane thickening ("wire-loop"lesions)
      b) Immunofluorescence: granular IgG and C3 in glomerular capillaries
   3. Mixed connective tissue disease: rare
   4. Polyarteritis nodosa (see Chapter 9)
      a) Renal involvement present in 80% of cases
      b) Clinical characteristics: hematuria, proteinuria, and hypertension; rapidly progressive renal failure common

    c) Light microscopic characteristics
       (1) Arcuate and segmental arteries show fibrinoid necrosis, inflammation, thrombosis, microaneurysms, rupture
       (2) Glomeruli show fibrinoid necrosis and proliferative changes; crescents common
   5. Wegener's granulomatosis: rare

M. Chronic glomerulonephritis
   1. The end stage of many diseases affecting glomeruli
   2. Clinical characteristics: chronic renal failure and hypertension
   3. Kidneys greatly reduced in size with a markedly narrowed cortex (granular contracted kidneys)
   4. Microscopic characteristics: marked sclerosis of glomeruli; intervening tubules show atrophy and dilatation ("thyroidization"); interstitium fibrotic
   5. Immunofluorescence and electron microscopy: variable electron-dense deposits containing IgG and C3

N. Other glomerular diseases
   1. Diabetic nephropathy (see Chapter 13)
   2. Amyloidosis (see Chapter 3)

IV. Tubulo-interstitial disease

  A. A group of renal diseases characterized by primary abnormality in the renal tubules and/or interstitium

  B. Infectious interstitial diseases
   1. Acute pyelonephritis
     a) Incidence: very common, particularly in females
     b) Etiology
       (1) An ascending bacterial infection; *Escherichia coli* in 75%
       (2) Abnormalities in the urinary tract leading to stasis of urine (any paralytic or obstructive lesion)
       (3) Vesicoureteric reflux of urine
       (4) Catheterization of the bladder
       (5) The onset of sexual activity ("honeymoon cystitis")
       (6) Pregnancy: effect of progesterone on ureteric muscle
     c) Clinical characteristics
       (1) Acute onset with high fever, flank pain, urinary frequency, and dysuria
       (2) Urine sediment shows neutrophils, white cell casts, and bacteria; culture positive
     d) Gross characteristics: involved kidney is enlarged and

shows abscesses in cortex and radial yellow streaks of suppuration in the medulla
   e) Microscopic characteristics: those of an acute suppurative inflammation; involvement characteristically patchy
   f) Prognosis: excellent with appropriate antibiotic treatment; in a few cases death occurs in the acute phase due to gram-negative bacteremic shock
2. Chronic pyelonephritis
   a) Infectious pyelonephritis: the most common cause of chronic interstitial nephritis; accounts for 15–20% of patients with chronic renal failure
   b) Etiologic factors
      (1) Chronic obstructive pyelonephritis
          i) Common; obstruction may be mechanical (calculi, prostatism, neoplasms) or functional (neurogenic bladder)
          ii) Associated with dilatation of pelvicalyceal system (hydronephrosis)
      (2) Chronic pyelonephritis associated with vesicoureteric reflux: occurs particularly in children
   c) Clinical characteristics: manifests as hypertension and chronic renal failure
   d) Pathologic characteristics
      (1) Irregular scarring of the kidneys, which are asymmetrically contracted; renal pelvis deformed and dilated
      (2) Microscopic characteristics: marked, but frequently patchy, interstitial inflammation and fibrosis; glomeruli show periglomerular fibrosis and global sclerosis
3. Renal tuberculosis: rare
   a) Kidney grossly enlarged; may show several yellow, crumbling, often large cavitary foci
   b) Microscopic characteristics: caseating epithelioid cell granulomas; acid-fast bacilli can usually be demonstrated
   c) Clinical characteristics: a combination of chronic inflammatory (low-grade fever, weight loss) and urinary symptoms (hematuria, frequency)
C. Toxic tubulo-interstitial disease
1. Analgesic nephropathy
   a) Excessive use of analgesics (phenacetin, aspirin) a rel-

atively common cause of chronic renal disease in Australia and Europe; rare in the United States
- b) Pathological characteristics: necrosis of the renal papillae followed by fibrosis and calcification
- c) Clinical characteristics: hematuria, ureteric colic, hypertension; and progressive renal failure
2. Radiation nephritis: rare
3. Drug-induced nephrotoxicity
- a) Acute tubulo-interstitial nephritis
    - (1) Most commonly caused by methicillin
    - (2) An immune hypersensitivity reaction
    - (3) Pathological characteristics: tubular degeneration and necrosis and marked inflammation of the interstitium
    - (4) Recovery usual when the drug is withdrawn
- b) Acute renal tubular necrosis: may be caused by aminoglycosides, amphotericin
- c) Nephrotic syndrome: may be caused by Troxidone, gold, mercurial diuretics
4. Heavy metal toxicity
- a) Mercurial compounds: cause proximal convoluted tubule damage
- b) Lead poisoning: damages the entire tubule
V. Vascular diseases of the kidney
- A. Nephrosclerosis (hypertensive renal disease)
    1. Benign nephrosclerosis: common
    - a) Occurs in most patients with essential hypertension
    - b) Pathological characteristics
        - (1) Mild, symmetric reduction in kidney size; finely granular surface
        - (2) Typical hyaline thickening of the walls of small arteries and arterioles
        - (3) Global sclerosis of glomeruli; atrophy of associated nephron, leading to interstitial fibrosis
    - c) Changes usually mild; chronic renal failure in fewer than 5% of cases
    2. Malignant nephrosclerosis: rare
    - a) Renal disease associated with malignant hypertension
    - b) Pathological characteristics
        - (1) Slightly enlarged smooth kidneys showing numerous petechial hemorrhages
        - (2) Fibrinoid necrosis of arterioles and glomeruli

          (3) Intimal cellular proliferation and fibrosis ("onion skinning") seen in interlobular arteries

     c) Clinical manifestations

          (1) Proteinuria with microscopic and macroscopic hematuria

          (2) Rapidly progressing renal failure

B. Renal artery stenosis

  1. Etiology

     a) Atherosclerosis: the most common cause

     b) Fibromuscular dysplasia of the renal artery: rare, occurring in younger patients (20–40 years)

     c) Post transplantation stenosis: rare

  2. Clinical characteristics: presents with hypertension caused by increased renin secretion

C. Renal changes in shock

  1. Shock of all types is associated with renal arteriolar constriction. This produces a series of renal changes.

  2. Prerenal uremia ("functional renal insufficiency")

     a) This is an appropriate physiologic response of the kidneys (to retain fluid and maintain blood pressure).

     b) Decreased glomerular filtration pressure results in the excretion of a small volume of highly concentrated urine.

     c) No morphologic changes are seen in the kidney. Reversal of shock leads to return to normalcy.

  3. Acute tubular necrosis (ATN)

     a) The result of continued renal vasoconstriction

     b) Characterized by necrosis of tubular epithelium, maximally affecting the distal convoluted tubule

     c) Clinical characteristics

          (1) Acute renal failure, with oliguria and azotemia

          (2) Oliguric phase: lasts 10–14 days

          (3) Oliguric phase followed by the diuretic phase, in which urine output increases but tubular function is still impaired

          (4) Complete recovery in 2–3 weeks

  4. Renal cortical necrosis: rare; characterized by necrosis of the entire renal cortex, including glomeruli; high mortality

VI. Neoplasms of the kidney

  A. Benign neoplasms

    1. Renal cortical adenoma

      a) Common, usually an incidental finding

b) Well-circumscribed, round, yellowish nodule in the cortex; usually less than 2 cm in size

c) Histologically composed of cytologically benign cells arranged in a papillary or solid pattern

2. Oncocytoma ("proximal tubular adenoma")
   a) A special kind of adenoma, believed to be derived from proximal tubular cells
   b) May be very large; no necrosis or hemorrhage
   c) Histologically composed of a uniform population of large cells having small round nuclei and abundant pink, granular cytoplasm

3. Angiomyolipoma
   a) Rare; may occur sporadically or in tuberous sclerosis
   b) May be solitary or multiple and bilateral; often large
   c) Benign
   d) Hamartomatous mass composed of mature fat, smooth muscle, and abnormal blood vessels

B. Malignant neoplasms
   1. Renal adenocarcinoma: synonyms: renal cell carcinoma; hypernephroma; clear cell carcinoma; Grawitz' tumor (Fig. 15-4, 15-5)
      a) The most common malignant neoplasm of the kidney; incidence increases with age
      b) Gross characteristics (Fig. 15-4)
         (1) Varies in size from small to massive; solid
         (2) Cut surface variegated with yellow-orange, hemorrhagic (red-black), and fibrous (gray) areas
         (3) Necrosis, cystic changes, and calcification common
         (4) Local invasion through the capsule and into the renal vein (Fig. 15-5) common
      c) Microscopic composition
         (1) Large clear cells (Fig. 15-5), granular oncocytic cells, and anaplastic cells
         (2) A solid, alveolar, or tubulopapillary arrangement
         (3) Highly vascular
         (4) Can be graded histologically: grade I (well-differentiated) to grade III (anaplastic).
      d) Clinical characteristics
         (1) Hematuria and renal mass
         (2) Evidence of metastases in bone, lung, liver, brain
         (3) A few renal adenocarcinomas secrete hormones, including

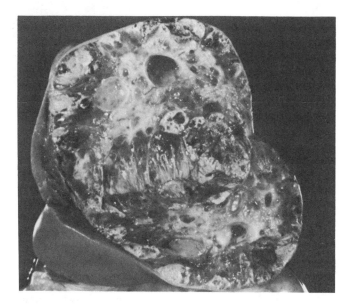

Fig. 15-4. Renal adenocarcinoma showing the typical variegated appearance. Note normal kidney to the left and below the large tumor mass.

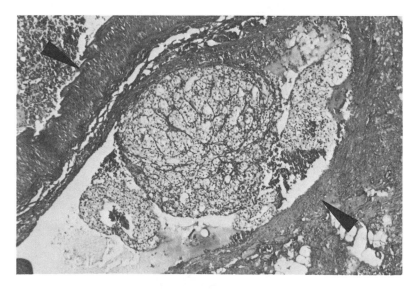

Fig. 15-5. Clear cell renal adenocarcinoma in lumen of renal vein at the hilum of the kidney. Renal vein indicated by arrows.

        i) parathormone: hypercalcemia, low serum phosphate

       ii) erythropoietin, causing polycythemia

  e) Clinical staging

    (1) Stage 1: limited to the kidney

    (2) Stage 2: infiltration outside renal capsule, but confined by Gerota's fascia

    (3) Stage 3: renal vein involvement or hilar lymph node involvement

    (4) Stage 4: extension ouside Gerota's fascia, or distant metastases

  f) Prognosis: 5-year survival about 40%

2. Nephroblastoma (Wilms' tumor)

  a) Constitute about 25–30% of cancers in childhood

  b) Abdominal mass present in most cases

  c) Gross characteristics: a large, firm tumor that often shows cystic change; bilateral nephroblastoma rare

  d) Microscopic characteristics

    (1) The most primitive nephroblastomas resemble renal embryonic mesenchymal tissue.

    (2) Differentiation may occur into epithelial tubular structures, primitive glomerular structures and mesenchymal (cartilage, smooth muscle, striated muscle, bone) tissue.

    (3) According to the degree of differentiation, three histologic grades are recognized.

  e) Prognosis: has improved dramatically with chemotherapy following surgery

3. Urothelial neoplasms: arise in the renal pelvis; uncommon

URETER

I. Congenital anomalies

  A. Congenital anomalies occur in about 2% of autopsies as incidental findings.

  B. They include abnormalities in position and number (double and bifid ureter).

  C. They may cause obstruction.

II. Urinary tract calculi (urolithiasis)

  A. Very common clinical problem, occurring in about 0.5–2% of the general population.

  B. Urinary calculi form in the renal pelvis or bladder.

  C. Etiology and types of calculi

1. Calcium oxalate stones (70%)
   a) These are hard, usually small (less than 5 mm in diameter), and may be smooth, round, or jagged; they are often multiple.
   b) Calcium oxalate precipitation occurs in
      (1) hypercalcemia associated with hypercalciuria.
      (2) idiopathic hypercalciuria without hypercalcemia.
      (3) hyperoxaluria: rare.
2. Phosphate stones (15%)
   a) These are composed of a mixture of phosphates: "triple" phosphate.
   b) Phosphate precipitation occurs in alkaline urine and is associated with infection of the urinary tract by urea-splitting bacteria (Proteus).
   c) They are grayish-white, soft with an irregular shape; they often become large, filling the renal pelvicalyceal system and taking its shape ("staghorn calculus").
3. Uric acid stones (10%)
   a) These are composed of urates, are yellowish brown, usually small, hard, and smooth. Multiple stones are common.
   b) They are precipitated in acidic urine.
   c) They are radiolucent, not visible on routine radiographs.
4. Cystine stones: rare and associated with cystinuria.

D. Clinical effects of calculi
   1. Hematuria
   2. Pain, typically severe renal colic, associated with the passage of small stones down the ureter
   3. Urinary tract obstruction with hydronephrosis
   4. A markedly increased incidence of urinary tract infection

III. Neoplasms of the ureters: rare, most commonly urothelial

URINARY BLADDER

I. Congenital anomalies
   A. Urachal abnormalities
      1. Persistence of the entire urachus causes a vesicoumbilical fistula.
      2. Persistence of parts of the urachus predisposes to infection leading to sinuses and fistulae.
      3. Urachal cysts and neoplasms occur rarely.
   B. Exstrophy of the bladder (ectopia vesicae)
      1. Very rare; present at birth

    2. Associated with failure of development of the anterior wall of the bladder and the overlying abdominal wall

II. Inflammatory lesions of the bladder
  A. Acute bacterial cystitis
    1. Common ascending infection caused by coliform bacteria, commonly *Escherichia coli, Proteus* ssp. and *Streptococcus faecalis*
    2. More common in females, and etiologically related to sexual intercourse, pregnancy, and instrumentation
    3. Clinical characteristics: presents with lower abdominal pain, frequent dysuria, pyuria, and fever.
  B. Acute radiation cystitis: occurs in cases where the bladder is included in pelvic irradiation for malignant neoplasms
  C. Cyclophosphamide: causes an acute hemorrhagic cystitis
  D. Tuberculosis: rare; complicates renal tuberculosis
  E. Schistosomiasis
    1. The perivesical venous plexus is the favored habitat of *Schistosoma haematobium*; it is common in Egypt and the Middle East.
    2. The ova pass through the bladder wall and are passed in the urine.
    3. In their passage through the wall, they cause marked inflammation, suppurative and granulomatous, with numerous eosinophils.
    4. The epithelium frequently shows squamous metaplasia. There is a greatly increased risk of squamous carcinoma.
  F. Malakoplakia
    1. A peculiar chronic inflammation characterized by yellowish plaques, nodules, or polyps in the bladder mucosa
    2. Composed of macrophages that have in their cytoplasm
      a) partially digested bacterial remnants
      b) small, round, calcified bodies (Michaelis–Gutman bodies)
    3. Believed to be due to a defect in macrophage removal of phagocytosed bacteria

III. Miscellaneous diseases
  A. Bladder diverticula
    1. May be congenital; occurs in childhood
    2. Acquired diverticula: commonly results from bladder neck obstruction by a hyperplastic prostate
    3. Predisposes to infection, calculi, and urothelial neoplasms
  B. Bladder fistulae
    1. May communicate with the skin, intestine, or the female reproductive organs

    2. Causes

       a) Trauma: obstetric trauma may cause vesicovaginal fistula

       b) Inflammation: diverticulitis of the colon: Crohn's disease

       c) Neoplasms: carcinoma of the cervix, colon, bladder

    3. Effects

       a) Vesicovaginal fistula causes constant dribbling of urine through the vagina.

       b) Vesicointestinal fistulae cause the passage of feces (fecuria) and gas (pneumaturia) with urine.

  C. Bladder Calculi

    1. May form in the bladder (primary) or descend from the kidney (secondary)

    2. Have the same composition and etiology as uretic calculi

IV. Neoplasms of the bladder

  A. Urothelial neoplasms

    1. Incidence

       a) Uncommon in the United States and Europe

       b) Very rare in Japan; very common in Egypt (complicates Schistosomiasis)

    2. Etiology

       a) Chemical carcinogens: aniline dyes containing benzidine and 2 alpha-naphthylamine

       b) Cigarette smoking: increases the risk

       c) Squamous carcinoma: complicates schistosomiasis

    3. Carcinoma in situ

       a) Usually occurs in males over 40 years; no symptoms

       b) Microscopic characteristics: epithelium shows disturbed maturation and cytologic evidence of malignancy

       c) Frequently multifocal; may extend into ureters and urethra

       d) Has a poor prognosis with rapid development of high-grade invasive carcinoma

    4. Gross characteristics

       a) The better-differentiated neoplasms are papillary, often large masses protruding into the lumen.

       b) Poorly differentiated neoplasms are ulcerative and frequently show evidence of infiltration of the bladder wall.

       c) Carcinoma in situ shows no gross alteration.

       d) Multiple neoplasms are common.

    5. Histologic characteristics

       a) Most bladder cancers are transitional cell carcinomas.

       b) Well-differentiated neoplasms are papillary with cytologically bland cells and a low mitotic rate. Cellularity of papillae determine grades I and II carcinoma.

    c) Grades III and IV carcinomas have solid growth patterns and show cytologic anaplasia and high mitotic rates.

    d) Squamous and glandular differentiation is common in high-grade carcinomas.

B. Other epithelial neoplasms
   1. Pure squamous carcinoma: rare
   2. Pure adenocarcinoma of the bladder: rare

C. Clinical characteristics
   1. Painless hematuria
   2. Involvement of the trigone, which may cause frequency and dysuria
   3. Involvement of the ureteric orifice, which may lead to hydronephrosis and pyelonephritis
   4. Rarely, development of fistulous tracts due to invasion into adjacent organs (colon, usually)

D. Clinical staging
   1. Stage 0: carcinoma in situ
   2. Stage 1A: tumors that shows no invasion of bladder muscle
   3. Stage 1B: tumors invade bladder muscle but do not extend through it
   4. Stage 2: tumors infiltrate full thickness of muscle wall into perivesical tissue
   5. Stage 3: regional lymph node involvement
   6. Stage 4: fixation of neoplasm to other pelvic structures or distant metastases

E. Prognosis
   1. Depends on clinical stage: with appropriate surgical resection, 80% of cases of stage II neoplasms survive 5 years. With extension outside the bladder, the 5-year survival drops to 20%.
   2. Depends on histologic grade: the better-differentiated the neoplasm, the better the prognosis.

16

The Reproductive System

MALE REPRODUCTIVE SYSTEM

I. Testis and epididymis
  A. Abnormal testicular descent
    1. Failure of descent (undescended testis; cryptorchidism): common; the undescended testis may be in the pelvic cavity (15%), in the inguinal canal (60%), or superficially in the inguinal region (25%).
    2. Abnormal descent of the testis (ectopic testis): rare; the testis is located outside its normal descent route, in the root of the penis, the upper thigh, or in the perineum.
    3. Extrascrotal testis
      a) Appears normal until about puberty. Placement in the scrotum before age 6–8 assures normal function.
      b) After puberty, a misplaced testis becomes atrophic and fibrous.
    4. Complications associated with an extrascrotal testis
      a) Greater susceptibility to injury and torsion
      b) Increased incidence of testicular malignant neoplasms
  B. Inflammatory lesions
    1. Acute epididymo-orchitis
      a) A common infection; caused by *Escherichia coli* and *Neisseria gonorrhoeae*
      b) Infection of the epididymis by organisms from the urethra
      c) Acute pyogenic inflammation of the epididymis, commonly extending into the testis
      d) Clinical characteristics: acute onset with high fever, pain, and tenderness of the scrotum
      e) Rapid resolution with antibiotics
    2. Tuberculous epididymo-orchitis
      a) Secondary to renal tuberculosis; bacilli reach epididymis via infected urine.
      b) Chronic granulomatous inflammation of epidiymis and testis with reactive fibrosis causes nodular enlargement.

      c) Caseous material may ulcerate and drain through the skin of the posterior scrotum in untreated cases.

   3. Mumps orchitis

      a) Mild acute inflammation of the testis is common in mumps.

      b) Very rarely, severe inflammation causes atrophy and fibrosis, leading to sterility.

   4. Syphilis

      a) Affects the testis in the tertiary (late) stage

      b) Characterized by the formation of a rubbery, firm mass of granulomatous inflammation (gumma)

   5. Granulomatous orchitis (idiopathic)

      a) Uncommon; uncertain etiology

      b) Microscopic characteristics

         (1) Destruction of the normal structure of the testis

         (2) Multiple epithelioid granulomas in relation to seminiferous tubules; caseous necrosis absent

      c) Gross characteristics: testis is enlarged, slightly painful, and firm

C. Vascular lesions: torsion of testis

   1. A common condition caused by twisting of the spermatic cord, leading to venous obstruction and infarction

   2. Occurs due to the presence of an abnormality of the testis or its ligaments; common in undescended testes

   3. Clinical characteristics: sudden onset of intense pain and swelling

D. Testicular neoplasms

   1. Germ cell neoplasms

      a) 95% of testicular neoplasms

      b) Age incidence

         (1) Seminomas: 25–50-year age group

         (2) Embryonal carcinomas and teratomas: children and young adults, decreasing in frequency after age 35 years

      c) Classification: according to their differentiation

         (1) Embryonal carcinoma: undifferentiated (20%)

         (2) Seminoma: seminiferous differentiation (30%)

         (3) Teratoma: somatic differentiation (10%)

         (4) Choriocarcinoma: trophoblastic differentiation (rare)

         (5) Yolk sac carcinoma: yolk sac differentiation (rare)

         (6) Mixed: different elements in various combinations (40%)

      d) Clinical characteristics

       (1) Usually present as a painless mass in the testis
       (2) Not uncommonly manifest as a metastasis (retro-peritoneum, lung, brain)

  e) Gross characteristics
       (1) Seminoma: firm, rubbery, homogeneous gray-white cut surface, resembling a raw potato (Fig. 16-1)
       (2) Teratoma: solid and cystic areas; cartilage and bone may be present
       (3) Embryonal carcinoma and yolk sac carcinoma: solid, fleshy lesions that show extensive hemorrhage and necrosis
       (4) Choriocarcinoma: extremely hemorrhagic

  f) Microscopic characteristics
       (1) Seminoma
           i) Sheets of uniform, round, germ cells resembling spermatogonia; a central nucleus and glycogen-rich clear cytoplasm
           ii) Fibrous septa infiltrated by lymphocytes
           iii) Granulomatous inflammation: present in 50%

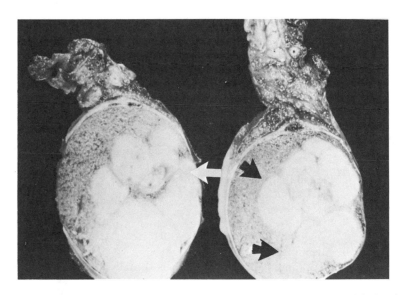

Fig. 16-1. Seminoma of testis. The cute surface shows a homogeneous lobulated white mass replacing part of the testis.

(2) Embryonal carcinoma: primitive, highly malignant appearing cells with numerous mitotic figures, necrosis, and hemorrhage; arranged in solid, glandular, and papillary patterns

(3) Teratoma

    i) Structures belonging to all three germinal layers: endoderm (gut, respiratory epithelium), ectoderm (skin, neural tissue), and mesoderm (cartilage, bone, muscle)

    ii) Elements may be mature, adult-type tissue (mature teratoma) or primitive embryonal-type tissue (immature teratoma)

    iii) Mature and immature teratomas of the testis biologically malignant

(4) Choriocarcinoma: presence of cyto- and syncytiotrophoblastic tissue; extensive hemorrhage is the rule; immunological stains for beta-HCG positive

(5) Yolk sac carcinoma: composed of primitive cells forming a fine, lace-like pattern; Schiller–Duvall (glomeruloid) bodies characteristic; stains positively for alpha-fetoprotein

g) Tumor markers in blood

(1) Beta-HCG is elevated in any neoplasm that has a choriocarcinoma component or syncytiotrophoblastic cells.

(2) Alpha-fetoprotein is elevated in embryonal carcinoma and yolk sac carcinoma.

h) All germ cell tumors of the testis are malignant

i) Treatment

(1) Seminoma is extremely radiosensitive.

(2) All germ cell neoplasms are highly sensitive to modern combined chemotherapeutic regimens. These have greatly improved the prognosis.

2. Gonadal stromal neoplasms: rare

  a) Leydig (interstitial) cell tumors: secrete androgens

  b) Sertoli cell tumor

3. Malignant lymphoma: rare; occurs in older (over 50 years) patients

4. Adenomatoid tumors

  a) Common benign neoplasm, usually occurring in the epididymis

  b) Gross characteristics: a circumscribed, firm nodule, usually small, with a homogeneous gray-white cut surface

      c) Microscopic characteristics: consists of mesothelial lined spaces and stroma composed of fibroblasts, collagen, and smooth muscle

      d) Also found in the pelvic cavity in females

II. Prostate

  A. Acute prostatitis

    1. Common causative bacteria are *Escherichia coli* and *Neisseria gonorrhoeae.*

    2. Clinically, it manifests as pain associated with urination and ejaculation. Marked tenderness is present over the organ, which is enlarged, firm, and infiltrated by numerous neutrophils, lymphocytes, plasma cells, and macrophages.

  B. Nodular hyperplasia of the prostate: synonym: benign prostatic hyperplasia (BPH)

    1. Incidence

      a) BPH is present in 95% of males over 70 years.

      b) Clinically significant BPH is very common, being present in about 5–10% of males over 70.

    2. Etiology

      a) Unknown

      b) Hormones: decline in androgens may be important

    3. Gross characteristics

      a) The lateral lobes and median lobe, which constitute the periurethral part of the gland, are maximally involved.

      b) The gland is enlarged, often reaching a massive size. It is firm, rubbery, and multinodular.

    4. Microscopic characteristics

      a) The nodules are composed of a variable mixture of hyperplastic glandular elements and hyperplastic stromal muscle.

      b) The glands are larger than normal and lined by tall epithelium that is frequently thrown into papillary projections.

    5. Clinical characteristics

      a) Obstruction of urinary outflow from bladder

        (1) Decreased flow

        (2) Incomplete emptying of the bladder, leading to increased frequency

      b) Complications

        (1) Dilatation and muscular hypertrophy of bladder caused by chronic retention of urine

        (2) Acute retention of urine due probably to sudden swelling associated with infarction of a nodule

    (3) Hematuria, also probably the result of infarction
    (4) Urinary infection because of stasis
    (5) Hydronephrosis and chronic renal failure
C. Neoplasms of the prostate
  1. Carcinoma of the prostate
    a) Incidence
      (1) Common
      (2) Most common in American Blacks, fairly common in Caucasions, very uncommon in Oriental races
    b) Etiology
      (1) Unknown
      (2) Androgens: prostatic cancer cells are androgen dependent
    c) Gross characteristics
      (1) The affected area is hard and gritty, appearing as an irregular, ill-defined, grayish-yellow area on cut section.
      (2) Nearly all cancers occur in the outer part of the gland. About 75% arise in the posterior lobe.
      (3) The size of the neoplasm varies from microscopic to massive.
    d) Microscopic characteristics
      (1) Prostatic carcinomas are adenocarcinomas arising in the glandular epithelium.
      (2) The cancer may be well differentiated, forming small or large glands, or poorly differentiated, with single malignant cells invading the stroma.
      (3) Histologic grading based on differentiation is useful in predicting prognosis.
    e) Dissemination
      (1) Local spread in the pelvis after extension through the prostatic capsule
      (2) Lymphatic spread to regional lymph nodes: common
      (3) Hematogenous spread to the lumbosacral spine: occurs early
    f) Clinical staging
      (1) Stage A: occult cancer, incidental finding; subdivided into A1 and A2 depending on quantity of cancer found
      (2) Stage B: confined within prostatic capsule
      (3) Stage C: extracapsular extension
      (4) Stage D: distant metastases

      g) Clinical characteristics
         (1) Urinary symptoms: dysuria, hematuria, frequency occur late because of the peripheral location of the tumor
         (2) Back pain due to vertebral metastases a common presenting feature
      h) Diagnosis
         (1) Digital palpation of the gland at rectal examination, followed by needle biopsy of a suspicious area
         (2) Serum prostatic acid phosphatase elevated in cancers that have infiltrated outside the capsule
      i) Prognosis
         (1) Depends on clinical stage and to a lesser extent on histologic grade
         (2) With early disease (Stage B): 80% survive 5 years following aggressive surgery
         (3) With stage D disease: only 20% survive 5 years
   2. Other prostatic neoplasms: rare

III. Penis
  A. Congenital anomalies
    1. Hypospadias: urethral opening situated on the ventral aspect of the penis at a variable distance from the tip
    2. Epispadias: opening of urethra on dorsal aspect of the penis
    3. Phimosis: an excessively small orifice in the prepuce that in extreme cases obstructs urinary outflow
  B. Neoplasms
    1. Condyloma acuminatum (venereal wart)
      a) Caused by a papilloma virus, is transmitted venereally
      b) Varies in size from 1 mm to several centimeters (giant condyloma of Buschke and Lowenstein).
      c) Appears as a papillary proliferation of benign squamous epithelium; virus causes vacuolation of the cytoplasm ("koilocytosis")
    2. Carcinoma in situ (Bowen's disease; erythroplasia of Queyrat)
      a) Appears as a red plaque on the glans or prepuce
      b) Has a high risk of subsequent invasive carcinoma
    3. Carcinoma of the penis
      a) Incidence
         (1) Uncommon in the United States; common in Oriental races

    (2) Incidence low in the circumcised male
  b) Gross characteristics
    (1) Common sites: glans and inner surface of the pre-
      puce
    (2) Early lesion: elevated, hard white papule followed by
      an ulcer with raised edges
    (3) A papillomatous or warty growth (less commonly)
  c) Microscopic characteristics: a squamous carcinoma of
    variable differentiation
  d) Behavior
    (1) Penile carcinoma shows slow growth locally.
    (2) Invasion of corpora cavernosa occurs early.
    (3) At the time of presentation, about 25–30% of patients
      have regional (inguinal) lymph node involvement.
    (4) Distant metastases occur only at a very late stage of the
      disease.
    (5) With adequate surgical removal of the primary and
      draining lymph nodes, 5-year survival approaches
      50%.

FEMALE REPRODUCTIVE SYSTEM

 I. Congenital anomalies
  A. These are commonly the result of abnormal fusion of the paired
    Müllerian ducts.
  B. Complete failure of fusion results in two completely separate
    uteri and double vagina.
  C. Lesser degrees of failure of fusion in decreasing severity lead
    to
    1. double uterus and cervices with a single vagina.
    2. a septate uterus, in which the endometrial cavity is divided
      but opens into a single endocervical canal.
    3. a bicornuate or subseptate uterus, in which the endometrial
      cavity is divided only in its fundal part.
  D. These congenital anomalies may be associated with sub-
    fertility.
 II. Ovaries
  A. Nonneoplastic lesions (sometimes mistaken for neoplasms)
    1. Follicular cysts: common; lined by granulosa cells; of no
      significance
    2. Corpus luteum
      a) May be large enough to be palpable, particularly if it is
        cystic or hemorrhagic

      b) Luteoma of pregnancy: appears as a mass, sometimes large, in the last trimester of pregnancy; involutes spontaneously after delivery

   3. Polycystic ovaries

      a) Polycystic ovaries are characterized by

         (1) bilaterally enlarged ovaries that show multiple follicular cysts in the outer, subcapsular region.

         (2) absence of corpora lutea (failure of ovulation).

         (3) hyperplastic ovarian stroma with thickening of the capsule.

      b) They are associated clinically with

         (1) amenorrhea, infertility, and virilism (Stein–Levinthal syndrome).

         (2) estrogen excess, causing endometrial hyperplasia and abnormal bleeding.

      c) The cause is probably an abnormal pattern of secretion of pituitary gonadotrophins.

   4. Endometriosis (see below)

B. Neoplasms of the ovary

   1. Incidence

      a) 75–80% of ovarian neoplasms are benign.

      b) Ovarian cancer accounts for about 5% of all cancers in females (the fifth most common cancer in American women).

   2. Classification of ovarian neoplasms (see Table 16-1)

   3. Serous tumors of the ovary

      a) Serous tumors comprise 30% of ovarian neoplasms; they are frequently bilateral.

      b) They occur in the 15–50-year age group, and tend to be benign in younger women

      c) Serous cystadenocarcinoma is the most common malignant ovarian neoplasm.

      d) Based on the microscopic appearance, three different biologic types are recognized:

         (1) Benign serous cystadenoma (Fig. 16-2)

            i) These vary in size from small cysts to large cystic neoplasms.

            ii) The larger cysts are multilocular, contain serous fluid, and have a smooth external surface; the internal surface is smooth or has delicate papillae.

            iii) Microscopically, the lining is a simple cuboidal or flattened epithelium that is cytologically benign.

Table 16-1. Classification of Ovarian Neoplasms

Neoplasms of celomic epithelium on surface (75% of ovarian neoplasms; 95% of ovarian malignancies)
  Serous tumors
  Mucinous tumors
  Endometrioid carcinoma
  Undifferentiated carcinoma
  Brenner tumor—benign
Germ cell neoplasms (15% of ovarian neoplasms; 1% of malignancies)
  Teratoma—mature and immature
  Dysgerminoma
  Yolk sac tumor (endodermal sinus tumor)
  Others
Stromal neoplasms (10% of ovarian neoplasms; 3% of malignancies)
  Granulosa-theca cell tumors
  Fibro-thecoma
  Sertoli-Leydig cell tumor (androblastoma)
Metastatic carcinoma

    (2) Borderline serous tumors (Fig. 16-3)
        i) Distinguished from benign serous cystadenoma
          by
          (*A*) exuberant papillary ingrowths
          (*B*) complex histologic pattern.
          (*C*) the taller, more active-appearing neoplastic
            cells lining the papillae having greater degrees of stratification and cytologic atypia
       ii) Distinguished from serous cystadenocarcinoma
         by the lack of infiltration of the stroma or capsule of the neoplasm
      iii) Behave in a low-grade malignant manner, metastasizing to the peritoneal cavity
      iv) Have a good prognosis (70% 10-year survival)
    (3) Serous cystadenocarcinoma
        i) Grossly, it shows extreme papillations and large solid, nodular masses in the wall of the cyst.
       ii) The serosal surface of the cyst may be irregular due to infiltrating papillary masses.
      iii) Microscopically, it has a highly complex papil-

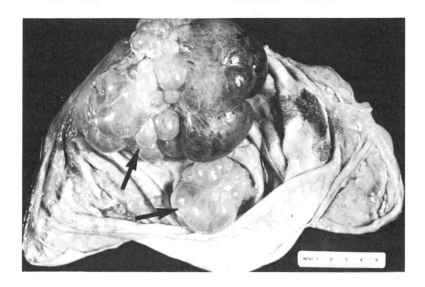

Fig. 16-2. Benign serous cystadenoma, ovary. The multilocular cyst has a smooth internal lining. Arrows = unopened locules distended with fluid.

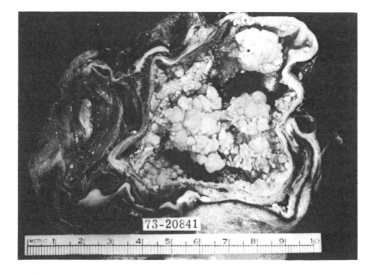

Fig. 16-3. Borderline serous tumor, ovary. The inner lining is thrown into numerous complex papillary masses.

lary pattern with marked cytologic atypia and stromal or capsular invasion.

iv) Calcification in the form of round, laminated psammoma bodies is commonly present.

v) Serous cystadenocarcinoma is a highly malignant neoplasm which infiltrates and metastasizes early in its course and has a bad prognosis: 10% 10-year survival.

4. Mucinous tumors
   a) Account for 20% of ovarian neoplasms
   b) Less frequently bilateral than serous tumors
   c) Benign, borderline, and carcinomatous mucinous tumors recognized using criteria similar to serous tumors
   d) Differ from serous cysts in that
      (1) they are filled with a glairy mucoid fluid
      (2) their epithelium is tall and columnar with basal nuclei resembling endocervical epithelium

5. Endometrioid carcinoma
   a) Accounts for 15% of ovarian cancers
   b) Defined by its microscopic resemblance to endometrial carcinoma
   c) May arise in foci of endometriosis
   d) Has a 50% 5-year survival rate

6. Germ cell neoplasms
   a) Benign cystic teratoma ("dermoid cyst")
      (1) Account for about 15% of ovarian neoplasms; bilateral in 10%
      (2) Cystic mass usually containing thick sebaceous material and hair in the cyst; may have teeth, cartilage, brain, and bone
      (3) Rare ovarian teratomas composed almost entirely of thyroid tissue ("struma ovarii")
      (4) Benign
   b) Immature teratoma (malignant)
      (1) Rare; usually in young (less than 20 years) patients
      (2) Grossly, solid neoplasms with minimal cystic change
      (3) Composed of immature elements derived from all three germ layers, with primitive neuroectodermal (neuroblastic) elements representing the most common immature elements
      (4) Behave like malignant neoplasms
   c) Dysgerminoma: rare

    (1) The ovarian counterpart of seminoma in the testis, having an identical appearance

    (2) Potentially malignant; 80% 5-year survival

  d) Yolk Sac tumor (endodermal sinus tumor)

    (1) Rare; occurs mainly in those under 20 years of age

    (2) Solid neoplasms with necrosis and hemorrhage

    (3) Histologically composed of a lacy pattern with Schiller–Duvall bodies; identical to its testicular counterpart

    (4) Produces alpha-fetoprotein

    (5) Highly malignant; bad prognosis

7. Stromal neoplasms

  a) Granulosa-theca cell tumors

    (1) Account for 5% of ovarian neoplasms; 5% bilateral

    (2) Composed of a variable mixture of granulosa and theca cells

    (3) Grossly, frequently have an irregular surface with extensive hemorrhage and cystic change

    (4) Microscopically, granulosa cells appear as small, uniform cells with small dark nuclei and scant cytoplasm; solid masses with small fluid-filled spaces ("Call–Exner bodies") typical

    (5) Secrete estrogens, causing endometrial hyperplasia

    (6) About 25% behave in a malignant manner; 5-year survival rate: 85%

  b) Fibroma (= fibrothecoma)

    (1) Account for 5% of ovarian neoplasms; 10% bilateral

    (2) Gross characteristics: solid, spherical, encapsulated whitish-yellow masses

    (3) Microscopic characteristics: composed of fibroblasts, collagen, and intespersed theca cells

  c) Sertoli–Leydig cell tumor (androblastoma; arrhenoblastoma)

    (1) Rare; resemble corresponding testicular neoplasms

    (2) Commonly produce androgens and cause virilization

8. Metastatic neoplasms of the ovary

  a) The ovary is a common site for metastases, particularly in carcinoma of the stomach and colon.

  b) Krukenberg tumor

    (1) Bilateral, solid ovarian masses

    (2) Signet-ring cell adenocarcinoma, commonly from stomach, with a prominent desmoplastic response

III. Fallopian tubes
   A. Acute salpingitis (pelvic inflammatory disease)
      1. This is a common complication of gonococcal infection.
      2. Pelvic inflammatory disease complicating abortion or delivery is usually caused by streptococci.
      3. It presents with fever and lower abdominal pain.
      4. Suppuration (tubo-ovarian abscess) occurs frequently.
   B. Chronic salpingitis (nonspecific): a common condition associated with fibrosis of the lumen, which causes infertility
   C. Tuberculous salpingitis: the fallopian tube is a relatively common site of tuberculosis
   D. Endometriosis
      1. The occurrence of endometrial tissue in a site other than the uterine cavity
      2. Sites of involvement
         a) Uterine myometrium (adenomyosis)
         b) Endometriosis externa: outside the uterus, occurs in
            (1) ovary, fallopian tube, parametrium
            (2) intestine: the sigmoid colon, rectum, and appendix
            (3) urinary tract (rare)
            (4) umbilicus (rare): skin at site of laparotomy (commonly caesarian section) scars
            (5) extra-abdominal endometriosis in the lungs, pleura, bones (rare)
      3. Pathologic characteristics
         a) Foci of endometriosis undergo cyclical changes with bleeding occurring at menstruation. They appear as areas of new and old hemorrhage ("chocolate cysts").
         b) Microscopically, cystic spaces are lined by endometrial epithelium and surrounded by stroma.
      4. Pathogenesis: theories include:
         a) Metaplasia of the celomic epithelium into endometrial foci
         b) Transport of fragments of normal menstrual endometrium along the lumen of the fallopian tubes and out through its peritoneal opening
      5. Clinical characteristics
         a) Functional foci of endometriosis bleed at the time of menstruation. In pelvic endometriosis, this is associated with pain ("dysmenorrhea").
         b) Fibrosis associated with bleeding may, if it involves the fallopian tube, cause infertility.

    c) Pregnancy causes decidualization of the endometriotic foci, leading to their involution in many cases.

  E. Neoplasms of the fallopian tubes

    a) Adenomatoid tumor: common benign neoplasm of mesothelial origin (see testis)

    b) Carcinoma of the fallopian tube: very rare

IV. Uterus (body and endometrium)

  A. The endometrial cycle: "dating" the endometrium

    1. Proliferative phase (preovulatory) endometrium

      a) Evidence of proliferation of both glandular and stromal cells: mitotic figures

      b) small, straight, endometrial glands having large nuclei with relative paucity of cytoplasm

      c) Stroma usually dense

    2. Secretory phase (postovulatory) endometrium

      a) 2–4 days after ovulation, subnuclear secretory vacuoles are present in the glands.

      b) Secretion becomes prominent in the cells and lumina on day 5–7 postovulation.

      c) Stromal edema appears on about the 7th day. Stromal cells enlarge and show predecidual change.

      d) The glands become progressively more tortuous.

      e) Spiral arterioles become prominent on the 9th day after ovulation

  B. Abnormal stimulation and response of the endometrium

    1. Exogenous progestational hormone effect

      a) Exogenous administration of progesterone or combined progesterone–estrogen oral contraceptives is characterized by

        (1) small glands showing minimal secretory activity.

        (2) abundant stroma showing decidual change and edema.

      b) Exogenous administration of estrogens causes hyperplasia of the endometrium.

    2. Unopposed estrogen effect

      a) This is caused by the following:

        (1) Anovulatory cycles (failure of ovulation) which occur

          i) irregularly at the extremes of reproductive life

          ii) in polycystic ovary syndromes

        (2) Estrogen-secreting neoplasms (e.g., granulosa cell tumor)

        (3) Exogenous estrogen administration

b) The result of unopposed estrogen effect is prolongation of the proliferative phase of the endometrial cycle. Different stages are recognized:
   (1) Cystic endometrial hyperplasia (mild hyperplasia): increased numbers of glands of varying sizes, many showing cystic dilatation; stroma is dense.
   (2) Adenomatous hyperplasia (mild-moderate hyperplasia): thickened endometrium shows a more marked increase in the number of glands showing epithelial proliferation.
   (3) Atypical adenomatous hyperplasia (severe hyperplasia): characterized by variable degrees of cytologic atypia. The most severe change is called adenocarcinoma-in-situ.
c) The risk of carcinoma is small (less than 1%) in cystic hyperplasia and great (15%) in severe atypical adenomatous hyperplasia.
d) Clinical characteristics
   (1) The prolonged estrogenic phase corresponds to a period of amenorrhea.
   (2) The hyperplastic endometrium is unstable and tends to breakdown with irregular bleeding.
   (3) Such irregular bleeding in the absence of a well-defined organic cause is known as dysfunctional uterine bleeding.
e) All of the changes of anovulatory cycles are reversed by progesterone, which induces secretory changes.

3. Inadequate luteal phase
   a) This is caused by inadequate functioning of the corpus luteum with low progesterone output.
   b) The secretory endometrium develops abnormally and breaks down irregularly, resulting in abnormal uterine bleeding.

4. Irregular shedding of menstrual endometrium
   a) At the end of the normal cycle, the menstrual endometrium is completely shed in 4 days.
   b) Rarely, the corpus luteum maintains low levels of progesterone secretion for a prolonged period, causing irregular and prolonged shedding of the menstrual endometrium.
   c) Clinically, the patient has regular periods with excessive and prolonged menstrual bleeding, frequently lasting 10–14 days.

C. Adenomyosis
   1. The presence of endometrial glands and stroma situated abnormally in the myometrium (at a depth of more than 3 mm from the base of the endometrium)
   2. Probably due to ingrowth of the basal layer of the endometrium; not associated with extrauterine endometriosis
   3. Distinct forms of the disease
      a) Diffuse, involving the entire uterus, and causing thickening of the muscle
      b) Focal, forming a nodular mass (adenomyoma)
   4. Clinical characteristics
      a) May be asymptomatic
      b) May cause painful menses (dysmenorrhea) or irregular bleeding
D. Inflammatory lesions of the endometrium
   1. Acute endometritis
      a) Rare.
      b) Occurs as a postabortum or postpartum infection or as an ascending gonococcal infection
   2. Chronic nonspecific endometritis
      a) Common
      b) Diagnosis depends on the finding of plasma cells in the endometrium
      c) Occurs with
         (1) retained products of conception
         (2) chronic salpingitis
         (3) intrauterine foreign body, such as an intrauterine device
   3. Tuberculous endometritis: usually associated with tuberculous salpingitis
E. Neoplasms of the uterine body
   1. Endometrial polyp (benign)
      a) Common; occurs at any age but are most common around menopause
      b) Polypoid masses that project into the endometrial cavity
      c) Composed of endometrial glands and stroma, which is frequently fibrous and contains thick-walled blood vessels
      d) Clinically, are frequently asymptomatic, but may cause excessive uterine bleeding
   2. Leiomyoma
      a) Benign neoplasm of uterine smooth muscle
      b) The most common neoplasm in females, being found in one of four women in the reproductive years
      c) May be solitary or multiple; often reach a large size

d) May be located
   (1) Submucosally, protruding into the uterine cavity. Such neoplasms may protrude through the cervix, undergo infarction, and be expelled (aborting myoma).
   (2) Intramurally, causing marked distortion of the uterus
   (3) Subserosally, these may be pedunculated and move in the abdominal cavity on a long stalk ("wandering leiomyoma").
e) Gross characteristics: circumscribed, round, firm, grayish-white, having a characteristic whorled appearance
f) Histological composition: a uniform proliferation of spindle-shaped smooth muscle cells
g) Degenerative changes frequent
   (1) Red degeneration, typically seen in pregnancy, where the neoplasm undergoes necrobiosis and develops a beefy-red color; associated with abdominal pain
   (2) Cystic change
   (3) Hyalinization (fibrosis)
h) Clinical characteristics
   (1) May be asymptomatic
   (2) Excessive uterine bleeding
   (3) Infertility

3. Leiomyosarcoma
   a) Rare, accounting for 3% of uterine malignant neoplasms; the most common uterine sarcoma; occurs in older, postmenopausal women
   b) Large, bulky, fleshy mass showing hemorrhage and necrosis
   c) Shows marked cytologic pleomorphism, atypia, and a high mitotic rate (over 10 mitoses per 10 high-power fields)
   d) Tends to recur locally and metastasizes via the blood stream; 5-year survival about 40%

4. Endometrial carcinoma
   a) Incidence
      (1) Accounts for 10% of cancers in women
      (2) Is a disease of older women; 90% occur in postmenopausal women, the most common age being 55–65 years
   b) Etiology
      (1) Prolonged estrogen stimulation. Endometrial hyperplasia precedes cancer in most cases.
      (2) Associated factors ("the corpus cancer syndrome")

       i) Obesity

      ii) Diabetes mellitus and glucose intolerance

     iii) Hypertension

     iv) Infertility: most patients are nulliparous

c) Gross characteristics

   (1) Polypoid, fungating mass in the endometrial cavity

   (2) Invasion into the myometrium

   (3) Uterus enlarged, often asymmetrically

d) Microscopic characteristics

   (1) Endometrial carcinoma is an adenocarcinoma. It is graded 1–3 according to differentiation.

   (2) Areas of squamous metaplasia are common:

      i) When squamous areas are well differentiated and extensive, it is called an *adenocanthoma*.

     ii) When poorly differentiated, the term *adenosquamous carcinoma* is used.

e) Clinical staging

   (1) Stage 0: carcinoma confined to the endometrium

   (2) Stage I: carcinoma confined to the uterine body; myometrial invasion present

   (3) Stage II: spread to the cervix

   (4) Stage III: extension of tumor outside the uterus into the parametrial tissue but not beyond the pelvic cavity

   (5) Stage IV: extension outside the pelvis or involvement of bladder or rectum

f) Clinical characteristics

   (1) Abnormal uterine bleeding is the earliest symptom.

   (2) Physical examination may be normal or show enlargement of the uterus.

   (3) Endometrial biopsy by curettage is diagnostic.

g) Factors in prognosis

   (1) Clinical stage: with adequate treatment 90% of patients with Stage I disease, 40% with Stage II and 10–20% with more advanced disease will survive 5 years.

   (2) Histologic grade. The overall 5-year survival is 70% in grade 1 lesions and 20% in grade 3 carcinomas.

5. Mixed mesodermal tumor (malignant mixed Müllerian tumor)

a) Rare, occurs in older women

b) Usually bulky, friable neoplasms involving the endometrial cavity and presenting as post-menopausal bleeding

c) Microscopic composition

(1) A malignant epithelial component, usually an adeno-carcinoma

(2) A malignant mesenchymal component. This may be entirely smooth muscle (homologous type) or show differentiation into striated muscle, cartilage, and bone (heterologous type).

   d) Highly malignant neoplasm that tends to metastasize early. Has an overall 5-year survival of about 40%.

6. Endometrial stromal neoplasms (rare)
   a) Benign stromal nodule
   b) Low-grade stromal sarcoma (endolymphatic stromal myosis)
   c) High-grade stromal sarcoma

V. Uterine cervix
  A. Inflammatory lesions
    1. Acute cervicitis
      a) Common
      b) Characterized by erythema, swelling, neutrophilic infiltration, and focal epithelial ulceration
      c) Causes
        (1) Veneral infections: gonococci, trichomonas vaginalis, Herpes simplex (see below)
        (2) Trauma of childbirth and surgical instrumentation
      d) Clinically, may cause vaginal discharge and pain
    2. Chronic cervicitis: the presence of detectable cervical abnormality—reddening, granularity, etc.—with "significant" numbers of chronic inflammatory cells is chronic cervicitis.
  B. Nonneoplastic proliferations
    1. Microglandular hyperplasia
      a) A polypoid lesion characterized by proliferation of endocervical glands
      b) Associated with oral contraceptive use
    2. Endocervical polyp
      a) Common; benign
      b) Gross characteristics: pedunculated or sessile, somewhat translucent polypoid mass; large polyps protrude out of the external os
      c) Microscopic characteristics: glands and vascular stroma
  C. Neoplasms of the cervix
    1. Condyloma acuminatum
      a) Caused by papilloma virus, transmitted venereally
      b) Occurs in two forms:
        (1) Wart-like papillomatous lesion
        (2) Flat condyloma

c) Characterized by hyperplasia of the squamous epithelium with marked vacuolation of cells (koilocytosis) and nuclear atypia
2. Squamous carcinoma (Fig. 16-4)
a) Incidence
(1) Common; 7500 deaths annually in the United States; ranks 6th as a cause of cancer deaths in females

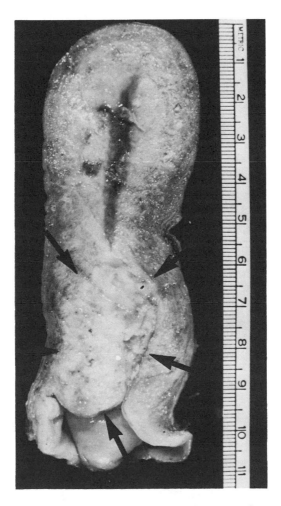

Fig. 16-4. Squamous carcinoma, cervic (arrows). The tumor arises at the squamo-columnar junction and has extended to involve the entire cervix.

       (2) Falling, owing partly to early detection by routine cytologic screening of cervical smears ("pap smears")

b) Etiology

    (1) Low socioeconomic classes

    (2) Increased risk with early onset of sexual activity, frequency of coitus, and number of sexual partners

    (3) Common in multiparous women who have married early

    (4) Common in prostitutes; vanishingly rare in nuns

    (5) Herpes simplex type II and papilloma virus have been suggested causes of cervical carcinoma; no proof for either

c) Precancerous changes in the cervix

    (1) Cervical carcinoma arises in a recognizable precancerous change in the epithelium. This change is known as dysplasia or intraepithelial neoplasia.

    (2) Dysplasia occurs at the squamocolumnar junction.

    (3) Diagnosis is made by cytology and cervical biopsy.

    (4) It is classified (in increasing severity) as mild, moderate severe, or carcinoma in situ (= intraepithelial neoplasia, grade 1–3).

    (5) The time span for progression of dysplasia is variable, but is generally measurable in years.

    (6) Dysplasia and carcinoma in situ produce no symptoms. Changes are visible in colposcopy.

d) Microinvasive carcinoma (Stage Ia)

    (1) A tumor that is clinically not apparent as a mass

    (2) Predominantly carcinoma in situ with microscopic foci of invasion across the basement membrane

    (3) May be diagnosed if the total depth of invasion is less than 3 mm from the basement membrane

e) Invasive squamous carcinoma

    (1) Occurs most frequently in the 30–50 year age group

    (2) Has a variety of gross appearances:

        i) An exophytic, fungating, necrotic mass

        ii) A malignant ulcer

        iii) A diffusely infiltrative lesion with only a minimal surface ulceration or mass

    (3) Microscopically, are squamous carcinomas of three different types:

        i) Large cell, nonkeratinizing squamous carcinoma: the most common, has the best prognosis

ii) Keratinizing squamous carcinoma with keratin pearls

iii) Small cell carcinoma: rare, has the worst prognosis

(4) Spread and clinical stage

i) Stage 0: carcinoma in situ

ii) Stage Ia: microinvasive carcinoma

iii) Stage 1b: invasive carcinoma confined to the cervix

iv) Stage II: extension beyond the cervix, but confined to the pelvic cavity

v) Stage III: extension to the pelvic side wall or involvement of the lower third of the vagina

vi) Stage IV: extension beyond the pelvis or involvement of bladder or rectum

(5) Clinical characteristics

i) Bleeding or vaginal discharge

ii) Diagnosis: by cervical biopsy

iii) Treatment: combination of surgery and radiation therapy, depending on the extent of disease

(6) Prognosis: depends primarily on the stage of the disease: stage 0, 100%, stage I, 90%, stage II, 75%, stage III, 35%, and stage IV, 10% 5-year survival

3. Endocervical adenocarcinoma

a) Accounts for 10–15% of cervical cancers

b) Arises in endocervical glands

c) Usually a well-differentiated lesion, often with a papillary appearance

d) Tends to have a less favorable prognosis than squamous carcinoma

VI. Vagina

A. Acute inflammation: vaginitis (nonvenereal)

1. After puberty, the vaginal mucosa is protected by the low pH produced by the Doderlein bacillus (*Lactobacillus acidophilus*).

2. Vaginitis is a common cause of vaginal discharge and discomfort; caused by

a) *Haemophilus vaginalis.*

b) *Trichomonas vaginalis*, a protozoan parasite.

c) *Candida albicans*, a yeast.

B. Vaginal adenosis

1. The occurrence of endocervical-type glands in the vaginal wall

    2. May form plaque-like, warty, nodular, or granular lesions
    3. Related to maternal exposure to diethylstilbesterol in pregnancy
    4. Probably represents the precursor lesion for clear cell adenocarcinoma; risk of cancer in vaginal adenosis small

C. Neoplasms of the vagina: overall rare; only 1-2% of cancers of female genital tract

    1. Squamous carcinoma
      a) 90% of vaginal cancers
      b) Occur in dysplasia and carcinoma in situ (vaginal intraepithelial neoplasia)
      c) Prognosis poor, with a 5 year survival of 30-40%

    2. Clear cell adenocarcinoma
      a) Rare, accounts for 10% of vaginal cancers
      b) Occurs in young women (10-35 years)
      c) Associated with maternal exposure to diethylstilbesterol in pregnancy

    3. Embryonal rhabdomyosarcoma (sarcoma botryoides)
      a) Occurs in the first 5 years of life
      b) Appears as a large, lobulated tumor mass that frequently protrudes from the vaginal orifice
      c) Microscopically, a highly anaplastic embryonal rhabdomyosarcoma
      d) Highly malignant

VII. Vulva

A. Vulvar dystrophies

    1. A group of epithelial changes of the vulva that present as opaque white plaques on the mucosal surface: leukoplakia

    2. Classified into two main types:
      a) Lichen sclerosus et atrophicus (atrophic dystrophy)
        (1) Presents as scaly, pruritic white plaques in postmenopausal women
        (2) Microscopic characteristics: atrophy of the epidermis, hyperkeratosis, and basal layer degeneration; upper dermis shows dense hyalinized collagen
        (3) Benign (not considered to be premalignant)
      b) Hyperplastic dystrophy
        (1) Affects postmenopausal women
        (2) Microscopic characteristics: hyperplasia of the epidermis and dermal lymphocytic infiltration
        (3) In the presence of epithelial dysplasia: it is precancerous

B. Neoplasms of the vulva
1. Condyloma acuminatum (venereal wart): common
2. Skin adnexal tumors occur in the vulva, commonly hidradenoma papilliferum.
3. Carcinoma in situ (Bowen's disease): the extreme of dysplasia in hyperplastic dystrophy
4. Squamous carcinoma
   a) Uncommon
   b) Usually occurs in women over 60 years
   c) Usually appears as an indurated plaque, progressing to a firm nodule that ulcerates; some are large
   d) Early lymphatic spread to inguinal and pelvic nodes
   e) 5-year survival: about 30%

VENEREAL (SEXUALLY TRANSMITTED) INFECTIONS

I. Gonorrhea
A. This is the most common venereal disease, with a reported incidence of over 300 per 100,000 population.
B. It primarily involves
1. the urethra in the male, producing urethritis: purulent urethral discharge with marked dysuria.
2. the cervix in the female, causing vaginal discharge and pain.
C. Gonococcal infection, in both females and males, may be asymptomatic (healthy carriers).
D. Infection of other sites in the genital tract is common.
1. In males: prostate, seminal vesicles, and epididymides, causing suppurative acute inflammation followed by fibrosis
2. In females: urethra, Bartholin's and Skene's glands, and Fallopian tubes
3. With varied sexual practices: gonococcal pharyngitis and anal gonorrhea
E. Entry of gonococci into the blood stream may cause
1. bacteremia with fever and a skin rash.
2. gonococcal endocarditis.
3. gonococcal arthritis, frequently monoarticular, affecting large joints, most commonly the knee joint.
F. Vaginal delivery of a fetus through a birth canal that has active gonococcal infection causes neonatal eye infection.

II. Syphilis
   A. Cause: *Treponema pallidum*, a spirochete
   B. Incidence: while the incidence of syphilis has increased, chronic disease has declined dramatically because of the effective antibiotic treatment of early disease
   C. Early syphilis (primary and secondary stages)
      1. The incubation period after infection is 9–90 days.
      2. The first lesion that appears is the primary chancre (primary syphilis); this is a painless, punched out; indurated ulcer at the site of treponemal invasion, usually the external genitalia. Spirochetes are present.
      3. The ulcer heals spontaneously in 3–6 weeks.
      4. Secondary syphilis
         a) This usually follows the primary stage after 2–20 weeks, but may begin before the chancre heals.
         b) It is characterized by fever, lymph node enlargement, a skin rash, and orogenital lesions (mucous patches, condyloma lata).
         c) Serologic tests for syphilis are positive.
         d) Microscopically, lesions show dense chronic inflammation with numerous plasma cells and spirochetes.
         e) Asymptomatic meningeal infection may occur, it is diagnosed by a positive serologic test in cerebrospinal fluid.
   D. Late syphilis (tertiary stage)
      1. Manifestations of late syphilis occur any time after 4 years from the primary infection.
      2. Tertiary syphilis takes one of three forms:
         a) Gumma
            (1) A localized area of granulomatous inflammation
            (2) May occur anywhere, but is common in the liver, bones, oral cavity, and testis
         b) Cardiovascular syphilis: causes aortic aneurysms, aortic valve incompetence, and coronary ostial narrowing due to the intimal scarring
         c) Nervous system syphilis (neurosyphilis): chronic meningovascular inflammation, tabes dorsalis, or general paresis of the insane
      3. The diagnosis in tertiary syphilis must be made by a combination of clinical, pathologic, and serologic findings. Organisms are not demonstrable except in general paresis.
   E. Congenital syphilis
      1. Transplacental infection of the fetus occurs in the last

trimester of pregnancy in a mother who has untreated early (first 4 years) syphilis.
2. Routine testing and treatment of pregnant women in early pregnancy has made congenital syphilis rare.
3. Congenital infection causes any of the following:
   a) Intrauterine death of the fetus.
   b) Neonatal or infantile congenital syphilis, which manifest lesions resembling lesions of early syphilis.
   c) Congenital syphilis may manifest in later childhood with
      (1) interstitial keratitis, leading to blindness.
      (2) nerve deafness, due to meningovascular inflammation.
      (3) abnormalities in permanent teeth (the incisors show a peg-shaped deformity (Hutchinson's teeth); the molars are abnormal (Moon's molars).

III. Herpes simplex type II (herpes genitalis)
   A. This is one of the current epidemic venereal infections.
   B. It causes lesions in the penis, vulva, and cervix. The lesions consist of very painful shallow ulcers that heal spontaneously but are recurrent and may be life-long.
   C. The main danger of herpes genitalis is infection of the fetus delivered through an infected birth canal. Neonatal infection is frequently fatal (encephalitis, disseminated viremia).

IV. Chancroid
   A. This is uncommon, and is caused by *Haemophilus ducreyi*, a gram-negative bacillus.
   B. It is characterized by the development of painful, shallow, necrotic, soft chancres at the site of inoculation on the external genitalia.

V. Lymphogranuloma venereum (LGV)
   A. This is uncommon, and is caused by a serotype of *Chlamydia trachomatis*.
   B. The acute phase is characterized by genital ulcers with enlarged inguinal nodes that show suppurative stellate granulomas.
   C. Chronic LGV is characterized by extensive fibrosis, which may cause rectal strictures and extensive lymphatic obstruction.

VI. Granuloma inguinale (rare)
   A. This is caused by *Calymmatobacterium donovani*, which may be identified in lesions as small coccobacillary forms (Donovan bodies). Silver stains are the best for identification.
   B. It is a chronic infection with large masses in the perineum associated with scarring.

PREGNANCY PATHOLOGY

I. Abnormal implantation
   A. Ectopic pregnancy
      1. The implantation of the fertilized ovum in a site other than the uterine cavity
      2. Common, occurring in about 1 in every 150 pregnancies
      3. Sites of ectopic pregnancy
         a) Ampullary part of the fallopian tube (majority)
         b) Isthmus of the fallopian tube in the interstitial part (common)
         c) Surface of the ovary (very rare)
         d) Abdominal cavity
            (1) Primary implantation (primary abdominal pregnancy) (very rare)
            (2) Secondary implantation after rupture of a tubal pregnancy (secondary abdominal pregnancy) (rare)
      4. Tubal pregnancy (Fig. 16-5)
         a) Usually ruptures, causing massive, potentially fatal intraperitoneal hemorrhage

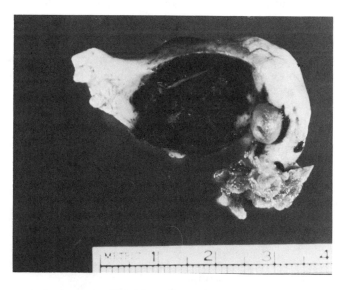

Fig. 16-5. Fallopian tube showing a hemorrhagic mass of a ruptured tubal pregnancy in the ampullary region.

b) May lead to death of the embryo in the tube, followed by
   (1) absorption of the products of conception
   (2) calcification of the fetus to form a lithopedion, which persists indefinitely
   (3) extrusion of the dead fetus through the fimbrial end of the tube, again associated with intraperitoneal hemorrhage
B. Placenta previa
   1. Low implantation of the ovum may lead to placenta formation in the lower uterine segment, sometimes overlying the internal os (placenta previa).
   2. Placenta previa causes problems in late pregnancy and early labor (antepartum hemorrhage).
C. Placenta accreta
   1. Placenta accreta is the absence of a line of separation between the villi and myometrium. The placenta fails to separate in labor, leading to severe postpartum hemorrhage.
   2. Placenta increta and percreta are further stages of this, where the villi actually penetrate the myometrium.
II. Gestational trophoblastic disease (trophoblastic neoplasms)
   A. Hydatidiform mole (grape-like mole)
      1. Incidence of molar pregnancy
         a) Occurs in 1 of every 2000 pregnancies in the United States.
         b) Has a much higher frequency (1:50) in India and the Far East.
      2. Etiology
         a) One theory is that hydatidiform mole is a benign neoplasm of trophoblastic tissue.
         b) An older theory was that hydatidiform mole was the result of a blighted ovum.
         c) A fetus is almost never present in a molar pregnancy.
      3. Pathologic characteristics
         a) The uterus is usually enlarged.
         b) The uterine cavity is filled with a mass of thin-walled, translucent, cystic, grayish-white grape-like structures.
         c) Microscopic characteristics include the following:
            (1) The villi are large and cystic, the interior being filled with an avascular, loose, myxoid stroma.
            (2) Trophoblastic proliferation produces sheets of cyto- and syncytiotrophoblastic cells. Cytologic atypia may be present.
         d) It is associated with greatly elevated levels of chorionic gonadotrophins.

4. Clinical characteristics
   a) Features of early pregnancy: amenorrhea, vomiting, positive pregnancy test
   b) Bleeding with passage of grape-like structures
   c) 2.5% lead to choriocarcinoma; in these, HCG levels do not return to normal after evacuation of the mole or rise subsequently

B. Chorioadenoma destruens (invasive mole): hydatidiform mole that invades the myometrium extensively, frequently reaching the serosa and producing hemorrhage and uterine rupture (rare)

C. Gestational choriocarcinoma
   1. Incidence
      a) Rare
      b) Most (50%) follow a hydatidiform mole; others occur after abortion (25%), normal pregnancy (23%), or ectopic pregnancy (2%)
   2. Pathologic characteristics
      a) Fleshy mass in the uterine cavity; extremely friable, showing extensive hemorrhage and necrosis
      b) Infiltrates the myometrium extensively
      c) Infiltrates blood vessels early in the course of disease, causing widespread metastases in lungs, brain, liver, bone marrow
      d) Microscopic characteristics
         (1) Choriocarcinoma is composed of cytologically malignant sheets of cyto- and syncytiotrophoblast cells associated with necrosis and hemorrhage.
         (2) Chorionic villi are absent.
      e) A highly malignant, rapidly growing neoplasm that rapidly causes death unless treated
   3. Clinical characteristics
      a) Bleeding occurring within a few months of a normal pregnancy, abortion, or hydatidiform mole
      b) Metastatic lesions almost invariably present at time of diagnosis
      c) Serum HCG markedly elevated; HCG level useful in monitoring treatment
      d) Chemotherapy remarkably effective

17

The Nervous System

INFECTIONS OF THE NERVOUS SYSTEM

I. Bacterial (pyogenic) meningitis:
   A. Etiology: agents of infection vary with the age of the patient.
      1. Neonatal period: *Escherichia coli, Streptococcus agalactiae* (group B streptococcus), and *Listeria monocytogenes*
      2. Under 5 years: *Haemophilus influenzae*
      3. In adolescents: *Neisseria meningitidis* (meningococcus)
      4. At all ages *Streptococcus pneumoniae* (pneumococcus)
   B. Route of infection
      1. Blood stream, the primary entry site being the respiratory tract (meningococcus and pneumococcus) or skin (neonatal meningitis)
      2. Direct spread from the middle ear or paranasal sinuses
      3. Inoculation by trauma, surgery, or lumbar puncture
   C. Pathologic characteristics
      1. Grossly, the leptomeninges (pia + arachnoid) are congested, opaque, and contain a purulent exudate.
      2. Microscopically, the leptomeninges are acutely inflamed with fibrin and neutrophils.
   D. Clinical characteristics: sudden onset, with high fever and signs of meningeal irritation: headache, vomiting, neck stiffness, and a positive Kernig's sign.
   E. Diagnosis: made by lumbar puncture, and examination of the cerebrospinal fluid (Table 17-1)
      1. The CSF is under increased pressure and appears cloudy.
      2. Presence of neutrophils, elevated protein, and decreased glucose is characteristic of bacterial infection.
      3. The specific agent is identified in gram-stained smears and culture.
II. Cerebral abscess
   A. Etiology
      1. Causes: a large variety of bacteria; commonly polybacterial anaerobic infection.

Table 17-1. Cerebrospinal Fluid Changes in Meningitis

	Pyogenic	Tuberculosis	Viral
Protein	elevated	elevated	sl. elevated
Glucose	v. low	low	normal
Chloride	low	v. low	normal
Appearance	turbid	clear; clot	clear
CELLS	neutrophils	mononuclears & neutrophils	lymphocytes
Gram stain	+	−	−
Acid-fast stain	−	usually −	−
Culture	bacteria	Mycobacteria	Virus

2. Common associated conditions
   a) Infection in the middle ear or mastoid air spaces (temporal lobe and cerebellar abscesses) and paranasal air sinuses (frontal lobe)
   b) Congenital cyanotic heart disease (parietal lobe)
   c) Acute bacterial endocarditis
   d) Penetrating brain injuries and cranial surgery
B. Pathologic characteristics: forms a mass with pus in the center surrounded by a fibrous wall whose thickness depends on duration.
C. Clinical characteristics
   1. Due to infection: fever, leukocytosis
   2. Due to a mass in the brain, which results in raised intracranial pressure.
   3. Due to destruction of brain: focal neurological dysfunction
III. Tuberculosis
   A. Tuberculous meningitis
      1. Etiology
         a) Secondary to disease elsewhere in the body, usually the lung
         b) Commonly occurs in the course of acute miliary tuberculosis
         c) May also occur in adults as an isolated condition, due to reactivation of a dormant meningeal focus of tuberculosis
      2. Pathologic characteristics

a) Tends to affect the base of the brain
b) Causes a chronic granulomatous inflammation with caseation, with neutrophils present in the acute phase
c) Fibrosis of the basal meninges
   (1) Causes cranial nerve palsies
   (2) Causes narrowing of small perforating arteries, leading to focal microinfarction in the brain
   (3) Causes obstruction of cerebrospinal fluid circulation with hydrocephalus
3. Clinical characteristics
  a) Insidious onset
  b) Diagnosis made by lumbar puncture (Table 17-1)
B. Tuberculoma of brain and cord (rare)
  1. An intraparenchymal caseous granuloma with extensive fibrosis
  2. Forms a mass, most commonly in cerebellum

IV. Neurosyphilis
  A. Neurosyphilis is a late manifestation of syphilis. Effective treatment of early syphilis has made neurosyphilis rare.
  B. Tertiary neurosyphilis manifests as one of the following:
    1. Chronic meningovascular syphilis: basal chronic inflammation with fibrosis; perivascular inflammation and obliteration of small vessels by endarteritis leads to microinfarcts.
    2. General paresis of the insane (GPI)
     a) Pathologically, it is characterized by
      (1) neuronal loss: cortical atrophy with gliosis.
      (2) *Treponema pallidum*, which can be demonstrated by special spirochetal stains.
     b) Clinically, patients manifest changes of cerebral cortical destruction: dementia and overt psychosis.
    3. Tabes dorsalis
     a) Spinal cord lesion characterized by degeneration of the dorsal nerve roots, dorsal ganglia, and posterior columns
     b) No spirochetes demonstrable in the lesions

V. Viral meningitis
  A. Etiology: several different viruses—enterovirus group, mumps, lymphocytic choriomeningitis (LCM) virus—can be isolated.
  B. In about 30% of cases, no virus can be isolated.
  C. Pathologically, there is acute meningeal inflammation; lymphocytes are predominant.
  D. Clinically, patients present with fever, headache, vomiting, and meningeal irritation. The disease is self-limited.

E. The diagnosis is made by lumbar puncture and CSF examination (Table 17-1).
VI. Viral encephalitis
  A. Etiology: several different viruses; "arboviruses" are a common cause of epidemic encephalitis.
  B. Pathological changes include neuron necrosis, microglial proliferation, and perivascular lymphocytic infiltration.
  C. Clinical characteristics include the following:
    1. Acute febrile illness, frequently with meningeal inflammation.
    2. Signs of neurologic deficit due to neuronal damage.
    3. Raised intracranial pressure due to cerebral edema.
  D. Specific forms of encephalitis
    1. Herpes simplex encephalitis
      a) Common in neonates (born to mothers with active herpes genital infection) and adults (common in immunosuppressed patients)
      b) Affects the temporal and inferior frontal lobes
      c) A severe, necrotizing, hemorrhagic acute inflammation, frequently causing death or severe brain destruction
      d) Specific diagnosis by brain biopsy
        (1) Cowdry A type intranuclear inclusions in neurons and glial cells
        (2) Virus demonstration by electron microscopy, labelled antibody staining or culture
    2. Poliomyelitis (Poliovirus)
      a) Poliomyelitis has become rare because of routine immunization in childhood.
      b) Poliovirus infection causes
        (1) meningitis
        (2) necrosis of anterior horn cells in the medulla and spinal cord. This produces a lower motor neuron paralysis of muscles.
    3. Rabies (rare): man is infected by animal bites.
    4. Cytomegalovirus encephalitis
      a) Occurs as a congenital infection
      b) Often associated with chorio-retinitis
      c) Causes microcephaly, hydrocephalus, and periventricular necrosis and calcification
    5. Progressive multifocal leukoencephalopathy (PML)
      a) Caused by papova viruses (JC virus and SV 40 virus)
      b) Usually occurs in immunocompromised patients (e.g., lymphoma; AIDS)
      c) Severe, commonly causing death

        d) Characterized by widespread focal demyelination of white matter

6. Subacute sclerosing panencephalitis (SSPE)
   a) Most commonly affects children several years after a known episode of measles
   b) Represents a prolonged measles virus infection
   c) Pathological characteristics
      (1) Neuronal degeneration with intranuclear inclusions
      (2) Diffuse demyelination and gliosis of white matter
      (3) Perivascular lymphocytic infiltration
   d) Clinical characteristics
      (1) Personality changes and involuntary myoclonic-type movements
      (2) Relentlessly progressive, causing extensive brain damage and death

7. "Slow" virus infections (rare)
   a) Creutzfeld-Jakob disease and kuru
   b) Slowly progressive, invariably fatal, diseases
   c) Pathological characteristics: neuronal loss, gliosis, and spongiform degeneration of the white matter; no inflammation
   d) Virus particles or inclusions not seen

VII. Fungal infections
   A. *Cryptoccocus neoformans* infection
     1. Usually occurs in immunocompromised hosts
     2. Pathological characteristics
        a) Microcysts in the brain substance containing masses of cryptococci with little inflammation
        b) Meningitis, typically basal
     3. Diagnosis
        a) Demonstrating the yeast in CSF by direct smear or culture
        b) Serologic detection of cryptococcal capsular soluble polysaccharide antigen in CSF and blood
   B. Other fungal infections (rare)

VIII. Parasitic infections
   A. Toxoplasmosis (*Toxoplasma gondii*)
     1. Acquired toxoplasmosis
        a) A common brain infection in Acquired Immunodeficiency Syndrome (AIDS)
        b) Produces mass lesions with necrosis, chronic inflammatory cells; toxoplasma pseudocysts and trophozoites can be seen
     2. Congenital toxoplasmosis

a) Transplacental infection occurs in the late stages of pregnancy.

b) The fetal brain shows extensive necrosis, calcification, gliosis, and microcephaly.

c) It is frequently associated with chorioretinitis.

B. Primary amebic meningoencephalitis (rare): caused by free living soil amebae of the genera Hartmanella–Acanthamoeba–Naegleria; infection occurs through the cribriform plate.

C. Cerebral malaria (rare): caused by *Plasmodium falciparum*, which is present in red blood cells in clogged brain capillaries; cerebral changes are due to diffuse ischemia.

D. African trypanosomiasis (sleeping sickness): caused by *T. rhodesiense* (East Africa) and *T. gambiense* (West Africa); transmitted by the tse-tse fly.

E. Cysticercosis

1. Caused by ingesting *Taenia solium* eggs (due to fecal contamination of food). The larvae enter the blood from the intestine and encyst (cysticerci) in muscle, brain, etc.

2. Cysticerci may occur in brain substance, ventricles, or subarachnoid space.

3. It causes epilepsy or hydrocephalus due to obstruction of CSF circulation.

4. Pathologically, the fluid-filled cyst contains the larva; a granulomatous inflammation with eosinophils, fibrosis, and calcification may surround the cyst.

TRAUMATIC LESIONS OF THE NERVOUS SYSTEM

I. Penetrating (open) injuries: often severe with a high incidence of infection

II. Nonpenetrating (closed) injuries

A. Cerebral concussion (commotio cerebri)

1. Transient loss of consciousness

2. No gross or histological lesions

3. Probably the result of relative motion between cerebral hemisphere and brain stem

B. Cerebral contusion and laceration

1. This is caused by movement of brain against bony prominences of the skull interior.

2. The simplest contusion is an extravasation of blood into the subpial region.

3. More severe injuries produce tearing of cerebral tissue (laceration).

C. Extradural hematoma (EDH)
1. This is an accumulation of blood between the skull and dura due to rupture of the middle meningeal artery.
2. Laceration of the vessel is commonly associated with a temporal region skull fracture.
3. After a variable lucid interval following the injury, patients show
    a) raised intracranial pressure: headache, vomiting, confusion, alteration in level of consciousness, and papilledema.
    b) tentorial herniation with oculomotor nerve palsy (pupillary changes) and brain stem compression (changes in heart rate, blood pressure, and breathing).
4. Progression is very rapid.
5. Emergency surgery is very successful.

D. Chronic subdural hematoma (SDH)
1. This is a common lesion, occurring commonly in elderly patients with cerebral atrophy; trauma required is minimal.
2. Blood collects in the subdural space, usually near the vertex.
3. Bleeding is slow, the result of rupture of veins passing from the cortex to the superior sagittal sinus.
4. The blood clot in the subdural space exerts an osmotic effect, drawing in fluid from the CSF and expanding slowly.
5. Clinical characteristics include:
    a) slowly developing increase of intracranial pressure.
    b) compression of underlying brain: hemiparesis, seizures.
6. Surgical evacuation of the fluid collection is curative.

E. Meningeal tears
1. Occur in base of skull fractures
2. Manifest as CSF fistulas through the nose (CSF rhinorrhea) and ear (CSF otorrhea)
3. Main danger: meningeal infection

F. Spinal cord injuries: due to forced movements ("whiplash" injuries of the cervical cord), vertebral fractures, or subluxations

CEREBROVASCULAR DISEASE

I. Cerebral ischemia
A. Causes of localized ischemia

1. Atherosclerosis
   a) Atherosclerosis is responsible for most cases of ischemic brain disease.
   b) It tends to involve the large arteries (Fig. 17-1).
   c) Occlusion distal to circle of Willis (end arteries) produces more severe changes than proximal occlusion.
   d) Effects of atherosclerosis
      (1) Narrowing: 75% occlusion required to cause a significant decrease in blood flow
      (2) Thrombosis
      (3) Emboli: may detach from fragmenting atheromatous plaques
2. Emboli
   a) Mural thrombi in relation to myocardial infarcts
   b) Vegetations of endocarditis
   c) Thrombi in relation to prosthetic cardiac valves
   d) Intramural thrombi developing in the left atrium in mitral stenosis and atrial fibrillation
   e) Emboli derived from atheromatous plaques

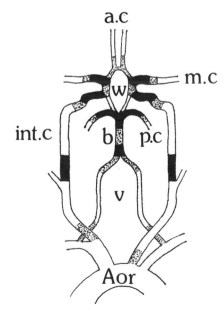

Fig. 17-1. Arteries of the brain showing distribution of atherosclerotic lesions. Dark areas are those most severely affected; stippled areas are less severely involved. Aor = aortic arch. int. c = internal carotid artery. v = vertebral arteries. b = basilar artery. w = Circle of Willis. a.c., m.c. and p.c. = anterior, middle and posterior cerebral arteries.

3. Arteritis: polyarteritis nodosa and giant cell arteritis
4. Spasm of cerebral arteries: migraine, hypertensive encephalopathy
B. Effects of localized ischemia
1. Cerebral infarction (Fig. 17-2)
a) This is the most common cerebrovascular "accident"
("stroke"), being responsible for 90% of such events.
b) It is most commonly the result of thrombosis.
c) Pathologic changes of infarction include the following:
(1) Gross and histologic changes are not demonstrable in
the first 6 hours.
(2) Liquefactive necrosis of gray and white matter occurs
(3) A fully formed cerebral infarct—48–72 hours—is a
pale, soft area composed of dead, liquefied cells. The
surrounding brain shows edema

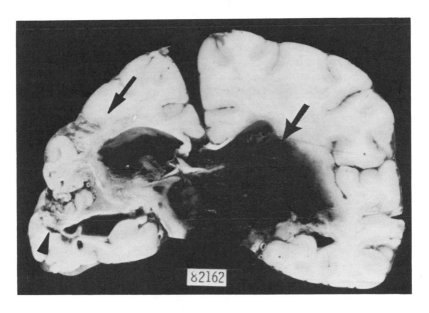

Fig. 17-2. Coronal section of brain showing an old cerebral infarct in the
distribution of the left middle cerebral artery and an acute spontaneous cerebral
hemorrhage on the right. Note the decrease in brain tissue and compensatory
dilatation of the lateral ventricle on the left. The hemorrhage has ruptured into the
right ventricle.

(4) 10–20% of cerebral infarcts are hemorrhagic.

(5) The healing phase shows numerous macrophages with foamy cytoplasm ("compound granular corpuscles").

(6) After 3 weeks cavitation begins and the area is converted to a cystic cavity.

d) Clinical characteristics

(1) A sudden loss of neurological function, corresponding to the area affected occurs.

(2) The associated cerebral edema may produce increased intracranial pressure and a neurologic deficit greater than that due to infarction.

e) Topography of cerebral infarcts

(1) The area of brain infarcted corresponds to the area supplied by the occluded artery (Fig. 17-2).

(2) Different clinical syndromes are caused by occlusions of different arteries.

2. Transient ischemic attacks (TIA)

a) This is caused in many cases by platelet or cholesterol emboli originating from ulcerated atheromatous plaques.

b) The attacks last a few seconds to 10 minutes.

c) The neurological deficit depends on the area of brain involved. Recovery is the rule. TIAs indicate the presence of severe cerebral vessel atherosclerosis; 30% of patients with TIAs will suffer cerebral infarction within 2–5 years.

3. Hypertensive encephalopathy

a) This is due to an acute arterial spasm (transient) precipitated by a sudden increase in blood pressure.

b) No necrosis occurs; it leads to cerebral edema.

c) Patients develop acute neurological dysfunction and raised intracranial pressure.

d) It requires emergency medical treatment; recovery is the rule.

C. Generalized cerebral ischemia

1. Causes

a) Marked hypotension or diminution of cardiac output

b) Severe generalized hypoxia as in respiratory failure or carbon monoxide poisoning

2. Effects

a) The decrease in oxygen supply interferes with energy (ATP) production.

b) Similar changes are produced in hypoglycemia.

c) Cortical neuronal necrosis frequently appears as a yellowish line in the deep cortical layer (laminar necrosis).

II. Spontaneous intracranial hemorrhage (nontraumatic)
   A. Cerebral hemorrhage (Fig. 17-2)
      1. Responsible for 10–15% of cerebrovascular accidents ("strokes")
      2. Causes
         a) Hypertension: over 80% of cerebral hemorrhages
         b) Vascular malformations: aneurysms, arteriovenous malformations
         c) Bleeding disorders
      3. Pathological characteristics
         a) Intraparenchymal arterial rupture leads to a rapidly expanding blood clot that destroys brain tissue.
         b) The clot can rupture into the ventricle or subarachnoid space.
      4. Clinical characteristics
         a) Very sudden onset ("cerebral apoplexy") with raised intracranial pressure
         b) Dense neurologic deficit (usually hemiplegia due to internal capsule hemorrhage), and loss of consciousness
         c) Has a high mortality
   B. Subarachnoid hemorrhage
      1. This results most commonly from rupture of a saccular aneurysm (Berry aneurysm) of the cerebral arteries.
      2. Rupture of aneurysms may occur at any time, usually after age 10 years. Frequency increases with age.
      3. Berry aneurysms are commonly located in arteries of the circle of Willis.
      4. Clinical characteristics include the following:
         a) Sudden onset, bursting headache, vomiting, extreme neck stiffness, and sudden loss of consciousness.
         b) The diagnosis is made by finding blood in the CSF.
III. Venous occlusion (rare)

DEMYELINATING DISEASES

I. Definition: a group of diseases in which demyelination occurs as a primary phenomenon
II. Multiple sclerosis
   A. Incidence
      1. The most common demyelinating disease
      2. A marked geographic variation; very common in northern Europe and Northeastern United States; rare in Asia

B. Etiology: measles virus is strongly suspected.
  1. Patients with MS have higher measles antibody titers in serum and CSF.
  2. Elevated levels of IgG are observed in CSF.
C. Pathology
  1. Plaques of demyelination in the white matter occur throughout the brain and spinal cord.
  2. Any area can be affected; sites of predilection are optic nerves, cerebellum, paraventricular region of brain stem, and spinal cord.
  3. Histologically, plaques show demyelination of neural processes, mild inflammation, and gliosis.
D. Clinical characteristics
  1. MS occurs most frequently in the 20–40-year age group.
  2. The common clinical course is episodic with relapses and remissions, progressing for many years.
  3. Common manifestations are visual changes, cerebellar incoordination, and spinal cord dysfunction.
III. Demyelination as a manifestation of immunologic injury
  A. Acute disseminated encephalomyelitis
    1. Occurs after viral infection (postinfectious) and immunization (postvaccinial)
    2. Demyelination due to the action of T lymphocytes against myelin protein
  B. Guillain–Barré syndrome
    1. Characterized by demyelination of cranial and spinal nerve roots and nerves, associated with lymphocytic infiltration
    2. Has a subacute clinical onset with lower motor neurone type paralysis, progressing for 1–2 weeks, then improving
    3. Follows a viral infection in 50% of cases
    4. CSF shows a normal cell count (less than $5/mm^3$) but has a markedly elevated protein level

DEGENERATIVE DISEASES

I. Affecting cerebral cortex
  A. Alzheimer's disease
    1. A common degenerative disease of unknown etiology characterized by progressive neuronal loss in the entire cerebral cortex
    2. Usually becomes clinically apparent after 50 years of age

    3. Clinical characteristics: cortical dysfunction (dementia) that slowly worsens over 5–10 years to death.

    4. Gross characteristics: diffuse thinning of the cortical gray matter; ventricles may show compensatory dilatation

    5. Microscopic characteristics:

       a) Neuronal loss

       b) Neurofibrillary tangles in the cytoplasm of the neurons

       c) Argyrophilic or senile plaques: extracellular collections of granular material

  B. Pick's disease: rare; causes presenile dementia

II. Affecting basal ganglia

  A. Parkinson's disease (paralysis agitans)

    1. Common, unknown etiology

    2. Caused by degeneration of the pigmented nuclei of the brainstem, especially the substantia nigra

    3. Depigmentation of the substantia nigra nuclei, which show cytoplasmic inclusions (Lewy bodies).

    4. Clinical characteristics: extrapyramidal dysfunction usually occurring after age 50 years; slowly progressive

    5. Other diseases or agents affecting the extrapyramidal system that produce a similar clinical syndrome

       a) Postencephalitic Parkinsonism

       b) Wilson's disease (hepatolenticular degeneration)

       c) Toxic agents: carbon monoxide and manganese

       d) Drug-induced Parkinsonism: phenothiazines, reserpine

       e) Atherosclerotic involvement of basal ganglia

  B. Huntington's chorea

    1. Inherited disease: autosomal dominant

    2. Characterized by atrophy of the caudate nucleus and putamen associated with neuron loss in frontal cortex

    3. Has its clinical onset in adult life (20–50 years); progressive with death in 10–20 years

    4. Clinical characteristics: dementia and choreiform involuntary movements.

III. Affecting cerebellum, brain stem, and spinal cord

  A. Motor neurone disease

    1. A very serious disease of motor neurones, both upper and lower, affecting older (50 years) individuals and progressing relentlessly to death in 1–5 years

    2. Unknown etiology; high familial incidence reported in Guam

  B. Inherited spinocerebellar degenerations (rare)

1. Friedreich's ataxia
2. Olivo–ponto–cerebellar degeneration

NUTRITIONAL DISEASES

I. Vitamin B_{12} deficiency: subacute combined degeneration of the cord (see Chapter 7).
II. Pellagra (dementia) (see Chapter 5).
III. Thiamine deficiency: Wernicke's encephalopathy, Korsakoff's syndrome (see Chapter 5).

CONGENITAL MALFORMATIONS

I. Defective closure of the neural tube
  A. Caudal end (spina bifida) (common)
    1. Located in the lumbosacral region
    2. Increasing failure of neural tube closure resulting in
      a) vertebral spine defect only (spina bifida occulta); may be associated with a dermal sinus
      b) meningocele: the meninges protrude through the vertebral defect forming a CSF-filled sac
      c) meningomyelocele: meningocele with spinal cord and nerve roots in the CSF-filled sac
      d) spina bifida aperta: a complete failure of fusion of the neural tube, which lays open, exposed to the surface
    3. Frequently associated with Arnold–Chiari malformation and hydrocephalus
  B. Cephalic end: (rare)
    1. Anencephaly: a complete failure of fusion of the neural tube at its cephalic end; there is no brain or skull
    2. Occipital meningocele and encephalocele
II. Trisomy 13–15 (Patau's syndrome): characterized by failure of development of the forebrain, leading to a single frontal lobe, single ventricle, and failure of development of olfactory bulbs
III. Posterior fossa malformations causing congenital hydrocephalus
  A. Noncommunicating hydrocephalus: due to the presence of an obstruction in the ventricular system
    a) Stenosis of the aqueduct: due to gliosis, usually secondary to an inflammatory process
    b) Dandy–Walker syndrome: caused by a failure of develop-

ment of the vermis of the cerebellum, with occlusion of fourth ventricle foramina.
  B. Communicating hydrocephalus
    1. Obstruction to CSF circulation distal to the fourth ventricular foramina
    2. Arnold–Chiari malformation
      a) Elongation of the medulla so that the fourth ventricle foramina open below the level of the foramen magnum
      b) Herniation of the cerebellum into the foramen magnum, obstructing upward flow of cerebrospinal fluid
IV. Syringomyelia
  A. Characterized by cavitation within the spinal cord, commonly cervical
  B. Cause uncertain; Arnold–Chiari malformation commonly coexists
 V. Phakomatoses: inherited diseases characterized by widespread malformations (hamartomas) involving nerves, skin, and blood vessels
  A. Von Recklinghausen's neurofibromatosis (common)
    1. Inherited as an autosomal dominant trait
    2. Skin lesions
      a) Café-au-lait patches
      b) Neurofibromas: may be massive (plexiform neurofibroma) ("Elephant man disease")
      c) Malignant neural tumors: occur in 5–10% of patients
    3. Tumors of the nervous system
      a) Large nerve neurofibromas; bilateral acoustic neuromas characteristic
      b) Meningiomas, often multiple
      c) Optic nerve gliomas
  B. Tuberous sclerosis (epiloia, Bourneville's disease) (rare)
    1. "Adenoma sebaceum" in the skin
    2. "Tubers" in the cerebral cortex: cause epilepsy and mental retardation
    3. Hamartomas composed of giant astrocytes occuring in the wall of the lateral and third ventricles
    4. Visceral lesions: rhabdomyoma of the heart, angiomyolipoma of kidney, pancreatic cysts
  C. Von Hippel–Lindau disease (rare)
    1. Retinal hemangiomas, visible on fundal examination
    2. Benign hemangioblastoma of the cerebellum: cystic vascular neoplasm, usually in adult life

3. Visceral cysts: notably in the kidneys and pancreas
D. Sturge-Weber disease (very rare)

NEOPLASMS OF THE NERVOUS SYSTEM

I. Classification
   A. Histogenetic classification: primary neoplasms of the nervous system are classified according to the cell from which they are derived.
   B. Topographic classification
      1. 70% of CNS neoplasms in childhood are infratentorial.
      2. 70% of CNS neoplasms in adults are supratentorial.
   C. Benign vs. malignant
      1. Criteria for malignancy in CNS tumors are somewhat different than those used in other sites.
      2. Even in the most malignant neoplasms, metastasis outside the central nervous system is very rare.
      3. Highly malignant tumors spread via the cerebrospinal fluid.
      4. Destructive infiltration of the brain is a criterion of malignancy.
      5. Many benign neoplasms such as meningioma and cranio-pharyngioma tend to recur after surgical removal.
II. Incidence
   A. 30% of all intracranial neoplasms are metastatic.
   B. Primary CNS neoplasms are not rare.
   C. 65% of primary CNS neoplasms are gliomas.
III. Clinical characteristics of CNS neoplasms
   A. Destruction by an infiltrating tumor produces irreversible focal neurologic deficits.
   B. Compression of neural tissue by an extraparenchymatous neoplasm produces reversible neurologic dysfunction.
   C. Mass effect causes increased intracranial pressure.
   D. Obstruction to CSF flow leads to hydrocephalus.
   E. Irritative effects (focal epilepsy) are caused by either infiltrating or compressing neoplasms.
IV. CNS neoplasms
   A. Glial neoplasms (gliomas)
      1. Astrocytomas: a wide range of neoplasms derived from astrocytes
         a) Cerebral hemisphere astrocytomas
            (1) Occur chiefly in adults (30–50 year group)

Table 17-2. Topographic Classification of CNS Neoplasms

	Extraparenchymal	Meningioma
Supratentorial tumors	Intraparenchymal	Glioma Metastases
	Sella turcica tumors	Pituitary adenoma Craniopharyngioma Chordoma
Infratentorial (posterior fossa) tumors	In adults	Acoustic schwannoma Cerebellar hemangioblastoma Brain stem glioma
	In children	Medulloblastoma Cerebellar astrocytoma
Spinal cord	Extradural	Bone tumors Metastases
	Intradural extramedullary	Meningioma Neurofibroma
	Intramedullary	Astrocytoma Ependymoma

(2) Firm, white lesions that may be grossly well-circum-scribed or diffusely infiltrative

(3) Composed of fibrillary and protoplasmic astrocytes; variably cellular

(4) Variation of rate of growth between slow (well-differentiated and rapid (anaplastic).

      b) Cerebellar astrocytoma (juvenile pilocytic astrocytoma)
        (1) Occurs in children
        (2) Presents as a well-circumscribed mass, often showing cystic change, situated within a cerebellar lobe
        (3) Microscopic characteristics: fibrillary astrocytes without atypia
        (4) Treatment: surgical excision of the tumor results in permanent cure in most cases
      c) Spinal cord astrocytoma: similar to cerebral hemisphere astrocytomas
    2. Glioblastoma multiforme
      a) The most common primary CNS neoplasm
      b) Occurs predominantly in the cerebral hemisphere
      c) Gross characteristics: large, infiltrative, and hemorrhagic (Fig. 17-3)
      d) Microscopic characteristics: highly cellular anaplastic astrocytic neoplasm with areas of necrosis; high mitotic rate
      e) Rapidly growing, destructive neoplasm that usually causes death within a year
    3. Oligodendroglioma
      a) Occurs in the cerebral hemisphere in adults
      b) Gross characteristics: well-circumscribed, with speckled calcification
      c) Microscopic characteristics: cellular, round oligodendroglial cells
      d) Prognosis after surgical removal is usually good
    4. Ependymoma
      a) Occurs at all ages; more frequent in childhood
      b) 60% of intracranial ependymomas occur in the fourth ventricle; 40% are supratentorial
      c) Account for 60% of spinal cord tumors; most commonly in the lumbar region
      d) Gross characteristics: well-circumscribed, nodular
      e) Microscopic characteristics: cellular ependymal proliferation with ependymal tubules and perivascular pseudorosettes
      f) Prognosis: varies from good (well-differentiated) to very bad (malignant)
  B. Medulloblastoma
    1. Derived from primitive neuroectodermal cells
    2. Occurs mainly in children

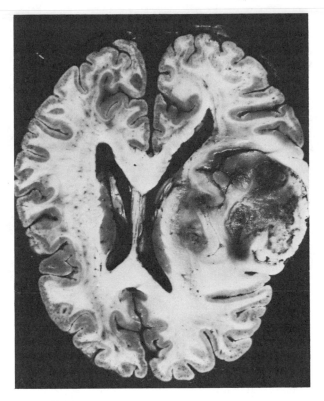

Fig. 17-3. Glioblastoma multiforme of cerebral hemisphere. The tumor appears circumscribed but has microscopic infiltration. The cut surface shows necrosis and hemorrhage. Note the shift of midline structures to the opposite side.

     3. Arises in the midline, commonly in the cerebellar vermis; grows rapidly, infiltrating extensively; spread through CSF common

     4. Gross characteristics: grayish-white fleshy mass

     5. Microscopic characteristics: highly cellular, composed of sheets of small primitive cells

     6. Prognosis: poor

  C. Meningioma (Fig. 17-4)

     1. A common CNS neoplasm derived from arachnoid cells

     2. Most common in middle-aged females

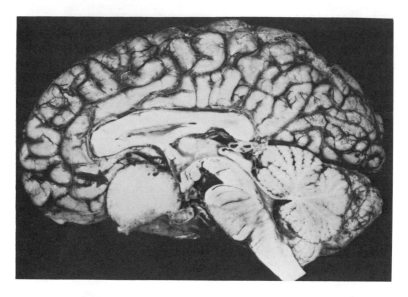

Fig. 17-4. Sagittal section of brain in midline, showing meningioma, basal (arrow). Tumor is extraparenchymal and encapsulated, compressing adjacent structures.

3. Usually slow growing, extraparenchymatous benign neoplasms that compress neural structures
4. Sites of predilection: convexity, parasagittal, base of skull, thoracic spine (extramedullary)
5. Gross characteristics: round, well-circumscribed, firm tumors attached to dura; infiltration of dura and bone common (not a sign of malignancy)
6. Microscopic characteristics: meningothelial cells, frequently forming whorls; calcified psammoma bodies common
7. Angioblastic meningioma: shows a vascular pattern; an aggressive neoplasm that may metastasize
8. Benign neoplasms; 10–15% of tumors recur locally after removal
9. Malignant meningiomas (rare): invade underlying brain
D. Pineal neoplasms (rare)
   1. Germ cell tumors: germinoma, teratoma, embryonal carcinoma, choriocarcinoma
   2. Pineal cell: pineocytoma, pineoblastoma

E. Neoplasms derived from embryonal remnants
1. Craniopharyngioma
   a) Derived from remnants of Rathke's pouch; most often seen in childhood
   b) Situated in the suprasellar region
   c) Gross characteristics: may be solid or cystic; may be extensive and infiltrative
   d) Cyst fluid oily; contains cholesterol crystals
   e) Microscopic characteristics: composed of stratified squamous epithelium
   f) Tends to recur after surgical removal
2. Epidermoid and dermoid cysts (very rare)
3. Colloid cyst of the third ventricle
   a) A cystic neoplasm of probable ependymal origin
   b) Contains thick mucoid material; lined by columnar epithelium
   c) Causes intermittent obstruction of the foramen of Monro, producing acute hydrocephalus
IV. Mesenchymal neoplasms
A. Cerebellar hemangioblastoma
1. Occurs either sporadically or in families with von Hippel–Lindau disease; benign
2. Gross characteristics: well-circumscribed mass; commonly cystic
3. Microscopic characteristics: numerous endothelial-lined small vessels separated by large stromal cells containing lipid in cytoplasm
4. Frequently associated with polycythemia, due to production of an erythropoietin-like substance
B. Primary malignant lymphoma (reticulum-cell sarcoma; microglioma)
1. Uncommon
2. Occur in the deep cerebral hemisphere; frequently multifocal
3. Gross characteristics: form ill-defined masses
4. Most commonly, aggressive large-cell B lymphomas (B-immunoblastic sarcoma)
5. Incidence increased in post-transplant patients and in Acquired Immunodeficiency Syndrome (AIDS)

18

The Musculoskeletal System

DISORDERS OF SKELETAL MUSCLE

I. Introduction
   A. Dysfunction of skeletal muscle is characterized by weakness of voluntary contraction.
   B. Causes of muscle weakness include:
      1. neurologic disease involving lesions of either upper or lower motor neurone.
      2. failure of neuromuscular transmission.
      3. primary muscle disorders
II. Primary muscle diseases
   A. Muscular dystrophies
      1. Definition: a group of rare primary muscle diseases
         a) Inherited; onset after birth at variable age
         b) Highly distinctive clinical features dependent on the distribution of involved muscles
         c) Nonspecific histologic changes in muscle
            (1) Irregular variation in size of individual myofibers
            (2) Displacement of myofiber nuclei to the center
            (3) Myofiber necrosis and phagocytosis
            (4) Accumulation of fat cells
      2. Types of muscular dystrophy
         a) Duchenne type: most common.
            (1) X-linked recessive: males are affected; females are carriers of the abnormal gene
            (2) Appears early in life; is rapidly progressive, leading to death by the end of the second decade
            (3) Symmetrical muscle weakness affecting the pelvic girdle muscles
            (4) Enlarged appearance of affected muscles—particularly calf muscles—due to increased fat content: "pseudohypertrophic" muscular dystrophy
         b) Facioscapulohumeral dystrophy

       c) Limb-girdle dystrophy

  B. Congenital myopathies: a group of very rare primary muscle disorders characterized by the following:

    1. Onset at birth or early infancy with weakness and decreased muscle tone ("floppy infant syndrome")

    2. Non-progressive with long survival being the rule

    3. Characteristic histologic changes that give the various diseases their names:

      a) Central core disease

      b) Nemaline myopathy

      c) Centronuclear myopathy

III. Disorders of neuromuscular transmission

  A. Myasthenia gravis

    1. Etiology

      a) Caused by failure of neuromuscular transmission

      b) Reduction of acetycholine receptors caused by IgG autoantibody against acetylcholine receptors

    2. Pathologic characteristics

      a) Electron microscopy shows simplification of the folds of the motor end plate.

      b) Antibody (IgG) can be demonstrated by immunologic techniques on the motor end plate.

      c) Thymic abnormalities include:

        (1) thymic hyperplasia in 70% of patients

        (2) presence of thymoma in 15% of patients

    3. Clinical characteristics

      a) Common disease; females aged 20–40 most commonly affected

      b) Characterized by weakness of muscles that is typically aggravated by repeated use.

      c) Muscles with the smallest motor units affected first (eye muscles).

      d) Course varies from mild (restricted to ocular muscles) to severe (generalized, fatal)

  B. Myasthenic syndrome (Eaton–Lambert syndrome)

    1. A paraneoplastic manifestation of cancer, most frequently oat cell carcinoma of the lung

    2. Weakness of muscles showing progressive improvement with repetitive stimulation

    3. Caused by impaired release of acetylcholine

DISORDERS OF JOINTS

I. Infectious arthritis
  A. Bacterial (pyogenic) arthritis
    1. The route of infection is hematogenous.
    2. *Staphylococcus aureus* is the most common agent; the gonococcus is common in homosexual males.
    3. It usually involves a single large joint.
    4. Clinically and pathologically, there is acute inflammation:
      a) Pain, tenderness, redness, swelling, warmth, and restriction of motion are present.
      b) The joint space is filled with pus.
      c) High fever and neutrophil leukocytosis.
    5. The joint space is cultured for diagnosis of agent.
  B. Tuberculous arthritis (rare): causes chronic pain and swelling, usually in a large joint
II. Immunologic diseases of joints
  A. Rheumatic fever (see Chapter 9)
  B. Systemic lupus erythematosus and progressive systemic sclerosis: frequently have joint involvement
  C. Rheumatoid arthritis
    1. Definition: a chronic disease of unknown etiology characterized by progressive, deforming, crippling arthritis
    2. Incidence and epidemiology
      a) Very common in the United States and Western Europe.
      b) Females 2–3 times more frequently affected than males
      c) Uncommon in tropical countries
      d) Age of incidence maximal between 30 and 50 years
    3. Etiology
      a) Unknown
      b) Immunologic injury currently favored etiologic factor
        (1) The synovium is infiltrated by lymphocytes, suggesting cell-mediated immunity.
        (2) Rheumatoid factor (present in 90%) is an auto-antibody (IgM commonly) reactive against IgG. This is not specific for rheumatoid arthritis.
        (3) Complement levels are reduced in synovial fluid.
    4. Pathologic characteristics
      a) The synovial membrane becomes swollen and congested with proliferation of inflamed granulation tissue (pannus).

    b) Pannus erodes articular cartilage, subchondral bone, and periarticular ligaments and tendons, causing progressive destruction of the joint.

    c) Fibrosis progressively increases.

5. Clinical characteristics

    a) Pain, swelling, and stiffness of joints

    b) Systemic symptoms such as low grade fever, weakness and general malaise common

    c) Joints usually affected symmetically

    d) Small joints of the hand typically involved

    e) Early occurrence of joint deformities

6. Extra-articular manifestation of rheumatoid arthritis

    a) Subcutaneous nodules

        (1) Occur in 10–20% of patients

        (2) Histologically composed of an area of necrosis surrounded by palisading histiocytes

    b) Vasculitis: commonly affecting skin of extremities, causing Raynaud's phenomenon, digital gangrene

    c) Pulmonary lesions

        (1) Rheumatoid nodules in the lung

        (2) Interstitial pneumonitis with fibrosis

        (3) Development of progressive nodular disease (Caplan's syndrome) in patients with anthracosis

        (4) Pleural effusion

    d) Amyloidosis

7. Course and prognosis

    a) 10–20% of patients have complete remissions after the first attack.

    b) Most others have relapses and remissions with slowly progressive disability from joint destruction.

D. Variants of rheumatoid arthritis

1. Felty's syndrome

    a) Occurs in older individuals with long-standing rheumatoid arthritis and high titers of rheumatoid factor.

    b) Associated with splenomegaly and pancytopenia due to hypersplenism.

2. Sjögren's syndrome

    a) Characterized by progressive destruction of salivary and lachrymal glands by an autoimmune lymphoid reaction, leading to:

        (1) xerostomia (dry mouth)

        (2) keratoconjunctivitis sicca due to absence of tears

b) Occurs in association with rheumatoid arthritis, collagen diseases, and as a separate entity
3. Juvenile rheumatoid arthritis (Still's disease)
   a) Rheumatoid arthritis occurring before the age of 16 years
   b) Characterized by an acute onset with high fever, skin rash, leukocytosis, and splenomegaly
   c) Rheumatoid factor negative
E. Ankylosing spondylitis
1. A common disease; affects young adult males predominantly
2. A very strong association with HLA-B27; present in 95% of patients (compared with 3-7% of controls)
3. Etiology unknown
4. Characterized by involvement of sacroiliac joints and low spinal articulations
5. Pathologically, inflammation is rapidly followed by fibrosis, calcification, and bony fusion (ankylosis) of joints.
6. Respiratory failure possible in involvement of thoracic spine and costovertebral joints
7. Rheumatoid factor negative
8. Extra-articular manifestations
   a) Aortic valve insufficiency
   b) Eye changes, commonly iridocyclitis
   c) Pulmonary fibrosis
9. Arthritis similar to ankylosing spondylitis: occurs in psoriasis, Reiter's syndrome, inflammatory bowel disease
III. Degenerative joint disease
A. Osteoarthritis
1. Incidence
   a) Radiological examination reveals 90% of patients over 50 years have osteoarthritis
   b) Though only a minority of these are symptomatic, osteoarthritis is the commonest cause of joint disability
2. Etiology: an unknown degeneration of articular cartilage
3. Pathological characteristics
   a) Joints affected are large, weight-bearing joints: vertebral column, hips, and knees.
   b) Articular cartilage shows microscopic clefts ("fibrillations") and becomes soft and eroded, exposing subchondral bone.
   c) Fragments of articular cartilage may break off into the joint space.

    d) Subchondral bone shows fibrosis, cystic change, and new bone formation (osteophytes or spurs).

  4. Clinical characteristics

    a) Pain, swelling of joints without inflammation; restricted joint movements

    b) Crepitus (grating sound) due to rubbing together of exposed bone

    c) Effects of osteophyte formation

      (1) Impingement of nerves, particularly in the spine

      (2) Heberden's nodes around distal interphalangeal joints

B. Gout (see Chapter 3)

C. Alkaptonuria (ochronosis) (rare)

CONNECTIVE TISSUE (COLLAGEN) DISEASES

I. Definition: a group of diseases characterized by
  A. multisystem involvement
  B. presence of autoimmune antinuclear antibodies
  C. small vessel vasculitis, frequently with fibrinoid necrosis

II. Systemic lupus erythematosus (SLE)
  A. Incidence
    1. A common, very serious disease
    2. Common in females; 20–40-year age group
  B. Etiology
    1. Etiology is unknown; infectious agents and genetic basis have been suggested but not proven.
    2. Immunologic abnormalities dominate.
      a) Serum antinuclear antibodies (ANA) are present in almost all patients.
      b) Antibodies against double-stranded DNA highly specific for SLE.
      c) Immune complexes formed with ANA and nuclear antigens produce a type III hypersensitivity autoimmune disease.
    3. Drug-induced SLE (hydralazine, procainamide hydrochloride) is identical to SLE; withdrawal of the drug reverses disease.
  C. Pathologic characteristics
    1. Small vessel vasculitis
      a) In the acute phase, the vessel wall is infiltrated with

inflammatory cells and shows fibrinoid necrosis; thrombosis may occur.

    b) In the chronic phase there is (onion skin) intimal fibrosis.

  2. Immune complex deposition with complement activation, leading to an acute inflammatory response

D. Clinical characteristics

  1. Systemic symptoms: fever, weight loss (80% of patients)

  2. Arthritis or joint pain without inflammation; usually without deformities (90%)

  3. Skin rash: butterfly rash on the cheek typical (70%)

  4. Hepatosplenomegaly and lymphadenopathy (60%)

  5. Cardiac lesions: pericarditis, endocarditis (Libman–Sachs)

  6. Renal involvement (55%): the most serious manifestation; renal failure: the most common cause of death

  7. Central nervous system lesions (25%): encephalopathy, nerve palsies

  8. Immune hemolytic anemia, thrombocytopenia, neutropenia

E. Course of the disease

  1. Extremely variable

  2. Acute progressive, uncontrollable disease (rare)

  3. Chronic disease with exacerbations and remissions (common)

III. Progressive systemic sclerosis (PSS; scleroderma)

A. Etiology: believed to be immune complex mediated autoimmune disease; many different antinuclear antibodies present

B. Pathologic characteristics: small vessel vasculitis associated with increased collagen deposition in many tissues

C. Clinical characteristics

  1. Commonly in females; onset between 20 and 50 years

  2. Onset insidious; course chronic; systemic symptoms uncommon

  3. Skin dominantly involved in most cases (90%)

    a) In the acute phase, there is a doughy edema.

    b) The epidermis becomes thin and shiny due to hair loss; enlarged vessels appear as telangiectases.

    c) Severe dermal fibrosis causes the face to appear taut and mask-like; claw-like contractures occur in the hands.

    d) Trophic ulcerations and calcification appear in the skin.

  4. Gastrointestinal tract involvement (60%)

    a) Esophageal fibrosis: dysphagia

    b) Small intestine: bacterial overgrowth and malabsorption due to stasis

5. Kidney involvement (60%) a common cause of death
   a) Vascular changes resemble those of malignant hypertension.
   b) Glomerular basement membrane thickening and mesangial hypercellularity causes nephrotic syndrome.
6. Lungs: diffuse interstitial fibrosis

IV. Polymyositis–dermatomyosis
   A. Uncommon disease; onset between 40 and 60 years
   B. Associated malignant neoplasm (most commonly lung and breast carcinoma) in 10–15% of patients with dermatomyositis
   C. Clinicopathologic characteristics
      1. Myositis (100%): edema, myofiber necrosis, and lymphocytic infiltration followed by atrophy and fibrosis; limb-girdle muscles maximally involved
      2. Skin changes (50%): typically a violaceous, edematous rash on the upper eyelids (heliotrope rash)

V. Mixed connective tissue disease (MCTD)
   A. A rare connective tissue disease having clinical manifestations that overlap with SLE, PSS, and polymyositis ("overlap syndrome")
   B. Diagnosed by high titer of antibodies against ribonucleoprotein (RNP)
   C. Runs a more benign course than SLE

SOFT TISSUE NEOPLASMS

I. Benign
   A. Fibromatoses
      1. Definition: disorders characterized by a benign proliferation of fibroblasts in the soft tissue
      2. Types of fibromatosis
         a) Musculofascial fibromatosis (desmoid tumor)
            (1) Slowly growing tumor in the abdominal wall muscles, most commonly in the rectus abdominis
            (2) Gross characteristics: large, rubbery mass that appears circumscribed
            (3) Microscopic characteristics: infiltrates along fascial planes; composed of benign fibroblasts and collagen
            (4) Has a very high (60–70%) incidence of local recurrence after wide surgical excision.
            (5) Does not metastasize
         b) Fibromatosis colli (sternomastoid tumor of infancy): causes torticollis (wry-neck) in infants

      c) Palmar fibromatosis (Dupuytren's contracture)

      d) Penile fibromatosis (Peyronie's disease)

      e) Mediastinal and retroperitoneal fibrosis

         (1) Characterized by extensive fibrosis of the retroperitoneum and/or mediastinum

         (2) Binds down the structures in the area, most frequently manifesting as ureteral obstruction

B. Lipoma

    1. The most common neoplasm of man; appears as an encapsulated mass of mature fat.

    2. Multiple lipomatosis (Dercum's disease): a rare, autosomal dominant disease characterized by numerous lipomas over the whole body.

C. Benign neural neoplasms (Fig. 18-1)

    1. Schwannoma (=neurilemmoma)

      a) Benign neoplasm derived from Schwann cells

      b) Occur most commonly in relation to large peripheral nerves e.g., eighth cranial nerve (acoustic neuroma)

      c) Encapsulated; compresses the nerve from which it arises

      d) Composed of Schwann cells only, arranged in two patterns.

         (1) Antoni A type: cellular spindle cell proliferation with the nuclei tending to form palisades

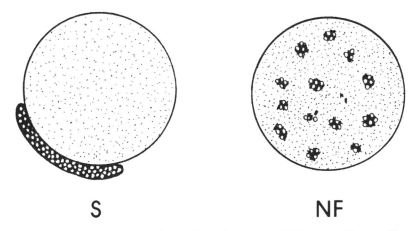

S   NF

Fig. 18-1. Benign neural neoplasms. S = schwannoma, NF = neurofibroma. The nerve is compressed in the schwannoma and incorporated in the neurofibroma.

(2) Antoni B type: a less cellular mass of Schwann cells with abundant myxoid stroma
        e) Malignant transformation very uncommon
    2. Neurofibroma
        a) An irregular proliferation of Schwann cells, fibroblasts, and an admixture of neurites
        b) Occurs both in relation to large peripheral nerves (e.g., spinal nerve roots) and small peripheral nerves (e.g., cutaneous neurofibroma)
        c) Nonencapsulated; expands the nerve from which it arises
        d) Increased mitotic activity suspicious for malignant transformation
    3. Generalized neurofibromatosis (von Recklinghausen's disease) (see Chapter 17)
        a) Multiple neurofibromas in skin, peripheral, and spinal nerves and viscera
        b) Occurrence of malignant transformation in 10% of cases
    D. Benign neoplasms of blood vessels (common)
        1. Hemangioma: capillary (composed of endothelial lined capillary-sized vessels) or cavernous (composed of larger vascular spaces)
        2. Lymphangioma (rare). The most common form, cystic hygroma: a cavernous lymphangioma that occurs in the neck in infants
    E. Benign fibrous histiocytomas
        1. Fibrous histiocytomas composed of varying amounts of fibroblasts and histiocytes
        2. In the skin: dermatofibromas and fibroxanthomas
        3. Common in relation to joints and tendon sheaths: giant cell tumor of tendon sheath
II. Malignant mesenchymal neoplasms (sarcomas)
    A. Sarcomas are malignant neoplasms derived from mesenchymal cells named according to the cell of origin (e.g., rhabdomyosarcoma, liposarcoma, malignant fibrous histiocytoma).
    B. The biologic behavior of sarcomas is extremely variable; it is divided broadly into the following categories:
        1. High-grade sarcomas
            a) These are primitive, highly cellular neoplasms, frequently showing marked cytologic pleomorphism and atypia and having a high mitotic rate.
            b) They may show little or no differentiation and are frequently difficult to classify exactly.

c) They tend to grow rapidly, recur locally after excision, and metastasize early.
d) They are rapidly fatal; treatment is rarely successful.
2. Low-grade sarcomas
a) These are better differentiated, less cellular, and show lesser degrees of cytologic atypia and a lower mitotic rate than high-grade sarcomas.
b) These neoplasms are characterized by
(1) slow rate of growth: often over years.
(2) a relatively low metastatic potential
(3) a high risk of local recurrence after surgical excision.
c) They have a lower fatality rate, with long survival after surgical removal being common.

DISORDERS OF BONE

I. Congenital diseases of bone
A. Achondroplasia
1. This is an autosomal dominant trait; failure of cartilage cell proliferation in epiphyses causes growth failure in long bones (dwarfism).
2. Membranous ossification occurs normally; the skull, face, and trunk are normally developed.
3. The individual is otherwise healthy.
B. Osteogenesis imperfecta (brittle bone disease)
1. This has an autosomal dominant inheritance with variable penetrance.
2. Defective synthesis of collagen and osteoid results in thin poorly formed bones that fracture easily.
C. Osteopetrosis (marble bone disease; Albers–Schonberg disease)
1. This is a very rare disorder.
2. Affected bones are greatly thickened with overgrowth of solid cortical bone.
II. Infections of bone
A. Pyogenic osteomyelitis
1. Etiology
a) Trauma: compound fractures
b) Spread from a neighboring focus of infection (e.g., mandibular osteomyelitis from a dental infection)
c) Hematogenous seeding
(1) Occurs in previously healthy, active individuals, mainly children and young adults

(2) Commonly caused by *Staphylococcus aureus*

(3) The metaphyseal region (the most vascular region of bone) most frequently involved

2. Pathological characteristics

a) There is acute inflammation in the bone, with abscess formation.

b) The abscess can rupture through the surface and form a subperiosteal abscess.

c) Rupture into the joint may cause suppurative arthritis.

d) Involvement of the medullary cavity causes spread of infection throughout the bone with extensive necrosis (sequestrum), leading to chronic suppurative osteomyelitis.

e) With effective, early antibiotic treatment, acute osteomyelitis resolves. Fewer than 10% of cases are complicated by chronic osteomyelitis.

3. Clinical characteristics

a) An acute onset, severe illness with high fever and severe pain in the involved bone

b) Neutrophil leukocytosis constant; blood culture positive in 70% of cases

B. Tuberculosis of bone

1. Rarely seen now in the United States

2. Reactivation of dormant foci in bone; in many cases, the lungs show no evidence of tuberculosis upon chest radiography.

3. Vertebral involvement (Pott's disease of the spine); the most common type of disease; characterized by

a) caseating granulomatous inflammation, leading to collapse of the vertebral body: may cause

(1) acute spinal cord compression

(2) vertebral deformity (kyphosis)

b) extension of the caseous material into

(1) epidural space, causing spinal compression

(2) groin and thigh along the psoas sheath

III. Metabolic bone disease

A. Osteoporosis (Fig. 18-2)

1. A decrease in the bone mass without abnormality in the structure of bone.

2. Etiology

a) Senile osteoporosis: very common, probably representing an aging phenomenon; more common in females (postmenopausal osteoporosis)

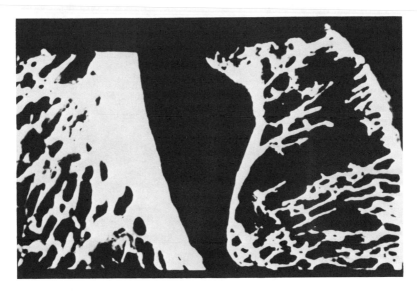

Fig. 18-2. Osteoporotic bone (right) compared with normal bone (left) showing the marked decrease in thickness of bony trabeculae.

      b) Associated with immobilization: form of disuse atrophy of bone

      c) Endocrine diseases

          (1) Cushing's syndrome

          (2) Thyrotoxicosis

          (3) Acromegaly

  3. Pathogenesis unknown; most patients in negative calcium balance

  4. Clinical and pathologic characteristics

      a) Osteoporosis affects all bones, most commonly

          (1) vertebral bodies: may cause compression fractures

          (2) femoral neck: predisposes to pathologic fractures of this region with minimum trauma

      b) Affected bones are normal in structure but the trabeculae are thinner and the total bone mass is decreased.

      c) Serum calcium, phosphate, and alkaline phosphatase are normal.

B. Osteomalacia

  1. A structural abnormality of bone in which there is defective

mineralization of bone, resulting in an increase in osteoid relative to calcium salts
2. Etiology: vitamin D deficiency (see Chapter 5).
3. Pathologic characteristics
   a) Histologic examination of undecalcified bone shows the presence of widened seams of uncalcified osteoid.
   b) Serum calcium levels are low, leading to secondary hyperparathyroidism (parathyroid hyperplasia). Serum phosphate and alkaline phosphatase maybe elevated.
C. Hyperparathyroidism (osteitis fibrosa cystica) (see Chapter 13)
D. Renal osteodystrophy
   1. Bone changes associated with chronic renal failure are highly complex.
   2. Failure of Vitamin D metabolism causes osteomalacia.
   3. The negative calcium balance may lead to changes of osteoporosis.
   4. Secondary hyperparathyroidism causes the changes of osteitis fibrosa cystica.
E. Paget's disease (osteitis deformans)
   1. Definition: a disease of unknown etiology characterized by thickening and disturbance in bone structure
   2. Incidence
      a) Very common in the United States and Western Europe
      b) Seen predominantly in patients over the age of 50 years
   3. Pathologic characteristics
      a) May affect a single bone (monostotic) or be generalized (polyostotic)
      b) commonly involved bones: pelvis, skull, spine, scapula, femur, tibia, humerus, and mandible
      c) Three stages of progression:
         (1) Osteolysis: irregular osteoclastic resorption of bone
         (2) Osteogenesis
            i) Osteoblasts actively deposit irregular bony trabeculae, balancing osteolysis.
            ii) Histologically, bony trabeculae are markedly thickened, irregular, and contain cement lines.
            iii) The bone is highly vascular, producing an effect similiar to that of an arteriovenous fistula.
         (3) Inactive sclerotic phase: osteogenesis continues, leading to marked thickening of bone.
   4. Clinical characteristics
      a) The early disease is asymptomatic.
      b) Pain, deformities, and fractures occur.

c) Thickening of bones may impinge on structures such as nerves leaving bony foramina.

d) Serum calcium, phosphorus, and parathormone levels are normal. Serum alkaline phosphatase is greatly elevated, reflecting the marked osteoblastic activity.

5. Complications

a) The arteriovenous fistula effect causes a hyperdynamic circulation with heart failure.

b) Malignant neoplasms, commonly osteosarcoma, develop in about 2–5% of cases.

IV. Bone cysts

A. Solitary bone cyst (unicameral bone cyst)

1. Uncommon; affects long bones in children and young adults

2. Metaphyseal, well demarcated; lined by connective tissue

B. Aneurysmal bone cyst

1. Rare; occurs in young adults

2. Affects vertebrae and flat bones more commonly than long bones

3. Radiologic characteristics: a large, cystic lesion causing eccentric expansion of the bone

4. Gross characteristics: a spongy hemorrhagic mass

5. Microscopic characteristics: hemorrhagic spaces lined by osteoclast-like giant cells and smaller cells; very similar to giant cell tumor

V. Neoplasms of bone (Table 18-1)

A. General

1. The most common neoplasms of bone are metastatic carcinomas.

a) In adults: most frequently from lung, prostate, breast, thyroid, kidney, and colon

b) In children: neuroblastoma

2. Common benign primary neoplasms are osteochondroma, enchondroma, and giant cell tumor.

3. Malignant primary bone neoplasms are most commonly osteosarcoma, chondrosarcoma, and Ewing's sarcoma.

B. Benign neoplasms

1. Osteochondroma (exostosis)

a) This is the most common benign bone tumor; it is common in long bones, and the pelvis.

b) The greatest majority are solitary. Rarely, multiple osteochondromas occur as a familial disease (diaphyseal aclasis).

Table 18-1. Classification of Bone Neoplasms

Cell of Origin	Benign	Malignant
Osteoblast	Osteoma	Osteosarcoma
	Osteoid Osteoma	
	Osteoblastoma	
Chondroblast	Enchondroma	Chondrosarcoma
	Osteochondroma	
	Chondroblastoma	
Uncertain	Giant cell tumor	Ewing's sarcoma
Medullary Cavity		Fibrosarcoma
		Leukemia/lymphoma/
		myeloma

c) The tumors are pedunculated and stick out from the cortex of the bone.

d) Histologically there is a bony base and a cartilaginous cap.

e) Malignant transformation (into chondrosarcoma) occurs very rarely in solitary osteochrondroma and commonly (10%) in multiple osteochondromatosis.

2. Enchondroma

a) This is a common benign neoplasm that occurs mainly in the hands and feet.

b) Multiple enchondromas may occur as a familial disease with autosomal dominant inheritance (Ollier's disease).

c) It is composed of firm, glistening hyaline cartilage that has a low cellularity on microscopic examination.

d) Malignant transformation does not occur.

3. Giant cell tumor of bone (osteoclastoma)

a) This is a common neoplasm; usually occurs in patients over 20 years.

b) Sites commonly affected are distal femur, proximal tibia, distal radius, and proximal humerus.

c) It is located in the epiphyseal end of long bones.

d) Lesions are frequently large, expanding the bone and thinning of the cortex; extension into soft tissue may occur.

e) Radiologically, it appears as an osteolytic radiolucent

mass traversed by thin sclerotic lines ("soap bubble" appearance).

f) Grossly, the tumor is fleshy, frequently showing areas of hemorrhage and cystic degeneration.

g) Microscopically (Fig. 18-3).

   (1) the critical cell is the stromal cell, which is a small spindle cell with very little cytoplasm.

   (2) numerous osteoclast-like multinucleated giant cells are seen.

h) It is benign, but displays malignant behavior with metastases in about 10%.

i) 50% of "benign" giant cell tumors recur locally after surgical excision.

C. Malignant neoplasms

  1. Osteosarcoma (Fig. 18-4)

    a) This is the most common primary malignant neoplasm of bone.

    b) It affects the 10–25-year-old age group.

    c) Etiology

     (1) Radiation

     (2) Thorotrast: a dye used in radiology in the past

     (3) Paget's disease of bone

    d) Osteosarcoma arises in the metaphyseal area in long bones. The lower femur, upper tibia, and upper humerus are most commonly involved.

    e) Grossly, the neoplasm is fleshy with necrosis and hemorrhage.

    f) As it grows, the tumor infiltrates

     (1) into the medullary cavity (common).

     (2) through the cortex into surrounding soft tissue.

    g) Elevation of the periosteum stimulates reactive new bone formation ("Codman's triangle").

    h) Radiologically, osteosarcoma appears as an expanding mass that has an irregular infiltrative edge.

    i) Microscopically,

     (1) malignant osteoblasts with anaplasia and a high mitotic rate are seen.

     (2) variable amounts of osteoid, which appears as a pink material between the cells and may become calcified (tumor bone), is found.

     (3) cartilage formation (chondroblastic osteosarcoma) and osteoclast-like giant cells occur in some cases.

    j) It is a highly malignant neoplasm that grows very rapidly and spreads early via the blood stream.

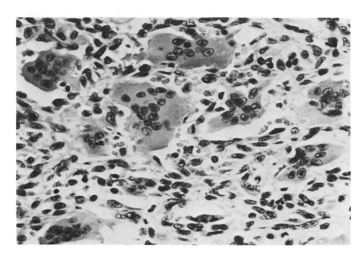

Fig. 18-3. Giant cell tumor of bone (microscopic) showing the osteoclast-like giant cells and the neoplastic small spindle cells.

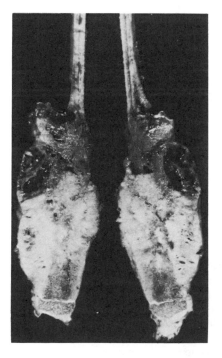

Fig. 18-4. Osteosarcoma (fibula). The neoplasm has destroyed the bone in the metaphyseal region and infiltrated through the cortex into the soft tissue.

k) It is radiosensitive and responds to several chemotherapeutic agents.

l) The 5-year survival rate is 20%.

2. Chondrosarcoma (Fig. 18-5)

   a) Chondrosarcoma accounts for about 20% of primary
   malignant bone neoplasms.

   b) It is a neoplasm of older individuals (30–60 years).

   c) Most cases occur without predisposing cause. A few cases
   occur in multiple osteochondromatosis and Ollier's disease.

   d) Pelvic bones, ribs, shoulder girdles, and long bones are
   commonly affected.

   e) Grossly, it forms large masses that expand and infiltrate
   the bone. Calcification is common.

   f) Microscopically, chondrosarcomas consist of malignant
   chondroblasts in chondroid matrix. The chondroblasts
   display varying degrees of cytologic anaplasia.

   g) On the basis of degree of cellularity and cytologic
   anaplasia, chondrosarcomas are graded histologically.

   h) It is a malignant neoplasm that tends to grow slowly,

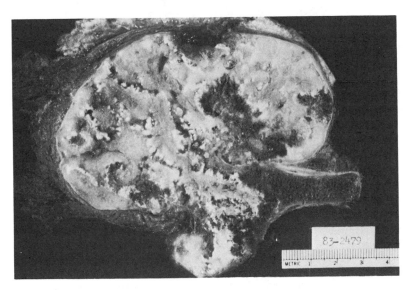

Fig. 18-5. Chondrosarcoma of rib.

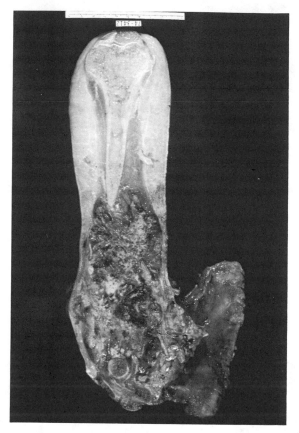

Fig. 18-6. Ewing's sarcoma of bone. The tumor is in the diaphyseal region, and has destroyed the bone with extensive infiltration of surrounding soft tissues.

forming large local masses. Metastasis occurs relatively late.
    i) Prognosis depends on the grade of the tumor. Grade I lesions have a 90% 5-year survival. For grade III, 5-year survival is 40%.
3. Ewing's sarcoma (Fig. 18-6)
    a) Ewing's sarcoma is an uncommon neoplasm of uncertain histogenesis.
    b) It occurs in children and young adults (5–30 years).
    c) It arises in the medullary cavity in the diaphysis of long bones, ribs, pelvis, and vertebra.

d) As it grows, it
   (1) extends in the medullary cavity.
   (2) destroys and expands the bone cortex.
   (3) extends outside bone into soft tissues.
e) Grossly, the tumor is soft, gray, and shows necrosis and hemorrhage.
f) Microscopically, it is characterized by
   (1) sheets of small, round cells with a hyperchromatic nucleus and a small amount of cytoplasm.
   (2) a high mitotic rate.
g) Ewing's sarcoma is a rapidly growing, highly malignant neoplasm. Its spread via the blood stream occurs early.
h) Its 5-year survival rate is about 10%.

19

The Skin

INFECTIONS OF THE SKIN

I. Bacterial infections
- A. Impetigo
  1. Impetigo is a superficial epidermal infection caused by *Staphylococcus aureus*.
  2. It commonly occurs in children, particularly on the face.
  3. It is characterized by an intraepidermal pustule. When the blister ruptures a typical thick, yellow, translucent crust forms.
  4. In neonates, extensive loss of epidermis may occur ("scalded skin syndrome").
- B. Hair follicle infections
  1. *Staphylococcus aureus*: the usual pathogen
  2. Furuncle: acute folliculitis with suppuration (boil, pimple)
  3. Carbuncle
     - a) Begins as a folliculitis but spreads laterally underneath deep fascial planes to form a large suppurative inflammatory mass
     - b) Occurs mainly in diabetics
- C. Erysipelas (rare)
  1. Caused by beta hemolytic streptococci
  2. An acute spreading inflammation of the dermis and epidermis, commonly occurring on the face or scalp
- D. Cellulitis
  1. Cellulitis is a spreading acute inflammation of the subcutaneous tissue, usually occurring as a complication of a wound infection.
  2. It is usually caused by *Streptococcus pyogenes*.
  3. A severe form of cellulitis characterized by extensive necrosis is sometimes caused by anaerobic bacteria.
     - a) Ludwig's angina: affecting the floor of mouth and neck
     - b) Fournier's gangrene: affects the scrotum
- E. Anthrax (rare)
  1. Caused by *Bacillus anthracis*

2. A strong occupational relationship to industries dealing with animal products and hides
3. Clinical characteristics: produces a malignant pustule, a large hemorrhagic blister that ruptures and leads to an ulcer having a black crust
F. Leprosy (Hansen's disease)
   1. Leprosy is common in tropical countries. In the United States, leprosy is seen in Southern California, Hawaii, and the southern states.
   2. It is caused by *Mycobacterium leprae*.
   3. Clinicopathologic characteristics are dependent on the immunological reactivity of the host to the leprosy bacillus:
      a) Lepromatous leprosy
         (1) This occurs in patients who have a low level of cellular immunity: the lepromin test is negative.
         (2) The bacillus multiples unchecked in skin macrophages, which form lepra cells, with large masses of acid-fast bacilli (globi).
         (3) Marked thickening and nodularity of the skin are seen.
         (4) The bacillus spreads via the blood stream, causing widespread lesions of the skin, eye, upper respiratory tract, and viscera.
      b) Tuberculoid leprosy
         (1) This occurs in patients who develop a relatively good T-cell response to the bacillus. The lepromin test is positive.
         (2) The organism is localized to the area of entry.
         (3) The skin lesion is characterized by the presence of epithelioid cell granulomas, numerous lymphocytes, and small numbers of leprosy bacilli.
         (4) Clinically, the skin lesion is a hypopigmented macule.
         (5) Nerve involvement is characteristic.
   G. Other mycobacterial infections (rare)
II. Viral infections
   A. Epidermotropic viruses
      1. Viral infection of the epidermal cells leads to degeneration and necrosis of epidermal cells, resulting in the formation of an intraepidermal vesicle.
      2. The identification of the virus causing the vesicle is by
         a) clinical examination: distribution of lesions.
         b) recognition of specific histologic changes.

     c) demonstration of virus by electron microscopy.
     d) culture.
  3. Small pox (variola): a triumph of preventive medicine. Once the scourge of the world, smallpox has now virtually disappeared.
  4. Chicken pox (varicella)
     a) This is a common childhood infection caused by *Herpes varicella* (also known as varicella-zoster).
     b) The virus enters via the respiratory tract and after an incubation period of 13–17 days, disseminates via the bloodstream, localizing mainly in the skin.
     c) The rash begins as a macule on the first day of fever and rapidly progresses to an intraepidermal vesicle.
     d) The disease is mild and self-limited.
  5. Herpes zoster (shingles)
     a) Caused by the varicella zoster (V-Z) virus, the same herpes virus that causes chicken pox.
     b) The virus reaches sensory ganglia during an attack of chickenpox, then remains dormant there for long periods.
     c) The disease represents reactivation of the dormant virus:
        (1) Ganglionitis, associated with the severe pain in the dermatome.
        (2) Spread of virus down the sensory nerves to the skin, where it produces vesicles.
     d) Involvement of the ophthalmic branch of the trigeminal nerve causes corneal lesions and may produce blindness.
  6. Herpes Simplex
     a) Two virus types: I and II. In general *H. simplex* type I causes oral lesions and type II causes genital lesions (see chapter 16).
     b) Primary herpetic infection by type I virus in children causes a severe ulcerative oral lesion with systemic symptoms known as acute gingivostomatitis.
     c) The primary infection is self-limited. The virus remains dormant in a nearby ganglion with repeated recurrences ("fever blisters").
     d) All herpesvirus blisters show giant cells with Cowdry type A intranuclear inclusions.
  B. Dermotropic viruses: measles and rubella cause inflammation around dermal blood vessels (an erythematous macular rash).
III. Fungal infections
  A. Dermatophyte infections (ringworm)

    1. Dermatophytes infect keratin of the stratum corneum, hair, and nails. They do not penetrate deeper.

    2. The three main species are *Trichophyton, Epidermophyton,* and *Microsporum.*

    3. Clinically, they cause circular, elevated, red, pruritic lesions.

B. Deep fungal infections

    1. Deep fungal infections of the skin may result from

        a) local inoculation (puncture wounds, etc.): chromoblastomycosis and sporotrichosis.

        b) bloodstream spread, usually from a primary focus in the lung: coccidioidomycosis, histoplasmosis, blastomycosis, paracoccidioidomycosis, candidiasis, and cryptococcosis.

    2. Clinically, the lesions may be papular, pustular, nodular, ulcerative, or verrucous (wartlike).

    3. Histologic sections show a mixed granulomatous and suppurative inflammation. The fungus can be demonstrated.

IV. Parasitic infections

A. Leishmaniasis

    1. The disease appears in the following forms:

        a) Cutaneous leishmaniasis (*L. tropica*): infection is localized, forming a chronic ulcer (oriental sore)

        b) Mucocutaneous leishmaniasis (*L. braziliensis*): affects the face, nose, and oral cavity, producing marked thickening with ulceration

        c) Visceral leishmaniasis or kala-azar (*L. donovani*): affects reticuloendothelial system (liver and spleen); skin involvement rare

    2. The parasite multiplies in macrophages, which accumulate in the affected area.

B. Filariasis

    1. Onchocerciasis (*Onchocerca volvulus*)

        a) Common cause of skin nodules and blindness in Africa

        b) Nodules (onchocercomas) in the subcutaneous tissue composed of a tangled mass of worms

    2. Lymphatic filariasis: due to *Wuchereria bancrofti* and *Brugia malayi*

        a) Common in South and Southeast Asia

        b) Lymphatic-dwelling filarial worms that cause lymphatic obstruction and chronic lymphedema ("elephantiasis")

C. Scabies

    1. Scabies is a common disorder caused by the mite *Sarcoptes scabiei.*

2. The mite burrows in the stratum corneum producing serpiginous burrows.
3. As it moves, it lays eggs, which cause pruritis.

IMMUNOLOGICAL DISEASES OF THE SKIN

I. Allergic dermatitis (eczema)
   A. A large number of allergens produce dermatitis, acting both externally or via the bloodstream.
   B. Type I and type III hypersensitivity mechanisms are involved.
   C. In the phase of acute dermatitis, there is
      1. marked intercellular epidermal edema (spongiosis) and vesicles.
      2. perivascular inflammation in the dermis.
   D. In the chronic phase there is epidermal hyperplasia, hyperkeratosis, and dermal chronic inflammation.

II. Pemphigus vulgaris
   A. This is a chronic, severe disease of middle age (40–60 years) characterized by bullae in the skin and oral mucosa.
   B. It is associated with IgG autoantibodies in the serum, which react against intercellular attachment sites of keratinocytes.
   C. Separation of keratinocytes from one another (acantholysis) leads to an intraepidermal (suprabasal) vesicle that contains rounded-up acantholytic cells.
   D. The attachment of the basal cells to the basement membrane is not affected; basal cells remain at the base of the vesicle like "a row of tombstones."
   E. Clinically, the vesicles are large and flaccid, and easily rupture.
   F. Systemic symptoms such as fever, loss of weight are prominent.
   G. Untreated, most patients die within 1 year. Treatment with steroids is effective in some.

III. Bullous pemphigoid
   A. This is a widespread bullous disease of the skin seen mainly in the elderly (60–80 years).
   B. It is associated with IgG antibody that is deposited in a linear fashion along the basement membrane.
   C. Basal cells separate from the dermis to produce a subepidermal vesicle. The vesicle contains a predominance of eosinophils.

D. The condition is benign.

IV. Dermatitis herpetiformis

  A. This is a chronic disease characterized by erythematous vesicles and severe itching. It cours in adults (20–40 years).

  B. It is associated with granular deposits of IgA at the dermo-epidermal junction, especially at the tips of dermal papillae.

  C. It is associated with gluten-induced enteropathy (celiac disease).

  D. Histologically, there are

    1. subepidermal vesicles containing predominantly neutrophils.

    2. microabscesses at the tips of dermal papillae.

V. Lupus erythematosus (see Chapter 18)

  A. Circulating immune complexes are deposited along the basement membrane of the skin and in small vessels: granular IgG and complement deposition.

  B. Skin lesions may occur either as isolated manifestations (discoid lupus erythematosus) or as part of systemic disease (SLE).

  C. Histologic examination shows

    1. atrophy of the epidermis with hyperkeratosis.

    2. liquefactive degeneration of the basal layers of the epidermis.

    3. a patchy lymphocytic infiltrate in the dermis.

INHERITED DISEASES OF THE SKIN

I. Epidermolysis bullosa: inherited disease of several different types characterized by onset in infancy and the formation of vesicles as a result of minor trauma

II. Darier's disease (keratosis follicularis)

  A. This is inherited as an autosomal dominant.

  B. It is characterized by slowly progressive skin eruptions consisting of hyperkeratotic, crusted papules.

  C. Histologic features consist of

    1. dyskeratosis (abnormal keratinization) with "corps ronds" in the granular layer.

    2. suprabasal acantholysis, leading to the formation of suprabasal clefts.

III. Familial benign pemphigus (Hailey and Hailey's disease)

  A. Inherited as an autosomal dominant.

  B. Characterized by localized eruption of vesicles.

  C. Histologically, acantholysis and suprabasal vesicle formation.

MISCELLANEOUS SKIN DISEASES OF UNCERTAIN ETIOLOGY

I. Psoriasis vulgaris
  A. This is a common chronic disease with remissions and exacerbations.
  B. It is characterized by sharply defined plaques covered by silvery scales.
  C. Histologically, it is characterized by
    1. regular acanthosis with parakeratosis.
    2. neutrophils in the epidermis, either in the stratum corneum (Munro abscess) or in the stratum malpighii (Kogoj pustule).
  D. The basic change in the epidermis is a markedly excessive rate of maturation.

II. Lichen planus
  A. This is a chronic disorder characterized by violaceous, itching papules and plaques in the skin, oral mucosa, and external genitalia.
  B. Histologically, there is
    1. irregular acanthosis with hyperkeratosis.
    2. liquefactive degeneration of the basal cell layer.
    3. band-like dermal inflammatory infiltrate that hugs the epidermis.
  C. There is a marked decrease in the rate of cellular proliferation.

III. Erythema multiforme
  A. This is an uncommon skin disorder of unknown etiology.
  B. It is associated with a large variety of diseases, including many infections, drugs, cancers, and autoimmune diseases.
  C. Clinically, there are macules, papules, and vesicles; target lesions are characteristic.
  D. Microscopically, there is epidermal cell necrosis and dermal inflammation.
  E. A severe form (Stevens–Johnson syndrome) has a high mortality.

IV. Erythema nodosum
  A. This is the most common type of panniculitis (inflammation of subcutaneous fat).
  B. It is associated with many diseases, including infections (beta-hemolytic streptococci, primary tuberculosis), sarcoidosis, acute rheumatic fever, and drug-related problems.
  C. It presents clinically as multiple, tender, red nodular lesions commonly occurring in the anterior tibial region.

V. Pityriasis rosea
   A. Common, self-limited condition occurring in adults (10-30 years)
   B. Suspected of being viral though an agent has not been isolated
   C. Clinically:
      1. Onset with a "herald patch," a sharply defined scaling plaque
      2. Followed by a generalized skin eruption consisting of oval salmon-pink papules covered by a thin scale.
   D. Histologically the features are those of a subacute dermatitis.

CYSTS OF THE SKIN

I. Epidermal
   A. Epidermal inclusion cyst (sebaceous cyst): very common; lined with squamous epithelium; filled with laminated keratin
   B. Pilar cyst: very common; lined by hair follicle epithelium (no granular layer)
II. Dermoid cyst
   A. Congenital cysts that occur at lines of embryonic skin closure and fusion
   B. Lined by an epithelium that shows various dermal appendages

NEOPLASMS OF THE SKIN

I. Benign tumors of keratinocytes
   A. Verruca vulgaris (common wart): very common; caused by a papovavirus; papillary squamous epithelial proliferation
   B. Condyloma acuminatum
      1. Similar to verruca vulgaris; caused by papovavirus
      2. Occurs in genital skin and mucosa and is sexually transmitted
   C. Molluscum contagiosum
      1. This is caused by a virus of the poxvirus group.
      2. Lesions are small, discrete dome-shaped papules having an umbilicated center.
      3. Histologically, the proliferating keratinocytes show large intracytoplasmic inclusions known as molluscum bodies.
   D. Seborrheic keratosis
      1. Very common lesion, often multiple, occurring in the trunk, extremities, and face, usually in elderly patients
      2. Sharply demarcated, brownish, soft, slightly raised lesions

3. Histological characteristics
   a) There is a variable mixture of squamous and basaloid cells.
   b) The lesion is above the level of the skin with no invasive tendency.
   c) Keratin-filled cysts (horn cysts) may be present.
   d) Melanin pigment may be present.
E. Keratoacanthoma
   1. Benign neoplasm, usually solitary, rarely multiple
   2. Occurs in middle age, usually on the face or upper extremities
   3. Characterized by rapid growth, reaching its maximum size in a few weeks
   4. Remains static for a variable period and then spontaneously involutes with scarring
   5. Histological characteristics
      a) The lesion is cup-shaped with an irregular keratin-filled crater in the center.
      b) Irregular epidermal proliferation extends into the crater and down into the dermis.
      c) Differentiation from squamous carcinoma is difficult.
II. Malignant tumors of keratinocytes
   A. Premalignant dysplasias and carcinoma in situ
      1. Actinic keratosis
         a) Caused by ultraviolet radiation of sunlight; occurs predominantly in fair-skinned individuals
         b) Appear as rough, erythematous, or brownish papules
         c) Histological characteristics
            (1) Dysplasia of the epidermis
            (2) Dermis shows myxoid degeneration of collagen (solar elastosis)
         d) Associated with the development of squamous carcinoma.
      2. Bowen's disease (carcinoma in situ)
         a) May occur either on sun-exposed or on nonexposed skin; also occurs on the vulva, oral mucosa, and glans penis
         b) Usually a solitary lesion that presents as a slowly enlarging erythematous patch
         c) Histological characteristics: complete loss of normal epidermal maturation with extreme dysplastic changes
   B. Basal cell carcinoma (basal cell epithelioma; BCE) (Fig. 19-1)
      1. This is a common lesion, occurring in sun-exposed areas of light-skinned individuals over the age of 40 years.

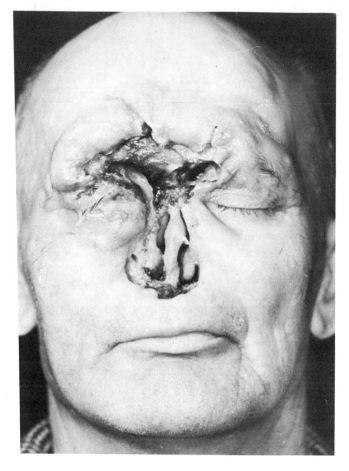

Fig. 19-1. Basal cell carcinoma of the face showing extensive local destruction.

    2. Rarely, multiple basal cell carcinomas arise in early life as part of an autosomal dominant inherited disorder.
    3. Clinical characteristics include the following:
        a) Commonly a pearly-gray, waxy papule.
        b) Later produces a punched out ulcer with rolled edged ("rodent ulcer").
        c) Sclerosing BCE presents as an indurated plaque without ulceration.

4. Histological characteristics include the following:
a) The tumor arises from the basal layer of the epidermis, infiltrating into the dermis.
b) The cells are small and arranged in nests and cords.
5. Basal cell carcinoma is a locally aggressive neoplasm, frequently invading deeply to involve bone and muscle. It does not metastasize.

C. Squamous cell carcinoma (SCC)
1. This most commonly occurs in sun-exposed skin in elderly, fair-skinned individuals. These SCC's are locally aggressive but metastasize very rarely (1%).
2. SCC may also occur in relation to chronic ulcers, burn scars, or sinuses. These have a much higher incidence of metastasis (20–30%).
3. Clinically, SCC presents as a shallow ulcer with a raised, everted, firm border.
4. Histologically, it is composed of malignant squamous cells that infiltrate the dermis.

III. Neoplasms of skin appendages: usually benign neoplasms that are identified by their distinctive histologic features and classified according to their differentiation.
A. With hair differentiation
1. Trichofolliculoma
2. Trichoepithelioma
3. Pilomatrixoma
B. With sweat gland (eccrine) differentiation
1. Syringoma
2. Syringocystadenoma papilliferum
3. Clear cell hidradenoma
4. Eccrine poroma
5. Eccrine spiradenoma
C. With apocrine differentiation
1. Hidradenoma papilliferum
2. Cylindroma
D. With sebaceous differentiation
1. Nevus sebaceus
2. Sebaceous adenoma

IV. Melanocytic tumors
A. Benign nevocellular nevus
1. Nevocellular nevi are hamartomas.
2. They are extremely common ("birth marks"); may be papular or pedunculated.
3. Nests of nevus cells may be found in the dermis (intradermal

nevus), in the junction between epidermis and dermis (junctional nevus), or in both locations (compound nevus).
4. Nevus cells in a compound nevus may show considerable pleomorphism and cytologic atypia (Spitz nevus). Differentiation from malignant melanoma can be difficult.

B. Congenital giant pigmented nevus
1. Present at birth; not inherited
2. Very large, pigmented, often hairy lesion occurring anywhere in the body (trunk, scalp and face, extremities)
3. Histologically, a compound nevus
4. Predisposes to malignant melanoma

C. Blue nevus
1. Common
2. Presents as a small, circumscribed bluish-black nodule composed of dendritic melanocytes in the dermis

D. Malignant melanoma in situ (i.e., noninvasive)
1. Lentigo maligna (Hutchinson's freckle)
   a) Mainly in sun-exposed areas of the skin in the elderly
   b) Presents clinically as an unevenly pigmented macule that becomes progressively larger
   c) Remains in situ for long periods (10–15 years)
   d) Histologically, a marked increase in spindle shaped, pigmented melanocytes in the basal epidermis
2. Superficial spreading melanoma (Pagetoid melanoma in situ)
   a) Small pigmented and slightly elevated lesion occurring regardless of exposure to sunlight
   b) In-situ phase much shorter than in lentigo maligna
   c) Invasion characterized by the development of ulceration and bleeding
   d) Histological characteristics: nests of large, rounded neoplastic melanocytes in the lower epidermis; cells have atypical hyperchromatic nuclei

E. Invasive malignant melanoma
1. Lentigo maligna melanoma: an invasion in a pre-existing in-situ lentigo maligna
2. Pagetoid malignant melanoma: develops in an in-situ Pagetoid melanoma
3. Nodular malignant melanoma (Fig. 19-2)
   a) Most cases (90%) arise de novo. A few cases arise in a pre-existing nevocellular nevus or in a congenital giant pigmented nevus.
   b) Clinically, nodular melanoma appears as an elevated

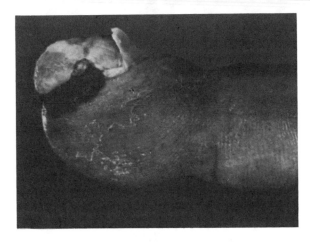

Fig. 19-2. Nodular malignant melanoma (toe, subungual). The nail is pushed up by the large nodular mass, the basal part of which shows pigmentation.

pigmented nodule that grows rapidly and tends to ulcerate.

c) Metastasis, by lymphatics and the blood stream, tends to occur early.

d) Histologically, malignant melanoma is characterized by
  (1) origin in the basal epidermis.
  (2) marked cytologic atypia, pleomorphism, nuclear hyperchromatism, and increased mitotic activity.
  (3) usual presence of melanin pigment. When no melanin is present the term amelanotic melanoma is used.
  (4) infiltration into the dermis.
  (5) a variable lymphocytic infiltrate around the invading melanocytes in the dermis.

e) Electron microscopy shows melanosomes in the cytoplasm.

f) Prognosis in malignant melanoma depends on
  (1) the type of melanoma: nodular melanoma is worse than invasive pagetoid melanoma and lentigo maligna melanoma.
  (2) the depth of invasion, determined by measurement: the most important factor.
  (3) the level of invasion (Clark). Level I: restricted to

epidermis; Level II: invading papillary dermis; Level III: invasion to junction of papillary and reticular dermis; Level IV: invasion of reticular dermis; Level V: invasion of subcutaneous fat.

(4) the number of inflammatory cells: the greater the number the better the prognosis.

(5) the clinical stage: the presence of lymph node metastases worsens the prognosis. When distant hematogenous metastases are present, 5-year survival is almost zero.

V. Tumors of dermal connective tissue
  A. Dermatofibroma (benign fibrous histiocytoma): firm, slowly growing, nodular dermal lesion composed of fibroblasts and collagen
  B. Atypical fibroxanthoma
    1. Common; benign, solitary lesion in a sun-exposed area of an elderly patient
    2. Histologically, a proliferation of fibroblasts and histiocytes with marked pleomorphism, bizarre multinucleated giant cells and numerous mitoses
    3. Lesion does not metastasize despite its malignant appearance
  C. Dermatofibrosarcoma protuberans (malignant fibrous histiocytoma)
    1. Slowly growing nodular lesion; may reach a large size and ulcerate the overlying epidermis
    2. Locally invasive; surgical removal without a wide margin followed by local recurrence
    3. Metastases rare, but may occur after many years
    4. Histological characteristics
      a) A highly cellular proliferation of fibroblasts
      b) Cytologic atypia and increased mitotic activity
  D. Tumors of blood vessels
    1. Capillary hemangioma (strawberry mark)
      a) Bright red, exophytic mass, sometimes reaching a large size, occurring in early infancy
      b) Spontaneously regresses in most cases
    2. Cavernous hemangioma (common)
      a) Occurs as a solitary lesion, commonly on the face, fingers, scalp, oral cavity
      b) Dull-red, soft, raised, ulcerated nodule; grows rapidly to its maximum size
      c) Histologically, numerous thin walled vessels
      d) Benign

3. Glomus tumor
   a) Common; usually in the extremities, most commonly under the nail bed
   b) Small, purple nodule that is extremely painful and tender
   c) Composed of vascular spaces surrounded by uniform, small round cells (glomus cells)

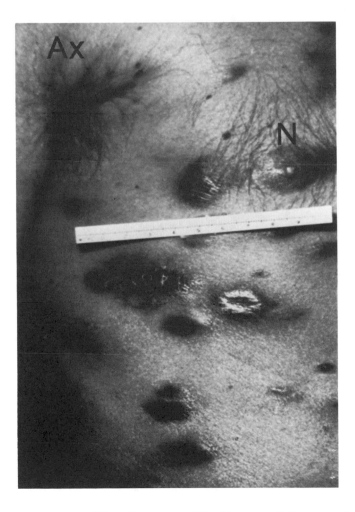

Fig. 19-3. Disseminated Kaposi's sarcoma of the skin in a male homosexual with the Acquired Immunodeficiency Syndrome. Ax = axilla; N = nipple.

   d) Benign
4. Kaposi's sarcoma (Fig. 19-3)
   a) Occurs in two distinct clinical settings:
      (1) Solitary: in the lower extremities in the elderly. Chronic, slowly progressive lesions that rarely metastasize
      (2) Disseminated: characterized by rapidly progressive disseminated disease involving internal organs and skin; occurs in
          i) Acquired Immunodeficiency Syndrome (AIDS) (see Chapter 2)
          ii) North and Central Africa
   b) Clinical characteristics: purplish and dark-brown papules and nodules that frequently become large and ulcerate
   c) Histological characteristics: spindle cell proliferation in which are numerous slit-like vascular spaces, extravasated erythrocytes, and hemosiderin pigment
VI. Malignant lymphoma
   A. This may occur primarily in the skin; the skin may also be involved in disseminated lymphoma, both Hodgkins (5%) and non-Hodgkins (15%).
   B. Mycosis fungoides is a T-cell lymphoma.
      1. It affects the skin primarily and predominantly with dissemination to lymph nodes and viscera occurring late.
      2. It is characterized by malignant T lymphocytes (mycosis cells). These are large cells with hyperchromatic, irregularly lobulated cerebriform nuclei.
      3. Cells are found in upper dermis and epidermis (Pautrier microabscess).
      4. The disease can be divided into three stages:
         a) Erythematous stage, where lesions are erythematous, scaling patches that itch severely.
         b) Plaque stage, characterized by well-demarcated, indurated erythematous plaques.
         c) Tumor stage, characterized by reddish-brown nodules that ulcerate.
   C. Sézary syndrome is a variant of mycosis fungoides that is characterized by:
      1. generalized erythroderma with intense itching.
      2. the presence of Sézary cells (indistinguishable from mycosis cells) in the peripheral blood.

VII. Mast cell lesions (mastocytosis) (rare)
  A. This is a group of diseases characterized by proliferation of mast cells in the skin.
  B. Release of histamine, 5 HT, and other substances from the mast cells causes urticaria and flushing.
  C. Types of disease include the following:
    1. Urticaria pigmentosa (common): benign
    2. Solitary mastocytoma: benign
    3. Systemic mastocytosis: malignant, disseminated disease

Index

Note: Page numbers followed by *f* denote figures; those followed by *t* denote tables.